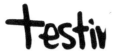

"This book is fantastic. Thoughtful and thor... any
levels and from so many perspectives. I ca... es
whose health and wellbeing are important t... any
conclusions from so many experiences as to c... ...have ever been asked
or asked myself. No longer any need to buy anything else because it is all here"
- *Jim Morris, Lifelong Fitness Fanatic and 80-year old vegan*

"What Leigh-Chantelle's book does is flip one of the central myths about veganism on its
head – that being vegan is about missing out on something (nutritionally speaking). On the
contrary, as these interviews show, it's a diet that's actually better for athletes, for people who
need to perform to the best of their physical abilities. That's a fantastic endorsement, and a
complete up-ending of one of the central myths of veganism."
- *Dale Vince, Founder of Ecotricity and Chairman of Forest Rangers Football Club (UK)*

"Expert Tips from Vegan Athletes, Fitness Fanatics & Exercise Enthusiasts is such an
inspiring read, I could not put it down. Diverse, fascinating athletes letting us into their
health and fitness secrets - this book is a treasure trove of information on what the
world's fittest vegans eat, how they work out and what they say when non vegans ask
the inevitable "Where do you get your protein?" If you want to feel better, look great and
help the world be a kinder place, this book is a bible on how to be your best self."
- *Alexandra Paul, Actress, Athlete and Vegan*

"While many people have the mistaken impression that vegans suffer a nutritional deficit,
professional athletes and weekend warriors around the world continue to excel in their
sports by fueling themselves with plant-based goodness. With Expert Tips from Vegan
Athletes, Fitness Fanatics & Exercise Enthusiasts, Leigh-Chantelle tells us how they keep
fit and achieve success, offering insights into their strengths and training routines as well
as their challenges and influences. Interviews here represent just about every imaginable
sport: long-distance running, cycling, body building, yoga, gymnastics, race car driving,
dancing, Olympic skiing, martial arts, ice hockey—even the little-known, highly physical
activity known as parkour. I can't think of a better book to demonstrate how a vegan diet
is not only the most compassionate, but the healthiest."
- *Mark Hawthorne, author of "A Vegan Ethic: Embracing a Life of Compassion Toward All" and "Bleating Hearts:
The Hidden World of Animal Suffering"*

"Do you think vegans aren't strong, fit and powerful? Think again! And let this book guide
you to greater health and personal power."
- *John Robbins, author Diet For A New America, President of The Food Revolution Network*

"I'm happy to count among my friends Germany's strongest man, Patrik Baboumian, a
vegan who could lift a library's worth of this book without breaking a sweat, and Clifford
Warwick, a UK bodybuilder who doesn't wrestle crocodiles but instead uses his wildlife
biology credentials to save them. It means I can go safely into alleyways on dark nights if
I can just get them to come along. Vegans seem to be taking over the world of sports, from
the Williams sisters to freerunner Tim Schieff to cyclist Catherine Johnson to Ironman
Brendan Brazier – even the world's memory champ, Jonas von Essen (remembering the
order of a deck of cards in under 30 seconds takes mind strength!). This book will help
make more vegan athletes, and that's terrific for animals, the Earth and arteries."
- *Ingrid Newkirk, President, People for the Ethical Treatment of Animals (PETA)*

Expert Tips from

VEGAN ATHLETES

Fitness Fanatics & Exercise Enthusiasts

Book Details

Epicentre Equilibrium Publishing

Copyright © 2015 by Leigh-Chantelle

Cover Illustrations by Weronika Kolinska (veganmisanthrope.tumblr.com)

Compiled by Leigh-Chantelle

Lettering by Leigh-Chantelle (leigh-chantelle.com)

Foreword by Robert Cheeke (veganbodybuilding.com)

Design by Bambi Wants Revenge (bambiwantsrevenge.com)

ISBN 978-0-9808484-6-5

epicentreequilibrium.com

The information in this book is presented solely for educational purposes. It is not intended to serve as medical advice, or a prescription, or to replace the advice and care of your doctor or health professional. Be sure to check with your doctor or health professional before adopting any of the methods and programmes mentioned within these pages.

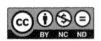

About the Book

Sometime in 2012, I read about a vegan bodybuilding champion from Berlin in Germany, Michael Griesmeier. I was fascinated about his story – as were many others online – and wanted to interview him for my vivalavegan.net website. I looked at other bodybuilding and fitness websites to see what questions people were asked the most, and added a few things I personally wanted to know. I sent this (quite long) list of questions to Michael and received a response back, with the help of a translator, soon after.

I found his answers interesting, informative and inspiring, and knew that there would be other vegan athletes who I could also interview and learn something from. I have many vegan friends from all corners of the world, many of whom I knew would be interested in being involved. I aimed to get 100 people to interview for this series, and if I could get that, I would release the interviews as a print book. I used Twitter to search for other vegan athletes, fitness fanatics and people who were exercise enthusiasts. I also searched vegan websites like greatveganathletes.com and the oft-mentioned veganbodybuilding. com for other vegan people who would be interested in being part of the series. I contacted a heap of people with a large majority of them included in these pages.

When I sent out the questions, I was very specific about what constitutes a vegan diet. In case you're not aware, a vegan is someone who chooses not to consume any animal flesh whatsoever (including chickens and sea creatures), animal products (including eggs, dairy and honey), and by-products (including gelatine.) Veganism is not just a diet however, it's a way of life that many of us have committed to, in order to not use, abuse, kill, or harm any animals. For ethical vegans - who are not just focused on plant-based food - this also includes not wearing animal skins (leather and fur) and animal products (silk and wool). Being vegan also means making compassionate choices with your fashion, cosmetics, household items, and not participating in events where animals will suffer or be exploited e.g. zoos and circuses.

Veganism is not a diet or a religion. Veganism is not about rules and regulations. It's not about constraints and fanaticism. It's about doing your part the best way you can to cause the least amount of suffering in this world. More Good and Less Harm is a great way of putting it. My main reason for becoming vegan over 18 years ago, was because I believe that we should not use, kill, or cause suffering to any (non-human) animals – especially when there are alternatives available. Veganism is the best thing that I can do, and the best way I know how to lead by example, to promote love, peace and compassion - and to stand against ALL injustices and exploitation that exist.

I started this athletes interview series in 2012, and had interviewed 137 people by early 2015. There are professional athletes, Olympians, personal trainers, coaches, and a variety of people who just love exercise and fitness. I have interviewed husbands and wives, business partners, life partners, brothers, best friends, and many who know – and adore – each other in this amazing vegan community we are part of. A few people didn't want to be involved with the book, a few couldn't be contacted, and a few more just simply didn't get back to me in time for the deadline. As of this book going to print at the end of 2015, all the people are to my knowledge vegan.

I follow a great Polish vegan artist, Weronica on Tumblr, who I asked to illustrate the cover for me. It's not her usual style, but I really love what she created. Another vegan artist had suggested that I may like the work of J.C. Leyendecker - which I do - and his illustrations of The Saturday Evening Post (from 1899-1943) inspired the cover. My go-to designer and good friend, Adele put these ideas and more into place, and I'm sure you love the style of this book as much as I do.

Here before you are the final interviews with 111 vegans who I've known for years, or had the pleasure to get to know over the past 4 years. I've met some of these new friends in person, and plan on seeing a lot more when I'm over their side of the world, or they're here in Australia. As I was editing the interviews – at every stage of the process – I would be constantly inspired, amused, and informed by these wonderful people who have shared their journeys with me and the Viva la Vegan! community. Some people have shared just a snippet of their life, some have shared it all – good and bad and in between. I hope you get something from what you read.

I see that a lot more people are aware of veganism, and that a lot more people (whether or not they're vegan) consume more veg meals than in the past. I am sometimes still shocked by this after almost 20 years of being vegan - especially when in remote areas travelling around Australia and seeing fully stocked health food sections with a large array of vegan goodies from all over the world. Another thing that is perplexing to me is just how many people still ask about protein - do vegans really get enough? Out of the 111 people featured in this book, 77 of them still get asked about where they get their protein - that's just under 70%. Vegans get protein from plants sources, yes, AND protein is in just about everything! Another thing I learned in this book was that a vegan diet makes recovery time faster, there's less downtime and therefore the best thing (for the athletes) is that this means more training!

Some of the interviewees are vegan (like I am) because of animal rights and ethics, whilst others are more focused on the environmental and health aspects of veganism. All have found that a vegan diet has helped them to excel in their own area of fitness. There are many reasons to be vegan – and many reasons to stay vegan. I hope the stories and choices this selection of vegans have shared informs, amuses and inspires you to be the best version of yourself – and the best vegan you can be.

Thanks to everyone who has supported this series,

Leigh-Chantelle

WANT TO SEE THE PHOTOS?

Please see the photo albums on the Viva la Vegan! FaceBook, Google+ and Pinterest Social Media pages.

Contents

Foreword by Robert Cheeke

On December 8, 1995, I attended an animal rights conference organized by my older sister, Tanya, in the agriculture town of Corvallis, Oregon, USA. That single event changed my life forever. After watching videos of large-scale factory farming and animal testing, listening to lectures and reading literature about animal rights, at the age of 15, I gave up all animal products for good. I didn't know then that my life would change so dramatically in ways that would impact human and non-human animals for decades. I grew up on a farm and naturally had a level of appreciation for farm animals and I had many farm animal companions who had first names just as a family dog or cat would have. Once I learned more about animal food production, the use of animals in clothing, for entertainment, in lab experimentation, and other areas of exploitation, I decided to dedicate the rest of my life to saving animals, preventing animal cruelty and suffering, and leading by a positive example.

I became vegan before the Internet came of age, and I worried about how I would get enough protein. I struggled with the perceived notion that I might not be able to get bigger and stronger without consuming animal foods. The general consensus by mainstream media, my family, and friends, was that I would not be able to achieve my muscle-building goals without consuming animal products. Boy, were they wrong! As a five-sport high school athlete, my nutrition program was essentially self-taught through trial and error. I fueled my athletic career exclusively with plant foods, and I powered my way to success in many different sports.

I was one of the fastest runners in my school, and our high school cross-country team was ranked #2 in the state. I wrestled, played basketball and soccer, and participated in more track and field events than perhaps anyone in my school history - completing every running, jumping, and field event, aside from the triple jump, 110 meter high hurdles, and pole vault. I won the Dan O'Brian award for the most complete and well-rounded track and field athlete in my school, and made a statement, loud and clear, that I could perform as well as anyone, just by eating plant foods and abstaining from all animal products.

I avoided foods and clothing that contained animal products as well as all products tested on animals. I was outspoken in my high school classes and even persuaded my gym teacher to order rubber basketballs rather than ones that had leather in them. I wore synthetic leather shoes from man-made materials, used synthetic leather soccer balls and basketballs, and gave presentations in school about animal rights. I was passionate and determined to make a difference for animals, using my athletic success to guide my activism.

Running was my strongest sport, which I pursued for a year in college - before I hung up my running shorts in favor of posing trunks and became a bodybuilder. Though I loved running, and I was naturally good at it, the idea of becoming bigger and stronger and fulfilling childhood dreams of being a muscle-bound individual like the cartoon characters He-Man and Captain Planet I looked up to, was intriguing and compelling.

I only weighed 120 pounds (54.5 kilograms) when I became vegan at age 15, and by the time I was 19 years old running cross-country in college I weighed 155 pounds (70 kg). When I decided to start lifting weights, I started small. I was a beginner, learning how to perform the exercises, using relatively light weights.

It was discouraging at first. Running came so easily to me - I had raw, natural talent that most runners would dream of having. Weightlifting took time to produce results, and I was forced to be patient. Allowing my consistent training to lead to adaptation, improvement, and eventual success was a process I embraced. Over the course of 12 weeks I gained 19 pounds (8.6kg), and gained 28 pounds (12.7kg) over a 10-month period. I added an additional 10 pounds (4.5kg) over the next two years, and by age 23 I weighed 195 pounds (88.5kg) - up 75 pounds (34kg) from when I became vegan less than 8 years prior. I had sufficiently put the animal protein argument to rest. I was a living example of someone without a predisposition to efficient muscle-building, based on my genetics, who gained an exceptional amount of muscle from eating plants.

After a few years of weight lifting, I created the website, www.veganbodybuilding. com, at age 22, and competed in my first bodybuilding competition at age 23 in 2003. I placed 4th, but the next time I would step on stage in 2005, I would place 1st and compete at the International Natural Bodybuilding Association (INBA) Natural Bodybuilding World Championships the following year in 2006, placing 2nd. I went on to win another bodybuilding competition, was a runner-up four times, and in 2010 I released a best-selling book titled, "Vegan Bodybuilding & Fitness – The Complete Guide to Building Your Body on a Plant-Based Diet".

By this time, the vegan athlete movement had come a long way and there were well-known vegans in many different sports. When I became vegan I didn't know any other vegan athletes, but by 2010, most of my friends were vegan athletes. After a full decade of weight training and eight years of competing in bodybuilding competitions, I decided to retire from competitive bodybuilding at age 30 and focus my energy on touring around the world, speaking about my journey going from a skinny farm kid to a champion vegan bodybuilder.

After ten years of appearing in magazines, on TV, on the radio, in newspapers, and all over the Internet, I stepped away from the spotlight and gave my support to the new generation of vegan bodybuilders and vegan athletes around the world. My website became a destination for those seeking to learn about the vegan athlete lifestyle and read about hundreds of successful vegan athletes interviewed and featured on our site. I worked behind the scenes and found new challenges to pursue, including writing another book. In 2014, I released the book, "Shred It!", and have been touring around the world from Australia to Canada, to the Caribbean, and all across the United States since its release.

As I sit back and reflect on the past two decades I have been a vegan athlete, I can't help but feel proud of the progress that has been made in this important movement. What was once a fringe idea that was not widely accepted is now going mainstream with Olympic and professional athletes in major sports embracing a vegan lifestyle. Athletes from all sports disciplines are coming to veganism for a wide variety of reasons, from the pursuit of improved athletic performance from eating whole plant foods, to those who no longer want to contribute to animal suffering. We're seeing a shift that is still small and still early, but on its way to a tipping point in the not-too-distant future. I am pleased to be part of a community that I believe will one day be considered to be on the right side of history regarding health, the environment, and ethics.

The bottom line is that all lives matter, because all beings can experience fear, pain, suffering, mourning and loss, and if we have no nutritional or other need to consume or use animals, it is wrong to make non-human animal lives suffer in ways we would not feel comfortable subjecting human lives to. The primary sources of nutrition: vitamins, minerals, amino acids, fatty acids, glucose, and all other essential nutrients, come in their original and optimal forms from plant-based whole foods; fruits, vegetables, nuts, grains, seeds, and legumes. Nutrition, science, environmental factors, and ethics are all in favor of a vegan lifestyle, and someday soon a vegan lifestyle will be part of mainstream culture and considered to be the norm.

This book will introduce you to more than 100 vegan athletes who have found success in their chosen craft - without the use of animal products - to find their own happiness in the pursuit of sport. Use this book as a source of inspiration and information. Mark Twain once said, "Twenty years from now, you will be more disappointed by the things that you didn't do, than by the ones you did do." This resonates with me and I hope it resonates with you too. Whether twenty years from now or two years from now, you don't want to be asking what might have been. We all have the capacity to create positive changes in the world. Remember that what is just a meal for us could cost an animal his or her life. Is it really worth taking an animal's life to satisfy a desire for a taste or texture of a food that isn't necessary for human health?

Leigh-Chantelle has been conducting interviews and assembling data for this book since 2012, and she has been a long-time friend to animals because she speaks for those who can't be heard. She has also been a friend of mine for many years. We met, quite appropriately, at The National Animal Rights Conference in the capitol city of the United States, Washington, DC in 2010. Since our initial meeting, we have since met up in numerous cities around America during her global travels to spread awareness about the vegan lifestyle. This book explores the realities inherent within today's plant-based athletes who are paving the way to a brighter future for all of us. I am proud to be part of this book and part of this important social justice movement.

Please join me in exploring the wonderful foods in the plant kingdom by keeping animal foods off your plate and animal by-products out of your body. Let real food fuel your ambitions and athletic pursuits. Strive for compassion, love, and selflessness, and I am confident you will be on the right side of history. Train hard, eat well, smile often, and lift others up. Follow your passion and make it happen.

Wishing you all the very best in health and fitness,
Robert Cheeke

Robert Cheeke is the best-selling author of Shred It! and Vegan Bodybuilding & Fitness, 2-time champion bodybuilder, and founder/president of Vegan Bodybuilding & Fitness.

www.veganbodybuilding.com

the Athletes

ALAN DUMOND
VEGAN LONG DISTANCE RUNNER

Muncie, Indiana, USA
Vegan since: 2004

alanvedge.com
SM: *Instagram*

Alan Dumond is a professional piercer and jeweler living and working in
Indiana, USA. He's been a runner for a few years now and vegan for a little over
a decade. He has mostly been interested in longer distance stuff, ran his first
100-miler in June 2014, and is looking forward to getting faster as he gains
experience.

WHY VEGAN?

How and why did you decide to become vegan?
I went vegan for ethical reasons - growing up using animal products just seemed like
a necessary evil, but learning that it was possible to abstain from them kind of opened
my eyes, and I knew I couldn't justify it anymore.

How long have you been vegan?
Over ten years.

What has benefited you the most from being vegan?
Veganism isn't really about benefitting myself - it's about putting my ethics into
practice in the real world. Even though my motivation was never for myself it did act as
a gateway for me into learning about other social justice movements so in that way it's
been very beneficial.

What does veganism mean to you?
Veganism is about equality and respect and not treating a living being like a product.

TRAINING

What sort of training do you do?
Primarily running. I do at least one long run a week, often back-to-back long runs. I
mix in various sorts of speed work with longer efforts as well. I do a little bit of cycling
mostly just for commuting purposes but it's a super fun active recovery for me.

How often do you (need to) train?
I usually have 1 day a week off from running that I'll either spend as a total rest day or
try to do some active recovery (bike ride, hike, walk, etc.). I run about 6 days a week
and during higher mileage weeks I do two runs a day.

Do you offer your fitness or training services to others?
Nope. I'm still new to this so I'm still learning myself.

What sports do you play?
I've never been good at sports. I'm not very competitive. I grew up skateboarding and

liked the self-competitive nature of always trying to get better that came with that. Since I can't really skateboard anymore, running and riding a bike have filled that gap in a lot of ways.

STRENGTHS, WEAKNESSES & OUTSIDE INFLUENCES

What do you think is the biggest misconception about vegans and how do you address this?

I think there's a lot of confusion about what "vegan" means. I largely blame misrepresentation in the media and the "celebrity vegan" phenomenon, but at this point the word vegan is so diluted and means so many different things to so many different people. I think the biggest misconception is the absolute lack of meaning the word really has. Ten years ago if someone told me they were vegan I knew what they meant. Now I really don't. That was really frustrating to me and I spent a lot of time fighting against it and trying to keep the term "pure" but at this point I guess I've realized that language changes and evolves, as do movements. I call myself vegan because it's the easiest way for me to describe that I don't want to contribute to animal use but I feel like I have more in common with a compassionate person who is dedicated to equality and justice and occasionally eats cheese or whatever than I do with a "vegan" who works against social justice movements or a "vegan" who cut out animal foods to try to lose weight.

What are your strengths as a vegan athlete?

I'm stubborn. The only way I'm quitting is if I get pulled from a course because I'm not making cut-off times.

What is your biggest challenge?

I'm not naturally athletic. A lot of ultra runners I encounter were athletes in high school and college and then just extended the distances they ran or switched from a different sport to running. I've only been running for a few years and prior to that was never very active or athletic.

Are the non-vegans in your industry supportive or not?

I can't say it's ever been an issue.

Are your family and friends supportive of your vegan lifestyle?

Totally. I don't think my family necessarily "gets" why I'm vegan and thinks it's a little strange but they're very accommodating and respectful.

What is the most common question/comment that people ask/say when they find out that you are a vegan and how do you respond?

I would say the most common question I get is the "What do you eat?" question, which I think is great because it gives me a chance to talk to them about veganism and to show them how familiar they probably already are with a lot of plant-based foods. A lot of people think their lifestyle would have to change radically to go vegan and in a lot of cases it's not as extreme of a change as they might think.

Who or what motivates you?

I'm pretty lucky to have some really awesome people around me who inspire me to be a better runner and a better person.

FOOD & SUPPLEMENTS

What do you eat for Breakfast?

I'm an oatmeal fiend after years of making fun of my sister for eating it every morning.

But if waffles are an option, I'm going with the waffles every time. Second-breakfast (which is important to ultra runners and hobbits) is usually a smoothie post-run.

What do you eat for Lunch and Dinner?
I don't really eat one particular thing for lunch and dinner. Because of my work schedule I end up eating out a lot more than I like, but I cook a fair amount too. I'm lucky to have a partner who is a vegan chef who is finishing up her masters in dietetics so she makes me some pretty amazing meals. When I have the time to prepare my food ahead I do a ton of lentils, brown rice, pasta, and huge salads. When I'm stuck eating out it's more burritos and pizza than I probably should eat.

What do you eat for Snacks - healthy & not-so healthy?
Cookies. Always cookies.

What is your favourite source of Protein?
I don't have a super high need for protein so I don't worry about it too much, but I eat a lot of beans and peanut butter so those are probably my favorites.

What is your favourite source of Calcium?
Leafy greens and fortified foods like soy or almond milk.

What is your favourite source of Iron?
Beans again and spinach. I don't really have a hard time getting enough iron.

What foods give you the most energy?
Coffee!

Do you take any supplements?
Daily I take a vegan creatine to help with hydration, a calcium/magnesium supplement to keep cramping in check, and B12 because you don't want to mess around with that. During long training runs and races I use electrolyte supplements and eat a ton of salt.

ADVICE

What is your top tip for Gaining muscle, Losing weight, Maintaining weight, Improving metabolism, and Toning up?
I am completely not qualified to answer these. I just run a lot and try to keep improving.

How do you promote veganism in your daily life?
I try to lead by example and be a positive influence on people.

How would you suggest people get involved with what you do?
I started with a run and walk program on my phone and just went from there. The biggest thing starting running that I learned was that you don't have to go out and run as hard and as far as you can every time. Take walk breaks. Slow down. Make it enjoyable. You'll build speed and endurance over time without even trying at first. Take it easy, stay injury-free, and just have fun exploring your surroundings and as you get comfortable you'll learn how much you can push your limits.

"Veganism isn't really about benefitting myself – it's about putting my ethics into practice in the real world. Veganism is about equality and respect and not treating a living being like a product."

ALAN MURRAY & JANETTE MURRAY-WAKELIN
VEGAN RAW ULTRA-ENDURANCE ATHLETES

Melbourne, Victoria, Australia
Vegan since: 1998

rawveganpath.com
SM: *FaceBook, YouTube*

Janette Murray-Wakelin & Alan Murray are Internationally-acclaimed Raw Vegan Ultra-Endurance Athletes and Motivational Speakers. They are originally from New Zealand, have travelled and lived worldwide and now live a conscious raw vegan lifestyle in Australia. In the year 2000, to promote "A New Environment for a New Millennium", Janette and Alan ran 2182.2km (1355.9 miles) - the length of New Zealand, 50 marathons in 50 days at beyond 50 years of age. During 2013, to inspire and motivate conscious lifestyle choices, to promote kindness and compassion to all living beings and to raise environmental awareness for a sustainable future; they ran 15,782 km (9806 miles), 366 marathons in 366 days at beyond 60 years of age while "Running Raw around Australia."

WHY VEGAN?

How and why did you decide to become vegan?
Having been vegetarian for several years we made a conscious choice to eliminate all animal products for our own health, the health and wellbeing of animals and for the health and sustainability of the planet.

How long have you been vegan?
We have been vegan for over 17 years and 100% raw vegan for over 11 years.

What has benefited you the most from being vegan?
We have benefitted from being vegan by attaining optimal health and physical fitness, but the conscious choice to be vegan has been as important to us mentally and spiritually.

What does veganism mean to you?
Veganism to us is not a means to an end, but rather a beginning, a beginning of conscious awareness for a kinder and more compassionate life for all human and animal kind, and for the earth that we share.

TRAINING

What sort of training do you do?
We run every day. We both run in barefoot Vibram shoes as a conscious choice to step lightly on the earth. We also do strength training and yoga on a daily basis.

How often do you (need to) train?
Every day.

Do you offer your fitness or training services to others?
Yes, both on a personal basis online, and during workshops and retreats available as announced on our website.

What sports do you play?
Ultra-Endurance Running.

STRENGTHS, WEAKNESSES & OUTSIDE INFLUENCES

What do you think is the biggest misconception about vegans and how do you address this?
The biggest misconception is that vegans may experience a health deficiency (i.e. protein, B12, calcium etc). We do not experience any health deficiencies by consuming sufficient fresh, ripe, organic fruits and vegetables, which give a highly nutritious balanced ratio of nutrients essential for optimal health and fitness, without harming animals or the planet.

What are your strengths as a vegan athlete?
Our strengths as vegan athletes are being optimally healthy and physically fit, having unlimited energy, clarity of mind and a positive attitude.

What is your biggest challenge?
Convincing others that what we are able to do physically and mentally is also available to them.

Are the non-vegans in your industry supportive or not?
Yes.

Are your family and friends supportive of your vegan lifestyle?
Yes.

What is the most common question/comment that people ask/say when they find out that you are a vegan and how do you respond?
A positive response is usually "I've always wanted to try it" and our response is "then now is the best time!"

A negative response is usually "Aren't you worried about getting enough protein?" and our response is "No, we're too busy enjoying life to be worried about anything, because we know that we're getting enough nutrients and our health and physical performance and endurance level attest to that."

Who or what motivates you?
We are motivated by the knowledge that by being vegan athletes we are living proof that the lifestyle we lead is the best for our health, for the health of the animals and for the health of the planet.

FOOD & SUPPLEMENTS

What do you eat for Breakfast?
Green smoothie of blended raw fruit and greens including bananas, pears, apples, berries and green leafy vegetables.

What do you eat for Lunch?
Large raw salad including greens, tomato, cucumber, etc with squeeze of lemon for dressing.

What do you eat for Dinner?
Whole raw large fruit (i.e. melon, papaya or pawpaw, pineapple) or multiple amounts of one fruit (i.e. banana, orange.)

What do you eat for Snacks - healthy & not-so healthy?
Fresh raw fruit or vegetables and/or freshly juiced fruit or vegetables - always healthy.

What is your favourite source of Protein?
Fresh dark leafy greens and juiced wheatgrass.

What is your favourite source of Calcium?
Fresh dark leafy greens and sesame seeds.

What is your favourite source of Iron?
Fresh dark leafy greens.

What foods give you the most energy?
Fresh, ripe fruit and fresh dark leafy greens.

Do you take any supplements?
No, not in the form of capsules etc. We eat only live foods.

ADVICE

What is your top tip for gaining muscle?
Use them.

What is your top tip for losing weight?
By eating only fresh ripe fruits and greens, you will regain the perfect weight for your body structure.

What is your top tip for maintaining weight?
Same as above, the body will maintain the perfect weight for body structure given the perfect diet.

What is your top tip for improving metabolism?
Eat nutritiously and exercise daily.

What is your top tip for toning up?
Strength training.

How do you promote veganism in your daily life?
By example of how we live, and what we achieved by Running Raw around Australia. We give lectures and workshops and speak in schools, at festivals and conferences worldwide. We are also making a documentary based on Running Raw around Australia and the message that it contains, "RAW: The Documentary."

How would you suggest people get involved with what you do?
Support the cause, go on our website and sponsor the documentary, like and follow our FaceBook Page, our blogs and YouTube videos - be inspired, be motivated. Together, we can make a difference!

"Veganism to us is not a means to an end, but rather a beginning, a beginning of conscious awareness for a kinder and more compassionate life for all human and animal kind, and for the earth that we share."

ALINA ZAVATSKY
VEGAN MARATHON RUNNER

Clinton, Washington, USA
Vegan since: 2013

veganrunnereats.com
SM: *FaceBook, Twitter*

Alina Zavatsky is a marathon runner, fitness enthusiast, and a vegan recipe developer. She created her blog, Vegan Runner Eats, to show that compassionate living can go hand in hand with being healthy and active. She also believes that a good workout doesn't have to belong to the gym, and challenges herself to exercise outside as much as possible.

WHY VEGAN?

How and why did you decide to become vegan?
The idea of being vegan always resonated with me. I've always loved animals, and for the most part of my life, it seemed illogical to love them and eat them at the same time, but I was just doing what everyone else around me was doing. I'd never met other vegans until I went vegan myself, so for a while I assumed that being vegan is extremely hard and unhealthy, especially for athletic people. In 2012-2013, I started educating myself about veganism and realized that my previous views on vegan nutrition were a misconception, so finally making a switch seemed logical. Now I can look at animals in peace, because I don't eat them anymore.

How long have you been vegan?
I went vegan in May of 2013 and never looked back. In November 2013, I ran a marathon as a newly vegan runner, and documented my training and racing on my blog.

What has benefited you the most from being vegan?
I am very impressed with the improvement in my athletic endurance. I can keep going even when it seems like there's nothing left, and I recover from workouts much faster. Plus, I enjoy having a lot of energy all day long, without midday crashes.

What does veganism mean to you?
Being vegan means exercising compassion towards all living beings – animals, other people, and ourselves. As much as we want to be kind to animals by not exploiting or killing them, we should remember to be kind to each other by leading by example, and not shaming. Kindness always works better than harassment.

TRAINING

What sort of training do you do?
I use a combination of running and high-intensity interval training (HIIT). I try to incorporate weights whenever I can to build muscle.

How often do you (need to) train?
Ideally, 5 days a week for 30-60 min.

Do you offer your fitness or training services to others?

I don't at the moment, but it's something that seems very appealing to me, so I may eventually decide to study and become a vegan fitness trainer.

What sports do you play?

Running is my primary sport, but I also do a little bit of cycling and swimming, as well as weight training and calisthenics. I've recently tried Pilates and liked it a lot.

STRENGTHS, WEAKNESSES & OUTSIDE INFLUENCES

What do you think is the biggest misconception about vegans and how do you address this?

Unfortunately, vegans are often considered to be preachy and judgmental. I try to show with my own example that it doesn't have to be that way. We can convince way more people to try out this compassionate lifestyle with our own kindness and support. Also, there's a misconception that a plant-based diet is deficient in a lot of nutrients - especially protein - so this is another thing that I try to disprove by my own example.

What are your strengths as a vegan athlete?

My improved endurance - great for long-distance running! - and the ability to recover quickly.

What is your biggest challenge?

Consuming plenty of calories to support my energy needs. Whenever I train a lot, especially for long-distance races, I tend to get hungry quickly, so I have to make sure to always have healthy snacks on hand.

Are the non-vegans in your industry supportive or not?

Generally, people are supportive. Every now and then, I hear concerns about my protein and nutrient intake, but I try to explain my position in a friendly manner, and that usually works well.

Are your family and friends supportive of your vegan lifestyle?

There was a lot of skepticism at first because my family and friends didn't know a lot about veganism, but once I showed them that it was working out great for me, they accepted it. At first, my husband was eating my vegan meals at home but ordered meat whenever we went out, but eventually he joined me after a couple months. I'm very proud of his progress.

What is the most common question/comment that people ask/say when they find out that you are a vegan and how do you respond?

The protein question must be the most popular one I hear. I try to explain that we don't need as much protein as we've been told by the meat and dairy industry. If someone says that they are afraid of becoming protein-deficient on a vegan diet, I tell them that I run marathons and do a lot of weight training as a vegan, and I have yet to experience any trouble from the lack of protein.

Who or what motivates you?

It's great to realize that not a single living being had to be killed or tortured in order for me to enjoy delicious and healthy meals every day. The longer I've been following this lifestyle, the more logical it seems to me.

FOOD & SUPPLEMENTS

What do you eat for Breakfast?

Overnight oats with nuts, dried fruit, ground flaxseed and sometimes, cocoa powder.

What do you eat for Lunch?
A lot of veggie wraps, baked potatoes topped with beans and salsa, or green salads.

What do you eat for Dinner?
Bean and lentil stews, soups, stir-fries, casseroles like my vegan moussaka, etc. I try out new recipes all the time.

What do you eat for Snacks - healthy & not-so healthy?
Hummus with veggies, homemade granola bars, all kinds of fruit. Not-so-healthy: I bake a lot, so here we go.

What is your favourite source of Protein?
Beans, tofu, tempeh, seitan.

What is your favourite source of Calcium?
Leafy greens.

What is your favourite source of Iron?
Beans, leafy greens, blackstrap molasses.

What foods give you the most energy?
Fruit, and starchy foods like potatoes and rice.

Do you take any supplements?
Only Vitamin B12.

ADVICE

What is your top tip for gaining muscle?
Eat protein with every meal, lift heavier weights, and do cardio in moderation.

What is your top tip for losing weight?
Eat a lot of fresh fruit and vegetables, eliminate all oils and vegan junk foods, incorporate longer cardio sessions into your workouts.

What is your top tip for maintaining weight?
Exercise regularly, and avoid long breaks between meals.

What is your top tip for improving metabolism?
Eat more veggies and minimally processed foods, combine cardio and weight training.

What is your top tip for toning up?
Don't be afraid of lifting heavier weights at the gym.

How do you promote veganism in your daily life?
I write about the benefits of a plant-based diet and vegan lifestyle on my blog. I try to include actionable tips anyone can follow to become compassionate, healthy and active. I focus on positive aspects of this lifestyle on my blog's Facebook page. As for the people around me, I try to be supportive and lead by example instead of preaching.

How would you suggest people get involved with what you do?
I'd love to convince people around me that the only boundaries we encounter are the ones we set for ourselves. We are capable of achieving so much more in life that the sky is truly the limit. A few years ago, I would have been shocked if somebody had told me that I would become a vegan marathoner spreading the word of compassion all over the world. It's time to stop being afraid, and start living life to the fullest.

"As much as we want to be kind to animals by not exploiting or killing them, we should remember to be kind to each other."

AMANDA MEGGISON
VEGAN MARATHON RUNNER

Melbourne, Victoria, Australia
Vegan since: 2009

tarianpantry.com.au
SM: *FaceBook, Instagram, Twitter*

Amanda Meggison is a cake-baking, marathon-running, certified nutrition specialist whose enthusiasm for living beautifully fuels her passion for a plant-based diet. Amanda and her website, Tarian Pantry are all about food and fitness.

WHY VEGAN?

How and why did you decide to become vegan?
After following a vegetarian diet for over 20 years, my husband Zac and I started to become more aware of our vegetarian food choices. We didn't drink milk or eat eggs but we did eat cheese and as our awareness grew, our questions regarding our choice to eat this product became more. There is still cruelty in the process of vegetarian products and this started to concern us. As a personal challenge, we decided to go vegan for 3 months to see how we would fare and over 5 years later we are still following a 100% vegan diet. There is no turning back now.

How long have you been vegan?
I have been vegan for over 5 years and have honestly never felt better. I know it sounds like a cliché but its true. I wouldn't follow any other lifestyle diet.

What has benefited you the most from being vegan?
My health, mindfulness and the ability to truly understand the origin of food. Food is not only something that stops the hunger pains, it fuels us to nourish our mind and body.

What does veganism mean to you?
It means becoming more aware of our food choices, to not only see the meal that sits in front of us but to know its journey, its story and to think beyond our own self. We are not the only being that has feelings, and I wish not to inflict any unnecessary pain on our animal friends just for a meal. We can survive without food that had a mother or a face and my journey of veganism is to help change people's perceptions that meat is not a fundamental part of our diet and we can live on plant-based fare alone.

TRAINING

What sort of training do you do?
I train in three main disciplines – swim, bike and run. Zac and I started our fitness journey with a pair of trainers participating in fun runs and half marathons. In November 2012 we purchased a bike and since then we found an interest in triathlons - so now we do all three (but running will always be our favourite).

How often do you (need to) train?

We train 6 days a week often twice a day with one session in the morning and another in the afternoon. In the lead up to races and events we train up to 15 hours a week and for our recovery weeks, we train around 7 hours. We always seem to be in lycra!

Do you offer your fitness or training services to others?

Soon, I am currently in training to become a spin instructor. For the moment, I offer motivation to get off the couch and start something! I have a coach who trains & supports us through our fitness goals, and we believe we have what it takes to help inspire and motivate others to love exercise and movement as much as we do.

What sports do you play?

Triathlons and marathons - are they classed as a sport?

"I set personal goals and work hard to achieve them but not every race is conquered with ease. My challenge is to back myself and believe I have what it takes to achieve greatness."

STRENGTHS, WEAKNESSES & OUTSIDE INFLUENCES

What do you think is the biggest misconception about vegans and how do you address this?

It has to be our lack of consumption of key nutrients such a protein, calcium and iron and that because we don't eat meat we are all fragile and weak. I addressed this by starting Tarian Pantry. I wanted an avenue to prove firstly that vegans are not weak or malnourished, plus vegans eat a diet rich in plant-based foods not just lentils and tofu. If you lead by example, those misconceptions will fade and our diet choice will be seen as nothing but a positive one.

What are your strengths as a vegan athlete?

My strengths are my personal and business message, Powered by Plants plus my determination to never give up when all I want to do it stop and rest. I'm not sure if I'm constantly trying to prove something to other people but if I am, then this gives me more strength and as I say when times are tough, 'my weakness is my strength'.

What is your biggest challenge?

Every training session and every race is my biggest challenge. I set personal goals and work hard to achieve them but not every race is conquered with ease. My challenge is to back myself and believe I have what it takes to achieve greatness. We must remember that we are always racing ourselves and not the people around us.

Are the non-vegans in your industry supportive or not?

We train with an extremely strong and motivated group of fitness conscious individuals and they are nothing but supportive, not to mention interested in our lifestyle diet choice. Our ability to train as hard as they do and recover without the help of a whey protein shake and steak is fascinating to them and we know our love of kale, pea protein and tofu is rubbing off on them so that's all the support we need.

Are your family and friends supportive of your vegan lifestyle?

Always, especially when I do the cooking! They say the proof is in the pudding. When the pudding is a raw cacao pudding with coconut ice cream and fresh berries they are 100% supportive. When we changed our eating habits, we also started to spend more time in the kitchen, as you can't adopt such a diet without getting your hands (and a few dishes) dirty.

What is the most common question/comment that people ask/say when they find out that you are a vegan and how do you respond?

"But where do you get your protein from?" We answer this one by simply replying, "From a varied and balanced diet rich in vegetables, grains, legumes, nuts, seeds and fruits." I am not sure the person who asked that question would be able to answer that with anything other than 'meat'.

When you follow a vegan or plant-based diet, suddenly everyone around you becomes an expert in nutrition. We wouldn't be able to do what we do lifestyle and exercise wise if we didn't eat a balanced diet.

Who or what motivates you?

Like-minded individuals and vegan athletes such as Rich Roll, Scott Jurek and Brendan Brazier are always inspiring me to push myself to the limits. Not only for their vegan lifestyles, but their ability to be able to train and race hard, and prove there are no limits to what the body can do.

I am also motivated by those closer to home, my vegan husband, my coach and my training partners, who each have a goal and work bloody hard to achieve it. Fitness is more than just getting muscles and being able to run a marathon, it's about mental strength and conditioning to believe you can do anything you set your mind to do.

FOOD & SUPPLEMENTS

What do you eat for Breakfast?

For breakfast on the go: Bircher muesli with coconut yoghurt and fresh fruit. When I have more than 5 minutes, a combination of Flip Shelton 5 grain porridge & Forage Quinoa porridge with stewed fruits and nuts.

What do you eat for Lunch?

Either a soup such as kale, tomato, lentil and quinoa; or a rye wrap with beans, spinach, carrot, sprouts, beetroot and avocado.

What do you eat for Dinner?

A dashi noodle broth with greens, zucchini, broccoli, kale and puffed tofu.

What do you eat for Snacks - healthy & not-so healthy?

Spirulina bliss balls or a chewy granola bar made with nuts, seeds and chia seeds.

What is your favourite source of Protein?

Greens such as kale, spinach, bok choy, broccoli and quinoa.

What is your favourite source of Calcium?

Tahini/sesame seeds, Brazil nuts, tempeh, figs and dates.

What is your favourite source of Iron?

Spirilina, wholegrains, nuts and lentils.

What foods give you the most energy?

As an endurance athlete, I have to fuel with foods that are going to give me lasting energy, so I eat foods that contain ingredients such as chia seeds, goji berries, Medjool dates and nuts. I also fuel with potatoes: roasted and mashed sweet potato.

Do you take any supplements?

I do take spirulina tablets for additional protein and aiding recovery, along with magnesium but as for Iron, Calcium or B12 supplements it's not necessary as we get ample enough in the foods we eat.

"Fitness is more than just getting muscles and being able to run a marathon, it's about mental strength and conditioning to believe you can do anything you set your mind to do."

ADVICE

What is your top tip for gaining muscle?
Swim! My arm muscles have never been so defined - plus the odd lifting of weights doesn't go astray.

What is your top tip for losing weight?
Eat a balanced diet - and yes this includes raw chocolate. If you want to lose weight then stay away from the sugar and heavily processed food-like products.

What is your top tip for maintaining weight?
Eat a balanced diet rich in fruits, vegetables, grains, legumes, nuts and seeds. Simple really, just bring your diet back to basics and stay away from 99% of the foods found on the supermarket shelves.

What is your top tip for improving metabolism?
Eat a balanced diet and portion control.

What is your top tip for toning up?
Squats, swimming, running and eating a balanced diet. Are you seeing a trend here? Eat a balanced diet rich in organic whole foods and stay away from the junk.

How do you promote veganism in your daily life?
Via my business Tarian Pantry – a business powered by plants. This website is a wealth of knowledge and weekly I write a blog about food, fitness, how to eat better, how to enjoy a plant-based diet, and generally how to really enjoy food, not to mention life.

I also offer Tarian nutrition coaching to help people feel more comfortable and confident about following a plant-based diet. I certainly don't want people to view this lifestyle diet as difficult, and I give tips and advice to make the transition to a vegan diet an enjoyable and tasty one.

How would you suggest people get involved with what you do?
Get in contact and start practicing what we preach. Shop local, eat better, and exercise more. Food is our fuel and what we eat helps power us for work, rest and exercise. Believing in the mindset "you are what you eat" will help you make better choices when it comes to what is served up on your plate each meal.

We would love to inspire more to follow in our footsteps of our powered by plants journey. It's one that keeps you full of life not to mention young in mind & body. Visit our website, find us on Facebook, Instagram, and Twitter.

"We are not the only being that has feelings, and I wish not to inflict any unnecessary pain on our animal friends just for a meal. We can survive without food that had a mother or a face and my journey of veganism is to help change people's perceptions that meat is not a fundamental part of our diet and we can live on plant-based fare alone."

Amber Zuckswert
VEGAN PROFESSIONAL DANCER

San Francisco, California, USA
Vegan since: 2010

epicself.com
meetup.com/organichealth
SM: *FaceBook, Google+, Instagram, Twitter, YouTube*

Amber Zuckswert is a professional modern/ballet dancer, the creator of Virtual Pilates, holistic to plant-based nutrition and lifestyle coach, yogi, minimalist, raw foodie, planet romping gypsy wrapped into one tall package.

WHY VEGAN?

How and why did you decide to become vegan?
For my personal health and environmental impact and my love of animals.

How long have you been vegan?
5 Years.

What has benefited you the most from being vegan?
My energy, focus and connection to the planet.

What does veganism mean to you?
It's a compassionate lifestyle choice that will radically change your health and protect your only home, Earth.

TRAINING

What sort of training do you do?
I'm a professional dancer, Pilates and yoga instructor who cross trains with weights and hiking.

How often do you (need to) train?
Every day at least.

Do you offer your fitness or training services to others?
Yes! I teach virtually, in my home base of San Francisco, and also teach retreats and workshops all over the globe.

What sports do you play?
Dance is my sport!

STRENGTHS, WEAKNESSES & OUTSIDE INFLUENCES

What do you think is the biggest misconception about vegans and how do you address this?
Lack of protein, muscle mass and angry ethical vegans. I share the facts about protein and lead by example.

What are your strengths as a vegan athlete?
I perform better and recover faster.

What is your biggest challenge?
Eating enough calories.

Are the non-vegans in your industry supportive or not?
Supportive for sure!

Are your family and friends supportive of your vegan lifestyle?
Yes, but they are not vegan.

What is the most common question/comment that people ask/say when they find out that you are a vegan and how do you respond?
Protein question is first.

Who or what motivates you?
Life.

FOOD & SUPPLEMENTS

What do you eat for Breakfast?
Green smoothies, apples and almond butter, chia seed porridge.

What do you eat for Lunch?
Massive salad or raw wraps.

What do you eat for Dinner?
Kelp noodle pasta, raw entrees, smoothies, salads, veggies.

What do you eat for Snacks - healthy & not-so healthy?
Fruit, nuts and seeds, salsa, guacamole and veggies, hummus, kale chips.

What is your favourite source of Protein?
Chia, flax or hemp seed, spirulina, greens.

What is your favourite source of Calcium?
Greens.

What is your favourite source of Iron?
Seaweeds.

What foods give you the most energy?
Quinoa, banana and almond butter, chia seeds.

Do you take any supplements?
B12 and Vitamin D.

"Veganism is a compassionate lifestyle choice that will radically change your health and protect your only home, Earth."

ADVICE

What is your top tip for gaining muscle?
Increase your workouts, eat more calories from cooked grains.

What is your top tip for losing weight?
Increase workouts, eat low fat raw vegan.

What is your top tip for maintaining weight?
Maintain balance in workouts, eat high raw vegan, no processed foods, no sugar or oils.

What is your top tip for improving metabolism?
Move more, drink more water, and eat healthy fats.

What is your top tip for toning up?
Lift weights, practice yoga/Pilates, move more in your day.

How do you promote veganism in your daily life?
I run the largest organic health and raw food Meet Up group in San Francisco and share my knowledge with everyone I know.

How would you suggest people get involved with what you do?
They can check out my website for over 500+ wellness articles, my YouTube channel and my MeetUp group.

Why Vegan?

The main reasons most people become vegan are:

- Animal rights and welfare concerns
- Environmental and sustainable living
- Ethical and moral reasons
- Health issues
- Spiritual and/or religious beliefs
- Weight loss or control

Be the Best Version of Yourself.

AMULYA
VEGAN INTERNATIONAL BELLY DANCER

Melbourne, Victoria, Australia
Vegan since: 2007

bellydanceramulya.com

Amulya Merrett is an international belly dance artist based in Melbourne who began belly dancing in Amsterdam when she was a teenager. She has performed in many European countries as well as Australia and has taught classes and workshops for many years in The Netherlands and Australia. Her repertoire consists of classical Egyptian belly dance, modern Egyptian, tribaret, tribal fusion and her own innovative artistic work. Amulya was part of BlackTop Circus Theater and was a regular performer at the Lucky Dip Show in Byron Bay.

WHY VEGAN?

How and why did you decide to become vegan?
Once I discovered the truth about the dairy industry. I already gave up eggs years before, when I found out about the baby male chickens going in the grinder alive.

How long have you been vegan?
Over 6 years.

What has benefited you the most from being vegan?
Knowing that I don't contribute to cruelty and better health - I used to have severe joint pains, and asthma - the asthma is completely gone now and the joint pain has lessened. After quitting dairy, the pain got less and the asthma completely disappeared within 5 weeks!

What does veganism mean to you?
A compassionate lifestyle that includes so many things, kindness to all beings, contributing less to climate change. I'm against specieism and being vegan is the only way to live a non-specieist life.

"Veganism is a compassionate lifestyle that includes so many things, kindness to all beings, contributing less to climate change. I'm against specieism and being vegan is the only way to live a non-specieist life."

TRAINING

What sort of training do you do?
Belly dancers tend to do regular stretches, I can recommend yoga to stay flexible. Flexibility is one of the most important things in belly dance, without this, one cannot dance. However, everybody can actually gain some flexibility, mostly I see students get more flexible already at the 3rd or 4th lesson. Besides stretching, turn on the music and just dance – it's the best way to exercise.

How often do you (need to) train?
Best would be daily, but I can be slack...

Do you offer your fitness or training services to others?
I teach belly dance.

What sports do you play?
No other sports, just dancing!

STRENGTHS, WEAKNESSES & OUTSIDE INFLUENCES

What do you think is the biggest misconception about vegans and how do you address this?
That we are unhealthy, are wasting away (awfully skinny or gaunt looking) and that vegan food is hard to cook. I try to be an example of a healthy looking vegan and post pictures of yummy food on FaceBook.

What are your strengths as a vegan athlete?
Flexibility, muscle strength and being fit. Belly dance is a bit of everything, but in a moderate version. It is perfect for all body shapes and ages.

What is your biggest challenge?
I have Ehler-Danlos Syndrome, a connective tissue disease. I was born with this and it is a huge challenge. It causes chronic fatigue, chronic pain, POTS and other issues. It causes chronic fatigue, chronic pain, Postural or Thostatitic Tachycardia Syndrome (POTS), and other issues.

Are the non-vegans in your industry supportive or not?
Yes they are. They love to come and watch me perform.

Are your family and friends supportive of your vegan lifestyle?
Sort of, they have accepted it but joke about it as well.

What is the most common question/comment that people ask/say when they find out that you are a vegan and how do you respond?
Actually, I rarely get comments, people just accept.

FOOD & SUPPLEMENTS

What do you eat for Breakfast?
Banana smoothie with orange juice.

What do you eat for Lunch?
Orgran crisp bread with avocado or Tofutti cream cheese on top.

What do you eat for Dinner?
Mostly Asian greens (bok choy etc) with tofu and rice, leafy green salads, sometimes a potato salad, pastas. I try to vary my dinners.

What do you eat for Snacks - healthy & not-so healthy?
Potato crisps.

What is your favourite source of Protein?
Tofu is one of my favorites - it is very versatile.

What is your favourite source of Calcium?
Again tofu, and green leafy vegetables.

What is your favourite source of Iron?
Green leafy vegetables.

What foods give you the most energy?
Bananas.

Do you take any supplements?
Yes vegan multi vitamins, and vitamin D.

ADVICE

What is your top tip for Gaining muscle, Losing weight & Toning up?
Since belly dance is a gentler type of exercise, don't expect to bulk up, but you will get fitter and more toned. Belly dance is mainly cardio so very good for weight loss and staying generally fit.

There are many different movements in belly dance you can practice at home. Shimmies are the hardest. They are perfect for cardio. However, if you want a more relaxing exercise type, you can practice the slower movements, they help with flexibility. Once you start belly dance classes, you will discover muscles you never knew you had. You can have a bit of muscle soreness after the first few classes, but not too much. My students never complain about a lot of soreness. A good teacher will build up each class gradually with a slow warm up.

How do you promote veganism in your daily life?
By showing how good the food is and by telling people about facts, those can be health facts, animal rights related facts and links to scientific publications.

How would you suggest people get involved with what you do?
Google for belly dance classes in your neighbourhood, or, even easier; have a look at my links page there are two websites in that that list classes in Australia, and outside of Australia.

Vegan Food Staples

The basic food staples for the vegan diet are:

- Fruits and Vegetable
- Whole grains
- Legumes, Pulses and Beans
- Nuts and Seeds

Focus on Reasons
Not Excuses.

Andrea Berman
VEGAN EXERCISE ENTHUSIAST

Boston, Massachusetts, USA
Vegan since: 2006

teaaddictedgeek.com
fitgeekfitness.com
SM: *FaceBook, Twitter, YouTube*

Andrea Berman is a P90X and INSANITY Certified Beachbody Coach in addition to being a Certified Life Coach. Her day job is a software engineering and she also enjoys writing, travel, and numerous geek loves including science fiction and fantasy. She blogs at Confessions of a Tea-Addicted Geek about her fitness journey, philosophy, and personal life, and can be reached for fitness coaching at FitGeek Fitness.

WHY VEGAN?

How and why did you decide to become vegan?
I had a bunch of food intolerances, and eliminating animal products got rid of them. Research made me go from dietary to lifestyle vegan.

How long have you been vegan?
Since February 2006, so over seven years now.

What has benefited you the most from being vegan?
In addition to health, mindfulness about the world around me and how my actions affect both it and others.

What does veganism mean to you?
It means to aim to harm none.

TRAINING

What sort of training do you do?
I run, walk, and do workout programs such as Les Mills Combat and Les Mills Pump.

How often do you (need to) train?
I work out 5-6 days per week.

Do you offer your fitness or training services to others?
Yes, I do. I have a variety of clients both local and long-distance whom I coach and offer my help to.

What sports do you play?
Not into sports, actually. I'm into other forms of fitness instead.

"We need more people to combat the nonsense that's out there. Nutrition and food should not be political, but unfortunately they are, which does not help the situation one bit."

STRENGTHS, WEAKNESSES & OUTSIDE INFLUENCES

What do you think is the biggest misconception about vegans and how do you address this?

That we are all crazy, religious fanatics. Too many people out there think you can out-exercise a bad diet and some can get away with it. I address this by being rational and mentioning my concerns with the abuse and corruption within the food industry and my desire not to support it, not to mention the environmental impact. By taking myself out of the system, I am casting my vote for a better world.

What are your strengths as a vegan athlete?

Better health, better recovery time, less likely to drop dead of a heart attack while jogging. Too many people out there who think you can out-exercise a bad diet and some can get away with it.

What is your biggest challenge?

Being told things such as I "need meat" and all sorts of very inaccurate statements about nutrition in general. It's very frustrating and I can only do so much to educate. We need more people out there to combat the nonsense that's out there. Nutrition and food should not be political, but unfortunately they are, which does not help the situation one bit.

Are the non-vegans in your industry supportive or not?

Some are and some aren't. I'm very happy to see Tony Horton and Shaun T (creators of P90X and INSANITY respectively) encourage people to drop meat and dairy. I absolutely love seeing that whenever they post to their pages.

Are your family and friends supportive of your vegan lifestyle?

Extremely, yes, I'm quite blessed to have a great family, which despite its meat-and-potato leanings, loves to make sure I'm fed "Andrea-friendly food". Not even my mom worries about how much protein I get, which says it all.

What is the most common question/comment that people ask/say when they find out that you are a vegan and how do you respond?

"Where do you get your protein?" My answer is usually "Food." Every source of natural food contains protein.

Who or what motivates you?

Prominent vegans in the fitness world such as Robert Cheeke, Giacomo Marchese, Scott Jurek, Brendan Brazier, all fighting the good plant strong fight.

FOOD & SUPPLEMENTS

What do you eat for Breakfast?

I usually do a quick fruit and protein smoothie, as I am frequently pressed for time. Typically it includes 1 scoop chocolate vegan Shakeology, 1/4 cup frozen strawberries, 1/2 banana, 1-1.5 cups of unsweetened chocolate flavored almond milk, and 2 TB of unsweetened cocoa.

What do you eat for Lunch?

Veggie wraps, quinoa and veggie salads, veggie burgers, any and all of the above. I do like to mix things up but during the weekday I usually have a bunch of different sandwich fillings prepared and stuff it in two slices of toasted Ezekiel bread or put into an Ezekiel wrap. I love Ezekiel. I can't do wheat too often, but sprouted wheat agrees with me and it's a very healthy carbohydrate.

What do you eat for Dinner?
Pretty similar to lunch. If it's a rest day or really hot outside, I'm pretty likely to make another smoothie and add more fruit to it, sometimes with a side salad.

What do you eat for Snacks - healthy & not-so healthy?
Hummus and veggies, Vega One or VegaSport protein bars, anything chocolate (it's my one vice you'll have to pry out of my cold, dead, rotting fingers). I like to keep this to a square or two of dark chocolate. Slice of toasted Ezekiel bread with natural peanut butter and sliced bananas on top.

What is your favourite source of Protein?
Tofu - I love tofu, especially pressed and marinated. Second favourite would have to be quinoa. Third would be lentils.

What is your favourite source of Calcium?
Also tofu. In addition, kale. I love, love kale.

What is your favourite source of Iron?
Quinoa, kale, spinach, lentils.

What foods give you the most energy?
Anything that's tasty and healthy!

Do you take any supplements?
Usually just Shakeology. On heavily active days, ones where I'm apt to burn 3000+ calories or more, I'll tack on Vega One and VegaSport products. I also love PlantFusion and Sunwarrior.

ADVICE

What is your top tip for gaining muscle?
Eat lots of nutritionally dense, healthy food.

What is your top tip for losing weight?
Eat clean, stay active. Avoid alcohol, processed foods, and fried foods as much as possible.

What is your top tip for maintaining weight?
Eat clean, stay active.

What is your top tip for improving metabolism?
Get active. Find small ways to increase your activity level as the day goes on. Want a real eye opener? Do what I did and invest in either a BodyMedia device or a FitBit.

What is your top tip for toning up?
Eat clean and do a good blend of cardio, strength training, and yoga.

How do you promote veganism in your daily life?
Living by example.

How would you suggest people get involved with what you do?
Just DO IT! Small steps over time can snowball. Don't be crazy and try to be perfect and do everything all at once, get a motivation or support group going and/or find one, and talk to others who have been where you're at!

Also, stay motivated. It's something you have to work on daily, and like all muscles needs a good workout. It's often said that motivation doesn't last but hey, neither does bathing.

Andrew Johnson
VEGAN EXERCISE ENTHUSIAST

Portland, Oregon, USA
Vegan since: 2007

jollygreenskitchen.blogspot.com
SM: *Instagram, Tumblr, Twitter*

Andrew Graeme Johnson is a 27-year old vegan athlete living in Portland, Oregon, USA. He is an engineer at a granola factory, a jack-of-all-trades, and an adrenaline junkie. You can see his recipes on Blogspot, and find him on Twitter and Instagram.

WHY VEGAN?

How and why did you decide to become vegan?
When I was much younger, my sisters went vegetarian, then vegan, before I knew what that even meant. They never pressured me to change my diet, but told me how to get information if I wanted to know about it. I put it off for years, until finally as a college freshman I dove into it and found the profound sadness in our treatment of other beings. I went vegan, and will stay vegan, because of my compassion for all beings.

How long have you been vegan?
I have been vegan since thanksgiving of 2007, so over 6 years. I was vegetarian for just over a year before that.

What has benefited you the most from being vegan?
I have never been healthier. My plant-based diet has helped me get and stay in great shape, recover more quickly, and feel better on a day-to-day basis than I had ever felt before.

What does veganism mean to you?
To me, veganism is an entire way of life built around compassion. It starts with the diet, yes, but it soon spreads into every other aspect of your life. My decisions about my clothing, my toiletries, my household supplies, they're all based on my belief that we as humans have no right to "use" animals for anything.

TRAINING

What sort of training do you do?
On an average week, I have about 4 work-out days. When it's a cold Winter, this consists mostly of running 10-15 miles per week, indoor rock climbing 3 days per week, a few yoga sessions, and volleyball. When the weather warms up, I will be increasing my running as well as including biking and swimming for triathlon training.

How often do you (need to) train?
I could probably get away with less than 4 sessions per week, but if I dip below that, I start to feel lazy.

Do you offer your fitness or training services to others?
I try to get as many friends involved as I can. Especially with long runs, rock climbing, and volleyball, the more people I can get interested the more beneficial. I used to work at the campus gym while in college, and I had friends who would come in for training sessions. I love to help people work on areas they'd like to improve, whether it is endurance, building muscle, or just feeling healthier.

What sports do you play?
All of them. Haha. Right now, I'm very active with running, climbing, yoga, indoor volleyball, and a little basketball. I also love ultimate frisbee, cycling, soccer, and football, so when the weather is good I'll start back with those. Swimming is a sport I've always struggled with, but I'm determined to keep improving.

"A body at rest will stay at rest, a body in motion will stay in motion."

STRENGTHS, WEAKNESSES & OUTSIDE INFLUENCES

What do you think is the biggest misconception about vegans and how do you address this?
I often hear that veganism isn't a healthy lifestyle. People will say, "Oh my friend went vegan for 6 months but they got really sick so they started eating meat and dairy again." It's difficult to fight ignorance, so I address these situations with information: talking about the health benefits of commonly known vegetables, fruits, and legumes, and stating how keeping a balanced diet of these foods is the key to staying healthy. The protein argument is a huge part of this misconception, but if you ask someone how strong a gorilla is, they'll catch on pretty quickly.

What are your strengths as a vegan athlete?
The biggest strength of all, I think, is that no other sentient being needs to suffer for me to succeed. That being said, I think that my plant-based diet helps to keep my body packed with naturally sourced vitamins and minerals, keeping my muscles, blood and bones ready for the exertion I put them through. I rarely get sick, so I don't miss any time with a cold or the flu. My body also seems to heal more quickly than it used to, so my recovery downtime is shorter.

What is your biggest challenge?
My biggest challenge is eating at the post-event parties. Whether it is a running race, a triathlon, or any other event, the food is generally laden with dairy and/or meat. Granted there is almost always a large portion of oranges, bananas, and similar fruit, but that's not enough for someone of my size (I'm 6'10") to curb their hunger after a race.

Are the non-vegans in your industry supportive or not?
In engineering, it seems to be 50/50. Some people are genuinely interested and made an effort to look for options if we go out to lunch or they bring food to the office, while the others just make jokes. As GM of an organic juice and smoothie bar, though, the majority of people are supportive. Many of my customers are vegan, vegetarian, or trying to increase their plant-based meals, so they are excited to come to a place that is mostly vegan and talk to a vegan behind the counter.

Are your family and friends supportive of your vegan lifestyle?
My family is extremely supportive, and I am so thankful for that. They are who I got my compassion from, and are all either vegetarian or vegan themselves. Holidays at home are a treat because now it's the non-vegan dishes that are the oddballs, not the vegan dishes.

What is the most common question/comment that people ask/say when they find out that you are a vegan and how do you respond?

"How do you do it?" or, "what do you eat?" are the most common questions I hear. I try to tell people that as a vegan I eat a wider variety of foods than I ate as an omnivore. People get set on this idea of a meat and potatoes meal, so they only think about the chicken, potatoes, and (maybe) green beans. They're missing out on so many wonderful vegetables, grains, legumes, and fruit. I tell them that going vegan opened my eyes to new foods, and encourage them to try it out for themselves.

Who or what motivates you?

Seeing other vegan athletes succeed in their fields is always a great motivation. Mostly, though, I find motivation in my family and friends. I'm lucky enough to know so many talented individuals, and when they share their passion for their sport with me, I get hooked and motivated to find my own passions. I suppose that is why I participate in and enjoy so many; I find love for sports extremely contagious. I'm also motivated by my own progress. Seeing myself improve at something I enjoy is richly rewarding.

FOOD & SUPPLEMENTS

What do you eat for Breakfast?

More often than not, is a veggie smoothie with spinach, kale, avocado, cucumber, apple, banana, ginger root, lemon, cinnamon and cayenne, mixed with ice, water, and some almond milk.

What do you eat for Lunch?

Generally a huge meal I make from scratch on Sunday and eat throughout the week. I love spinach lasagna, black bean empanadas, asparagus quiche, soup and bread – basically, what most people eat for dinner.

What do you eat for Dinner?

I tend to work out at night, so when I get home my dinner consists of a big protein shake and small snacks. The protein shake is generally frozen banana, an apple, oatmeal, cannellini beans, protein powder, peanut or almond butter, and cinnamon, mixed with ice, water, and almond milk.

What do you eat for Snacks - healthy & not-so healthy?

I eat about 6 times a day, so snacks are a necessity. I tend to make a lot of muffins, homemade hummus with veggies or triscuits, banana buckwheat pancakes with peanut or almond butter and agave instead of syrup, couscous salads with plenty of nuts and veggies, and if I have no time to cook a snack myself I'll grab a Clif bar and a banana.

What is your favourite source of Protein?

I like to use a combination of protein-rich foods and protein powders throughout the week. For foods, I like cannellini, black, and mung beans, almonds, and lentils. For powders, I like hemp seed, Vega, Sun Warrior, and PlantFusion.

What is your favourite source of Calcium?

I eat a large quantity of leafy greens and beans on a daily basis for my calcium.

What is your favourite source of Iron?

I eat a lot of beans, tofu, and spinach.

What foods give you the most energy?

I think my vegetable smoothie in the morning is my greatest energy-boosting meal. I'll drink one of those (roughly 30 oz.) before work, and I'll have all the energy I need for hours.

Do you take any supplements?
Last year I took a B-12 supplement because a friend recommended it, but I honestly did not notice any benefit while taking it. Currently the only supplements I take are protein powders.

ADVICE

What is your top tip for gaining muscle?
Do anything Robert Cheeke says! Eat a healthy, balanced diet, with about 1 to 1.5 grams of protein per pound of bodyweight, and do plenty of weight training. I noticed that when I did a very intense workout 3 times per week, focusing on a different set of muscle groups each session and increased my protein intake to 200 g per day, I had noticeable gains.

What is your top tip for losing weight?
Stay active. Especially early in the morning, so that you boost your metabolism and it stays high throughout the day. Run often. If you can't run, jog. If you can't jog, walk. Never take the elevator or escalator up a few flights; take the stairs. Cut out as much added sugar from your diet as you can. When I stopped drinking soda and store-bought juices at 19, I lost a lot of weight. If you make a few small adjustments, and do these every day, you'll notice a big change over time. I lost 60 pounds (27 kilograms) by following the suggestions I just mentioned.

What is your top tip for maintaining weight?
I can't say this enough: eat a balanced diet. Don't overload on one type of food, eat plenty of fruits, vegetables, grains, and legumes. These foods are nutrient-dense, so you get full without consuming too many calories. Also, try not to sit for too long. Get up and move around, even if it's only a short walk down the street. A body at rest will stay at rest, a body in motion will stay in motion.

What is your top tip for improving metabolism?
I've noticed that a quick workout in the morning does a great job at boosting my metabolism. I like to go for a short run or do yoga, but anything that raises your heart rate for 20 minutes or more will work. I also eat a lot of spicy foods like peppers, ginger, and cinnamon, and drink green tea. These are all shown to increase metabolic rate.

What is your top tip for toning up?
I highly suggest yoga. It's helped me not only tone my shoulders, obliques, and legs, but also to improve my balance and state of mind. It's hard to find a practice more beneficial than yoga, in my opinion.

How do you promote veganism in your daily life?
As I mentioned before, I manage a meat- and dairy-free juice and smoothie bar. I'm also an animal rights activist, and take part in peaceful protests against Yum! Brands (headquartered in Kentucky), McDonalds, leather and fur stores, and other businesses that promote abuse against animals. Much of my social media presence is also dedicated to veganism.

How would you suggest people get involved with what you do?
Drop in on a NorthWest VEG event. NW VEG is a great non-profit here dedicated to educating and encouraging people to adopt plant-based diets. You can also get involved with the Columbia chapter of the Sierra Club, as we fight to protect animals and their homes in the wild.

ANDREW KNIGHT
VEGAN EXTREME SPORTSMAN

Winchester, England, UK
Vegan since: 1993

extremevegansports.org
andrewknight.info
SM: *YouTube*

Andrew Knight is an Australian-British bioethicist and European veterinary specialist in welfare science, ethics and law. He has authored over 80 academic and 50 popular publications on animal issues, including an extensive series examining the contributions to human healthcare of animal experiments. These formed the basis for his 2010 PhD, and his 2011 book "The Costs and Benefits of Animal Experiments" (hardback 2011; paperback 2013).

WHY VEGAN?

How and why did you decide to become vegan?
When I was 23 my girlfriend and I both went vegan at the same time in an attempt to impress each other. It must have worked because we're still good friends many years later.

How long have you been vegan?
Too long (because I'm ancient), but not long enough (because I wasn't smart enough to start from birth).

What has benefited you the most from being vegan?
Hard to say as the list is so long. I have the satisfaction of knowing my life inflicts the least harm reasonably possible on other sentient creatures, the least adverse environmental impacts, and the least inequitable consumption of limited global food, water and land resources. I don't have much body fat and am much fitter. My animal advocacy career has taken me around the world and I've met some wonderful, inspiring people. And like I said, it impressed my girlfriend, which was very important at the time.

What does veganism mean to you?
I don't consume or use animal products or those tested on animals to the extent reasonably possible. Of course virtually everything in the world is linked to everything else in some way, and it's impossible to walk the Earth without participating in abuse of others to some degree (every footstep squashes microbes, for example). But I try to do the best I can. Perfection is unrealistic.

"Virtually all plants have protein, just to differing degrees. If you want a lot of it, you just have to pick the right foods. It's not hard – massively strong animals like elephants and gorillas manage just fine."

TRAINING

What sort of training do you do?

I very rarely iron, but I cross train regularly by running. However, when training for my last mountaineering challenge, I was knocked from my bike after riding home from weightlifting at the gym, and had surgery to fix my fractured elbow. This was sufficient proof that weights are bad for my health, so I'm staying away from them. At least until my arm recovers. I'm not too keen on bikes either.

How often do you (need to) train?

When fit and not working I run nearly every day, or I start to get frustrated.

Do you offer your fitness or training services to others?

If anyone wants to try anything extreme and possibly foolish then I'm more than happy to advise them. Other than one brilliant English lad who went sky diving in a banana costume to publicise the vegan diet, unfortunately no one has asked – or taken – my advice.

What sports do you play?

Ironing. The more extreme kind. Combining "the thrill of a danger sport with the satisfaction of a well-pressed shirt" the popularity of extreme ironing has risen spectacularly. International championships now exist, with the English recently beating the Australians by having the greatest number of people ironing underwater at the same time, in a flooded quarry. The waters were so freezing they desperately hoped they'd never have to win back the title.

As a native Australian though, I rather hope otherwise. Maybe I can make the Aussie team someday with sufficient training. But Aussies are tough, so I realise this will have to be hard-core. This was why in late 2011 I carried my mountaineering ironing board to the summit of Wales' highest mountain, Mt Snowdon (1085m/3720 feet). I was almost blown off the top by 50mph (80kph) winds, but for a few seconds on the summit I was the highest ironer in all of England and Wales. The photos of this amazing adventure are on my website.

One year later, I returned from an ironing trip to the French alps. I ironed above 3000m (1.86miles) in temperatures as low as -20C (-4F). A wilderness snowstorm even enabled me to practice survival ironing. My shirts got seriously crisp that day!

STRENGTHS, WEAKNESSES & OUTSIDE INFLUENCES

What do you think is the biggest misconception about vegans and how do you address this?

That vegans must endure grim and joyless lives of self-denial: "Doubtless we dream of little more than our own untimely deaths, as we feebly stagger through our days, made pale and weak by lack of essential animal proteins..." Personally, I've tried to address this by establishing the Extreme Vegan Sporting Association, which exists to showcase vegan fitness, and to demonstrate just how much fun the vegan lifestyle can actually be!

What are your strengths as a vegan athlete?

Probably a certain stupidity. I ski black slopes in the Alps my friends don't like. I think I'm just less aware of the potential consequences, or a lot more foolish. Whatever it is, it seems to work!

What is your biggest challenge?

Figuring out how to transport sufficient vegan cheesecake for my very substantial needs to the tops of the mountains I sometimes climb.

Are the non-vegans in your industry supportive or not?
I don't discuss my expeditions a great deal with my co-workers. For some reason they seem to think I'm mad.

Are your family and friends supportive of your vegan lifestyle?
My family are mostly not vegan, and oddly seem to prefer not to discuss food with me too much! And my friends are mostly vegan anyway.

What is the most common question/comment that people ask/say when they find out that you are a vegan and how do you respond?
Q: Where do you get your protein? A: Virtually all plants have protein, just to differing degrees. If you want a lot of it, you just have to pick the right foods. It's not hard - massively strong animals like elephants and gorillas manage just fine.

Who or what motivates you?
I just want to try to be the best person I can be, which means doing the most good, and the least harm, that I reasonably can, to sentient others.

And I'd also like to make the Australian extreme ironing team, and beat the British. A lot.

FOOD&SUPPLEMENTS

What do you eat for Breakfast?
2 pieces of toast, large bowl of porridge, and fruit.

What do you eat for Lunch?
2 sandwiches, and fruit.

What do you eat for Dinner?
Rice, pasta, couscous or other carbohydrate-rich base, plus stir-fried veggies with one of the fake meat products (burgers, sausages, tofu, nut roast, etc), and vegan cheesecake or yoghurt.

What do you eat for Snacks - healthy & not-so healthy?
Flap jacks (Australian: 'muesli bars').

What is your favourite source of Protein?
Vegan cheesecake.

What is your favourite source of Calcium?
Vegan cheesecake.

What is your favourite source of Iron?
Vegan cheesecake.

(You said favourite source – not densest source!).

What foods give you the most energy?
Vegan chocolate.

Do you take any supplements?
Vegan multivitamin (including B12) and flax oil (for the omega 3 fatty acids) pills/capsules daily.

ADVICE

What is your top tip for gaining muscle?
Lift weights very regularly, and eat plenty of healthy, vegan food. Don't burn too many calories, e.g. by jogging too much. Get plenty of rest.

What is your top tip for losing weight?
Jog very regularly, eat moderate amounts of healthy vegan food. Don't be lazy. I've recently discovered that Latin dancing can also be a very good cardio workout.

What is your top tip for maintaining weight?
Balance your intake of healthy vegan food and calories, with those you burn in exercise, in order to increase, decrease or maintain your weight as desired.

What is your top tip for improving metabolism?
To increase metabolic rate, exercise!

What is your top tip for toning up?
Again – very regularly exercise. Salsa may be only moderately helpful, but can be awfully good fun!

How do you promote veganism in your daily life?
Often, through example. By staying fit and healthy, trying not to be (publicly, at least) unwell, and by having fun vegan adventures people enjoy hearing about!

How would you suggest people get involved with what you do?
Go to a large department store with a backpack. Try on a range of ironing boards until you find one you can carry between your pack and your back. Take it mountaineering, and send the photos to me via my website. In fact, any extreme ironing would do. I would particularly like to encourage someone to go extreme ironing, while skydiving, while wearing a banana costume...

Of course, I'm open to other extreme vegan sports too (the website includes numerous galleries including yodelling and cooking, as well as conventional sports like body building), but it's hard to imagine anything more extreme than ironing! The Mt Snowdon climb nearly killed me.

"I have the satisfaction of knowing my life inflicts the least harm reasonably possible on other sentient creatures, the least adverse environmental impacts, and the least inequitable consumption of limited global food, water and land resources. I don't have much body fat and am much fitter. My animal advocacy career has taken me around the world and I've met some wonderful, inspiring people."

You get what you Work For

ANNE-MARIE CAMPBELL
VEGAN TAE KWON DO BLACK BELT

Toronto, Ontario, Canada
Vegan since: 2011

meatfreeathlete.com
SM: *FaceBook, Google+, Instagram, Pinterest, Twitter, YouTube*

Anne-Marie Campbell is a vegan athlete and animal rights activist. She has been a competitive athlete since the age of 9, and currently trains in martial arts, with a Black Belt in Tae Kwon Do. A big part of her mission is to spread awareness and information about the vegan lifestyle while leading by example. She is the Founder of MeatFreeAthlete.com, a Vegan Resource and Blog. Her motto is "Eat Kind, Be Strong."

WHY VEGAN?

How and why did you decide to become vegan?
I saw a post online about factory farms and the cruelty that comes with it. Before that point, I never thought about where my food came from. I didn't know any vegetarians or vegans, or anyone who spoke about animal welfare issues that concerned those raised for food. For the first time I was seeing terrible pictures and reports of cruelty, and that marked the beginning of my personal journey to making the connection. I started seeking out information online and I was horrified. I didn't want any part of it.

How long have you been vegan?
Since May 2011.

What has benefited you the most from being vegan?
The benefits have been both physical and spiritual. Living a vegan lifestyle has given me a deeper connection with my relationship to the world around me and has given me a greater sense of appreciation and respect for my life and those I share this earth with. I find that when you truly love yourself, you will want to extend that love to others, and you can't do that by exploiting and causing harm to others. As an athlete, there's been a definite improvement to my athletic performance since becoming vegan. I have more energy to train longer and harder, and I recover faster.

What does veganism mean to you?
Living a lifestyle where my actions match my morals. Veganism is much more than what I eat. It represents a way of living that shows my respect for all life, and consciously making the decision to cause no harm. Veganism is my rejection of the traditional elitist attitude that humans are somehow superior or more important than other animals.

TRAINING

What sort of training do you do?
I'm a Black Belt in Tae Kwon Do, and currently working on earning my 2nd Degree. I also train in Mixed Martial Arts (MMA), and love yoga. Hockey is also a sport that I played competitively for many years, and I'll still play recreationally when I have the time.

How often do you (need to) train?
Ideally, I aim to train 3-4 times a week.

Do you offer your fitness or training services to others?
I'm not a trainer, but I assist teaching Tae Kwon Do at my dojo, and I am interested in taking on more of an instructor role in Tae Kwon Do in the future.

What sports do you play?
Tae Kwon Do, Hockey, Yoga, MMA, and Roller Hockey.

STRENGTHS, WEAKNESSES & OUTSIDE INFLUENCES

What do you think is the biggest misconception about vegans and how do you address this?
A lot people still think you need meat for protein, and that you can't be active and healthy as a vegan. I lead by example to bust those myths when I train, and also on my website.

What are your strengths as a vegan athlete?
My passion is my strength. I have been a competitive athlete since I was 9 years old (starting with gymnastics). I have always loved sports and my passion for athletics keeps me focused on always improving myself and enjoying every minute of it.

What is your biggest challenge?
Injuries are always a challenge, physically and mentally. Being a competitive athlete for so many years, and in full contact sports, I've had pretty much every injury from head to toe, from concussions, dislocated ribs, broken nose, torn muscle, broken feet, ACL, MCL, and other not so fun injuries. The injury cycle is a big challenge, but worth it.

Are the non-vegans in your industry supportive or not?
The people around me are really open to the concept of being vegan and how it helps performance. I just lead by example, and if people are interested, I am more than happy to answer their questions and guide them in any way.

Are your family and friends supportive of your vegan lifestyle?
My family has been very accepting and really embraced it themselves.

What is the most common question/comment that people ask/say when they find out that you are a vegan and how do you respond?
Some people seem surprised because I am an athlete, and they wonder how I do it. Also, people will ask about what I eat or how I do it. Most people seem overwhelmed by the idea of being vegan. I like to show by example how easy it really is, and that being vegan really isn't as hard as it sounds. I will usually suggest some great foods to try that replace meat and dairy, and let them know they should enjoy trying new stuff, and not to get overwhelmed by the idea of being vegan. I realize most people won't go vegan over night, so I approach it as a journey, and everyone has their own journey to take.

Who or what motivates you?

I love seeing vegan babies and kids. It's so inspiring and gives me a great feeling of hope for the future. I absolutely love when parents give their children the gift of an early start at a healthy, compassionate lifestyle.

For my activism, I always remember the animals out there being exploited and killed for unnecessary human use. Every single one of them matters. My voice is for them. For my athletics, my motivation comes from my drive to be a better version of myself. I am my only true competition.

FOOD & SUPPLEMENTS

What do you eat for Breakfast?

Lots of juicy fruits, like oranges and grapes. I find those types of fruits to be really hydrating in the morning. I also like flax oatmeal with organic unsweetened soy milk.

What do you eat for Lunch?

Raw veggies with hummus, tofu summer rolls, mixed bean salads, quinoa veggies stir-fry, cereal with banana, or mixed nuts and fruit.

What do you eat for Dinner?

Mexican refried beans with homemade pico de gallo, guacamole, organic Textured Vegetable Protein (TVP), and organic corn chips. Homemade soup with lots of onion, garlic, kale, mushrooms, and lentils. Firm organic tofu or tempeh, with potatoes (sweet or red skin), lots of veggies. Hearty four bean chili, with corn chips and avocado. Whole grain pasta with fresh mushrooms. Quinoa tabouli. Brown rice, beans, and lots of steamed veggies. To name a few!

What do you eat for Snacks - healthy & not-so healthy?

Organic popcorn with nutritional yeast (some brands are a great source of B12), apples and peanut or almond butter, mixed nuts and fruit, granola, nachos and salsa, and homemade chocolate chip cookies.

What is your favourite source of Protein?

Quinoa, black beans, chickpeas, kidney beans, lentils, brown rice, organic soy milk, tofu, and tempeh.

What is your favourite source of Calcium?

Kale, almonds, flax seeds, broccoli, bok choy, and soy milk.

What is your favourite source of Iron?

Lentils, quinoa, fortified cereal, chickpeas, tofu or tempeh, and chia seeds.

What foods give you the most energy?

Before training, I keep it simple. Beans, raw mushrooms, and spinach drizzled with balsamic vinegar is a great combination for me. Also, raw veggies and hummus, or quinoa with black beans or chickpeas with green veggies.

Do you take any supplements?

No. I don't find that I need them.

ADVICE

What is your top tip for gaining muscle?
After training, fuel your body with what it needs to build and repair muscle. Eat clean proteins, like quinoa, beans, tofu or tempeh, for example, with veggies, and hydrate with water.

What is your top tip for losing weight and maintaining weight?
Listen to your body. Eat when you're hungry, and eat foods that nourish your body. Eat unprocessed foods, and avoid junk foods that are loaded with sugar and fat.

What is your top tip for improving metabolism?
Listen to your body. If you feel sluggish after you eat something, it's probably stunting your metabolism too. Also, avoid processed foods with sugar and high fat. Eat fresh foods that look closest to the way they were grown. The more natural the food is, the more your body knows how to digest it and thrive from it.

What is your top tip for toning up?
Be active and eat clean, unprocessed foods. It takes work, but put in your time and you'll see the results. Find activities you enjoy or are passionate about. Being active shouldn't be a chore - it should be time with yourself that you enjoy.

How do you promote veganism in your daily life?
I launched my website, which is a vegan resource and Blog. There are featured contributors, including myself, all writing on topics of experience relating to vegan health, fitness, food, and lifestyle. I also feature different vegan athletes and vegan recipes. I write a blog, lead by example, give tips, and help guide and support people transitioning or living a vegan lifestyle.

How would you suggest people get involved with what you do?
Get social: There's such a great vegan community online and it's an amazing source of support and information.

Be vocal: Share your experiences, it may just inspire others.

Reach out: You can reach me at my website, Instagram, Twitter, Facebook, and YouTube.

"Living a vegan lifestyle has given me a deeper connection with my relationship to the world around me and has given me a greater sense of appreciation and respect for my life and those I share this earth with. I find that when you truly love yourself, you will want to extend that love to others, and you can't do that by exploiting and causing harm to others."

More Good, Less Harm.

ANTHONY MANN
VEGAN BODY BUILDER & TRAINER

Northampton, England, UK
Vegan since: 1990

physicalpt.co.uk

Anthony Mann is a fully qualified personal trainer, a vegan bodybuilder and he is very passionate about fitness and boxing. He believes anyone can achieve their goals with hard work and guidance, whatever your fitness background.

WHY VEGAN?

How and why did you decide to become vegan?
I became vegan after being a vegetarian for a few years at 15 years old because of my brother Keith Mann who opened my eyes to the suffering of animals.

How long have you been vegan?
I've been vegan for over 23 years.

What has benefited you the most from being vegan?
Knowing I'm not eating animals or contributing to the plight against them.

What does veganism mean to you?
Veganism means everything to me - proving at 45 years I can be as good physically as a meat eater.

TRAINING

What sort of training do you do?
I weight train 4-5 times a week on different muscle groups. I'm also a personal trainer so I run with clients as and when needed from 2 miles to training clients up to 22 miles for marathon training. I sometimes box or spar 1-2 times a week.

How often do you (need to) train?
4-5 times a week.

Do you offer your fitness or training services to others?
Yes, I'm a personal trainer.

STRENGTHS, WEAKNESSES & OUTSIDE INFLUENCES

What do you think is the biggest misconception about vegans and how do you address this?
That we don't get enough protein - my answer is to train with me, look at me, that shuts them up.

What are your strengths as a vegan athlete?
I wouldn't say I have particular strengths as such, I'm just me but I can hold my own against any meat eater whatever their age.

What is your biggest challenge?
Finding clean, healthy, high-protein food if I'm out and about so often I have to carry food with me.

Are the non-vegans in your industry supportive or not?
Some people don't understand why I don't consume animals etc. I had a recent comment from a personal trainer in the gym I train at - I'd just had 3 months off with disc and nerve damage so lost over a stone - was "So are you going to eat meat now to help you put weight on?" I was flabbergasted at his ignorance.

Are your family and friends supportive of your vegan lifestyle?
Family and friends either say nothing or love to comment about how nice meat is etc. I used to get angry but now I'm quite calm and either ignore it or try to educate them.

What is the most common question/comment that people ask/say when they find out that you are a vegan and how do you respond?
The main question is "What do you eat?" and "Why are you vegan?" Both easy answers: anything that hasn't being murdered and because I care and don't think it's right to eat animals.

Who or what motivates you?
I am self-motivated. I strive to try to look good, be fit and prove people wrong. Plus with fitness being my job it's important to me also from a work perspective.

FOOD & SUPPLEMENTS

What do you eat for Breakfast?
Oats, and banana protein shake.

What do you eat for Lunch?
Brown rice, sweet potato, spaghetti with tofu, veg mince, mock duck, soya chunks, plus asparagus, broccoli and peas.

What do you eat for Dinner?
Mixed beans tofu salad, Shephard's pie plus green veg. Oats, cinnamon, protein shake. Tempeh stir fry with brown rice, lentils, chick peas, mixed with vegetables and any food from lunch.

What do you eat for Snacks - healthy & not-so healthy?
Rice cakes with peanut butter, homemade protein oat bars, banana, apples, vegan yoghurt, oat cakes, celery, weetabix, mixed nuts, blueberries, homemade apple pie and soya custard.

What is your favorite source of Protein?
Tempeh and tofu.

What is your favorite source of Calcium?
Soy milk and broccoli.

What is your favorite source of Iron?
Spinach.

Do you take any supplements?
B vitamins, Vitamin C and Zinc.

ADVICE

What is your top tip for gaining muscle?
Eat, eat, eat, and lift heavy weights.

What is your top tip for losing weight?
Train 4-5 days a week at a minimum of 30 minutes per day, varying the workouts. Eat three small main meals and two snacks aiming for approx 1200 calories.

What is your top tip for maintaining weight?
Don't lose sight of your diet - keep training intensely, avoid sugar, but have a cheat day.

What is your top tip for improving metabolism?
Eat small and often and don't find excuses not to train.

What is your top tip for toning up?
Don't avoid the weights as some women do thinking they will get big muscles, but in turn the more muscle you have the more calories you will burn. Combine that with a sensible diet and a good cardio routine, variety is the key and avoid alcohol or cut right back. Drink lots of water and avoid salt.

How do you promote veganism in your daily life?
I don't really promote it as I found preaching got me nowhere. I just use my physique as my tool. Most people are scared of change and think eating meat and dairy are important for nutrition and calcium without realising what is in our food, so if asked, I just educate and try to advise on how to eat for what they want.

"One farmer says to me, 'You cannot live on vegetable food solely, for it furnishes nothing to make bones with;' and so he religiously devotes a part of his day to supplying his system with the raw material of bones; walking all the while he talks behind his oxen, which, with vegetable-made bones, jerk him and his lumbering plow along in spite of every obstacle."
- Henry David Thoreau

The Only Bad Workout is the one You Didn't Do.

ATSUYUKI KATSUYAMA
VEGAN BAREFOOT ULTRA-MARATHONER

Bangkok, Thailand
Vegan since: 2009

facebook.com/bonita.c.sc
krunusa.wordpress.com

Atsuyuki Katsuyama (K) is a Japanese vegan barefoot ultra-marathoner. He has run 100 full-marathons in his life, including 18 ultra-marathons, and 77 full/ultra-marathons in the last 77 months. From 25 April to 12 July 2015, K completed a 5030km (3125miles) running adventure in 79-days from Los Angeles to New York. By running ultra distance with his barefoot (and natural) running style, he is sharing his ideas of "Run naturally, gently and sustainably on our earth." He currently lives in Thailand, and owns a small vegan restaurant, Bonita Cafe and Social Club in Bangkok, Thailand, with his Thai wife. This place has become a popular social club for those who care about good life, where lots of vegans, athletes and animal rights activists gather from all over the world.

WHY VEGAN?

How and why did you decide to become vegan?
It was a very simple and sudden start. Four years ago, when I was living in California, I had a chance to listen to an American vegan couple, my best friends, April and Chris, who are also runners, talk about being vegan. Three minutes later, I said, "OK! From now on, I am vegan!"

My mother has been a cooking teacher in Japan for 50 years. I have been watching her and I have been running a lot. Therefore, I have always cared about my food, trying many different diet styles. That was my first time to talk with vegan people, but, with my background, I felt that the plant-based diet is quite reasonable and that it is very ethical way of living life. I suddenly became vegan. Since then, I never want to get back to non-vegan. And, I really appreciate April and Chris. Without them, I would not be who I am now, and our vegan cafe, Bonita Cafe and Social Club, would not be here.

How long have you been vegan?
Over five years.

What has benefited you the most from being vegan?
Before, I ate everything. Especially since I lived in the southern part of China for eight years. So, I ate all the four-legs, except desks, and all the flying things, except airplanes. At that time, I believed those fresh animal-based things could give me power. So, it was a 180 degree change to become vegan. But, nothing happened. I still feel powerful, running 100 mile races. Actually, I feel much more powerful now. Before, I could feel my inner temperature going up and down, therefore I needed lots of effort to adjust my temperature. But, nowadays, I feel my inner temperature is quite stable, and I do not need to use unnecessary

energy to adjust my temperature. Thanks to being vegan, I feel so calm and powerful now. And, one more important thing is I am feeling that I am living in calm cruelty-free world.

What does veganism mean to you?
It is not just the way of eating. It is my lifestyle. Veganism brings healthy and ethical lifestyle to me.

TRAINING

What sort of training do you do?
When preparing for running across the USA, I ran half marathon distance (21km) most days in 2013. In 2014, I ran full marathon distance (42km) most days. This is just running quantity. I am also improving my running quality, with my barefoot running technique.

How often do you (need to) train?
I train every day.

Do you offer your fitness or training services to others?
When I was one of the managers of Bangkok Barefoot Run Club, I was teaching barefoot running and natural running. Natural running is the idea of running naturally, with our own body, not depending on things, provided from outside. We can run with our own body, and not depend on high-tech gadgets. In this way, we can run effectively (faster, longer, farther) and sustainably, without injury, for a long time in our life. Now, I teach some friends, too, when my friends are interested in this natural running.

What sports do you play?
I run.

STRENGTHS, WEAKNESSES & OUTSIDE INFLUENCES

What do you think is the biggest misconception about vegans and how do you address this?
Many people misunderstand and are afraid and think that avoiding animal-based products may reduce our energy or power. But, I say, "I feel very powerful and I can run 100 miles." That is enough for them to start to consider their diet.

What are your strengths as a vegan athlete?
Two points: 1. I do not need to waste unnecessary power for digesting heavy animal-based foods, therefore I feel so energetic, and I can use that power to perform well in my running. 2. Compared with when I ate everything, being vegan has given me a lot faster recovery. In this way, I can keep on running, while the others need to take rests.

What is your biggest challenge?
I do not find any difficulties being a vegan ultra-runner. I just enjoy it.

Are the non-vegans in your industry supportive or not?
There are very few people, who try to attack my vegan lifestyle. Probably, that comes from their jealousy, so I just do not worry about them. However, on the other hand, most of my friends are really interested in and curious about the combination of veganism and ultra-running. Many of them are not satisfied with their diet either. With these people, I love discussing co-relation of good diet and good sport performance.

Are your family and friends supportive of your vegan lifestyle?
Yes, they are.

What is the most common question/comment that people ask/say when they find out that you are a vegan and how do you respond?

People: "How do you take protein?"

I: " Many kinds of plant based foods. How do you take YOUR protein?"

People: "Meat."

I: "Do you know how much protein you need in one day?"

People: "No"

I: "If you do not know it, how can you say that you are taking enough protein?"

People: "?"

I: "I know how much protein I need to take in one day, and all the vegetables and fruits can cover that amount. And, I run 100 miles, too!"

Who or what motivates you?

All kinds of people. I especially love a humble person.

FOOD & SUPPLEMENTS

What do you eat for Breakfast, Lunch, Dinner and Snacks?

I do not have any set pattern for what I eat in a day. I eat all kinds of vegan foods and drinks. Most of what I eat is what we serve in our vegan restaurant. I love our foods. That is why they are in our menu and served for our customers. They are so delicious, so I eat them everyday.

This is what I do: I drink three liters of water every day, each one an hour before each meals. Then, 30 minutes later, I eat lots of fruits. Then, another 30 minutes, I eat meals. When I eat fruits and meals, I choose whole food.

What is your favorite source of Protein, Calcium and Iron?

I do not pick up some specific foods. I just eat many kinds of vegetables, fruits and grains, as I know which vegan foods contain what amount of protein, calcium, iron and other essential things.

What foods give you the most energy?

I believe the combination of eating various kinds of foods, especially whole foods, gives us energy. But, I want to emphasize one point. Certain food does not bring energy and health to us. Our good health is brought by the combination of good food, good exercise, good rest, good mind and good breathing.

Do you take any supplements?

Vitamin B12.

ADVICE

What is your top tip for gaining muscle?

Run. Eat properly.

What is your top tip for losing weight?

Run. Eat lots of whole foods.

What is your top tip for maintaining weight?

Run. Eat lots of whole foods.

What is your top tip for improving metabolism and toning up?

Run.

How do you promote veganism in your daily life?

For my case, I own a vegan restaurant in Thailand. This is big enough to promote veganism. Every day, many kinds of people, from all over the world, visit our place, and I am very happy to exchange our ideas and wisdom. I also run with many running friends. Many of them are interested in improving their performance, so they are interested in good diet, too. When they ask me for my opinion, I open my mouth and share my thoughts.

How would you suggest people get involved with what you do?

For veganism, I never say, "You must be a vegan!" We are all different, and people will move, when they want to move. When they are willing to listen to my thoughts, I will open my mouth. For running, I never say, "Run strong!" As a vegan natural runner, I do not show that I am strong. On our great earth, a human being is just a weak piece. I love running naturally, gently, lightly and softly. In this way, I believe we can enjoy running sustainably, without injury, and effectively. In this way, with my veganism and natural running, I am sharing my ideas of a sustainable way of living on our earth.

"I believe the combination of eating various kinds of foods, especially whole foods, gives us energy. Certain food does not bring energy and health to us. Our good health is brought by the combination of good food, good exercise, good rest, good mind and good breathing."

"I am only one, but I am one. I cannot do everything, but I can do something. And I will not let what I cannot do interfere with what I can do."
- Edward Everett Hale

Don't make excuses, make changes.

AUSTIN BARBISCH
VEGAN PERSONAL TRAINER & BODYBUILDER

Austin, Texas, USA
Vegan since: 2012

austinbarbisch.com
veganfasterstronger.com

Austin Barbisch is a full-time personal trainer and massage therapist and has been since 1996. He is interested in pretty much anything involving the human body including nutrition, postural correction and how the body adapts to different training techniques. He loves running, completing his second 100-mile ultra-marathon in February 2013 and winning a 24 hour race December 2012 with 115.32 miles (185km). He also won this race the next year by over 9km over the 2nd place finisher. Austin does bodybuilding shows as well, with two completed shows in 2013 resulting in four 2nd place trophies and winning his bodybuilding class in 2014. He also finished in 1st place in his division in the Concept 2 world database in the 500 and 1000m in indoor rowing distances. Other hobbies include sculpture, photography, and reading. His main passion right now is to show how a vegan lifestyle can support our personal health, the health of our fellow animals and the world we all live in.

WHY VEGAN?

How and why did you decide to become vegan?
I switched to a plant-based diet for ethical reasons. I had seen factory farming atrocities in the media long ago, but somehow managed to displace that reality from my everyday life. I met a few vegan friends, and started to realize that in order to live in ethical truth, just being kind to my neighbor was not going to cut it. Being vegan makes me feel like I am doing something kind for the world and the beautiful life forms running, flying and swimming on it. If my instincts don't lead me to kill an animal, then I have no place eating one.

How long have you been vegan?
Since July of 2012.

What has benefited you the most from being vegan?
My recovery after strenuous work is much faster and I seem to thrive on one less hour of sleep (that's 15.2 days of conscious life a year.) I have had increased cardiovascular endurance, taking 35 minutes off my last 100 mile run as well as finally getting 1st place in bodybuilding competitions.

What does veganism mean to you?
It means treating the world as you would like to be treated.

"If my instincts don't lead me to kill an animal, then I have no place eating one."

TRAINING

What sort of training do you do?
I run, lift weights and row. I train and compete in ultra-marathons in the cooler part of the season and switch to competitive bodybuilding as it warms up. I row throughout year.

How often do you (need to) train?
I train on a five-day split with chest, back, shoulders, arms and legs each having their own day. I train pretty intensely, trying to break prior weight or rep records every time if possible. Starting with a few warm up sets, I get up to my heavy lifting with low rep sets, finishing up with lots of drop sets or high rep burnouts.

Do you offer your fitness or training services to others?
Yes, I do online and telephone Personal Training and dietary plans.

What sports do you play?
I compete in ultra-marathons, bodybuilding shows and indoor rowing competitions.

STRENGTHS, WEAKNESSES & OUTSIDE INFLUENCES

What do you think is the biggest misconception about vegans and how do you address this?
When I first started this journey into a plant-based diet, I was fairly sure that my running would probably get better, but my bodybuilding would suffer. I feel that most people currently feel that vegans are not very athletically competitive, and will go back to eating meat after they get tired of being weak and lethargic. I have been breaking all of my previous running and lifting records since turning vegan.

What are your strengths as a vegan athlete?
My recovery after strenuous work is much faster and I seem to thrive on one less hour of sleep. I have had increased cardiovascular endurance, taking 35 minutes off my last 100 mile run as well as placing higher in bodybuilding and rowing competitions.

What is your biggest challenge?
To continue to increase my running and rowing endurance while gaining more lean muscle mass.

Are the non-vegans in your industry supportive or not?
Many fellow trainers gave me grief about my decision. They said I would run my muscle off with too much running and a plant-based diet, but are now starting to respect my decision based on proven muscular gain and running performance.

Are your family and friends supportive of your vegan lifestyle?
My awesome family is supportive in any endeavor I pursue. Most of my friends know I'm crazy, but not stupid, so they are also supportive.

What is the most common question/comment that people ask/say when they find out that you are a vegan and how do you respond?
The ever popular "How do you get your protein?" to which I answer, "It's in the plants."

Who or what motivates you?
I am extremely motivated to prove the performance improvements that can be obtained from a vegan diet, under the guise of my selfish desire to help the animals who don't have freedom or a voice to stop their senseless slaughter.

FOOD & SUPPLEMENTS

What do you eat for Breakfast?
I usually start my day with a Proto-mocha-latte. This is a breakfast concoction that I have been relying on for the last 10+ years to start my day. It is comprised of 2-4 cups of coffee, a cup of almond milk and protein powder. Sometimes I add a ½ cup of oatmeal for additional carbohydrates.

What do you eat for Lunch?
I try to get one or two nice big salads into the day (mixed greens, chopped apples, pears, steamed cauliflower, broccoli, nuts and a good dressing tossed with lots of nutritional yeast.) I usually make a smoothie with protein powder, frozen bananas, strawberries, blueberries, and some type of green like kale, spinach or frozen broccoli after my workouts.

What do you eat for Dinner?
Usually whatever is vegan at the salad bar at Whole Foods, or a repeat of lunch.

What do you eat for Snacks - healthy & not-so healthy?
I very occasionally have an almond or coconut-based ice cream at parties, but keep it out of my fridge. I do keep a bag of chips and hummus handy most of the time though. The sweetness of my protein powders seems to quench the sweet tooth most of the time.

What is your favourite source of Protein?
Tofu (non-GMO and sprouted), Seitan, soy milk and a quality protein powder.

What is your favourite source of Calcium?
Green salads, nuts and fortified nut milks.

What is your favourite source of Iron?
Greens, nuts and hemp protein.

What foods give you the most energy?
My proto-mocha-latte of course!

Do you take any supplements?
I will occasionally take creatine when preparing for a bodybuilding show.

ADVICE

What is your top tip for gaining muscle?
To train with total intensity using 8-15 rep sets. I love to reach failure in a set and feel the burn, because that's when the muscle is forced to adapt by growing. Just make sure you don't work the same body part more than every six days or you may not allow your body enough time to heal the damage in order to grow bigger and stronger.

What is your top tip for losing weight?
Dropping processed food out of your vegan diet and reducing the daily caloric input slightly. I also recommend fasting a couple of hours before bedtime. Cardio 3-6 days a week in 30 min bouts helps me finalize my stage conditioning.

What is your top tip for maintaining weight?
If it ain't broke don't fix it. If, however, you want to replace your fat weight with muscle, then I would refer to the gaining muscle advice and drop all processed foods as a starting point.

What is your top tip for improving metabolism?

Eating consistently throughout the day with high intensity weight training sessions and short, fast cardio sessions.

What is your top tip for toning up?

Cut out processed foods, with 2-5 weekly workouts and 3-5 20-minute cardio sessions.

How do you promote veganism in your daily life?

I try to promote it by example. If I can look healthy and do well in races and shows, the results will speak for themselves.

How would you suggest people get involved with what you do?

For non-vegans, I would recommend they go vegan for a month just to see how much improvement they feel in their energy levels. For fellow vegans, I would love to see them at bodybuilding shows, running events, or some other sport that I'm not involved in yet! Anything to spread the plant-based message. We have animals to save!

Get Creative!

Try a Different Food Type each week
- Grains/Seeds e.g. quinoa, millet, amaranth, teff, wild rice, chia
- Milks e.g. soy milk, rice milk, oat milk, almond milk
- Legumes e.g. chick-peas, tofu, tempeh, red kidney beans

"Our tools for effecting change are knowledge and understanding; persistence and hard work; love and compassion and respect for all life."
- Dr Jane Goodall

BELINDA JANSEN
VEGAN RUNNER

San Francisco Bay Area, California, USA
Vegan since: 2012

belindajansen.com
SM: *Instagram, Twitter*

Belinda Jansen is a runner by morning, Graphic Designer by day, and an experimental vegan cook by night. She began running six years ago as a way to help her lose weight, but has since fallen in love with the sport. She is currently training for her third half marathon and has various fun-runs and one marathon under (fuel) belt. She also loves weight training and outdoor activities, like hiking and kayaking. You can follow her "runventures" and cooking experiments on Instagram and Twitter.

WHY VEGAN?

How and why did you decide to become vegan?
Like most, I started out as a vegetarian. In 2001, I saw a video of an indigenous tribe killing a rabbit for food and that's when I made the connection - the only difference between my cat who I love like a child and the animals on my plate are norms dictated by society. From then on, I could not benefit from the death of any creature. At this point, I did not realize the implications of the egg and dairy industries. Then, a few years ago, I started having violent stomachaches after eating eggs and dairy. While my doctor advised me just to take antacid, I decided that my body was telling me that it no longer wanted these things inside it. So, I went vegan. The decision was originally based on health, but once in the community, I learned more about the dark side of animal husbandry - things that I can't turn a blind eye toward - and knowing what I know, I could never use anything from an animal again.

How long have you been vegan?
I have been vegan since 2012.

What has benefited you the most from being vegan?
My mind and spirit has benefited most. I had a lot of dark tendencies growing up—a lot of mental anguish. Living a compassionate life has helped me heal.

What does veganism mean to you?
It means valuing all life and living selflessly to help make a better world for all creatures.

TRAINING

What sort of training do you do?
I run and weight train. I'm a bit of an anomaly in that I like to do both. Too often runners hate weight lifting and weight lifters hate running. Running is my thing - I am a runner - but I love how powerful weightlifting makes you feel. I love the benefits of both sports.

How often do you (need to) train?

I train 6 days a week, sometimes twice a day. Depending on if I'm training for a race, the balance of weight training and running shifts. I'm currently training for my third half marathon, so I run 5 days a week and two of those days feature a weight-training workout later in the day. The 6th day is cross training - either stationary bike or swimming and a core workout. If I'm not training for a race, I cut back on running and focus more on building strength.

Do you offer your fitness or training services to others?

I love sharing what I've learned and spreading the love of being active to anyone who asks, but don't offer services in any official capacity.

What sports do you play?

Only running.

STRENGTHS, WEAKNESSES & OUTSIDE INFLUENCES

What do you think is the biggest misconception about vegans and how do you address this?

I hate the stereotype of the "preachy vegan." I have never met a vegan who tried to impose their beliefs on anyone else, but I've met plenty of omnivores that immediately question my choices. I'm sure that there are some vegans that do get a little "preachy," and I get it - we are a passionate lot. If you give me the opportunity, I will talk your ear off, but I only do it when the message is well received. I prefer to concentrate on the positives - the benefits that I experience - and steer clear of negative, condemning language. Sort of the "you catch more flies with [vegan] honey" mentality.

What are your strengths as a vegan athlete?

A vegan diet is perfect for endurance sports. I love my carbohydrates, and I put them to good use on long runs. A plant-based diet also helps you recover faster. Two days after my marathon, I was running again, where omnivores might have to take two or three weeks before thinking about hitting the pavement.

What is your biggest challenge?

My weight is my biggest challenge. I lost over a 100 lbs (45kg) a few years ago, and while I would like to lose more, my body just isn't ready to give it up. It's both mentally and physically challenging. On the mental side, I feel like I am not a proper representation of a vegan lifestyle, and that fellow vegans assume I must be a junkfoodatarian - I have trouble getting respect in the weight room. It's difficult to work so hard - eating clean and working out - not to have it reflected in my outward appearance. On the physical side, excess weight makes every mile I run harder and physically inhibits some things in the gym. Other ladies set goals like "to do an unassisted pull-up in a month," but I would either need to lose so much weight or gain so much muscle to do the same, these types of goals seem impossible to me.

Are the non-vegans in your industry supportive or not?

There are so many examples of vegans excelling in running and other endurance sports - it would be hard for anyone to argue against it.

Are your family and friends supportive of your vegan lifestyle?

For the most part, yes they are supportive. Sometimes there are concepts that they can't quite understand (abstaining from honey is a big one), but they never make me feel bad about my decision.

What is the most common question/comment that people ask/say when they find out that you are a vegan and how do you respond?

So many times people say, "No eggs, no dairy, and no meat. What do you eat?" People think all we eat is salad and tofu, but vegans often have a more varied diet than omnivores. I'll explain how switching to veganism makes you rethink what you eat, leading you to explore new foods, and end up eating a greater variety of foods than before.

Who or what motivates you?

The memory of my grandfather motivates me. Growing up, we were very close. He was a very outgoing and loving man. I owe so much of who I am today - my education, my compassion, and my I-can-do-anything attitude - to him. Every Sunday morning long run, his spirit accompanies me in my heart.

FOOD & SUPPLEMENTS

What do you eat for Breakfast?

Fruit, oatmeal, green smoothies, muesli, tofu scramble and country potatoes (if I have a lot of time), Clif or Lara bar (if I'm on the go).

What do you eat for Lunch?

All kinds of different salads, soup, sandwiches and leftovers.

What do you eat for Dinner?

I usually just make something up, so it's rare that I eat the same thing twice. I like to pair a green veggie (favourites include broccoli, Brussels sprouts, green beans, and asparagus) with a starch (potato, sweet potato, brown rice, farrow) and a protein source (tofu, beans, lentils). I take whatever I have on hand, toss it with some seasoning (my go tos are: garlic, onion, parsley, basil, chives, paprika, red pepper flakes, and Mrs. Dash), and cook by either baking or sautéing. Otherwise, I'll eat a veggie burger (with no bun because I just kind of like it that way) with baked fries or Protein Pancakes (recipe from of Rawmazing website) with fruit.

What do you eat for Snacks - healthy & not-so healthy?

I like having leftover Protein Pancakes with grapefruit after a workout, protein shakes before a gym workout, open-face peanut butter sandwich, just peanut butter on a spoon, veggies with hummus, fruit, edamame, and, again, Clif or Lara bar if I'm on the go. My indulgences include Tofu Pie (usually made for a family gathering), vegan marshmallows, dark chocolate, Newman's sandwich cookies, and I usually get Skittles around Halloween and Easter because it's the only candy my mom knows I can eat.

What is your favourite source of Protein?

Tofu, beans and lentils. Occasionally I'll employ a mock-meat if I'm short on time or supplies.

What is your favourite source of Calcium?

Tofu, broccoli, fortified almond milk and kale.

What is your favourite source of Iron?

Edamame, tofu, lentils and spinach.

What foods give you the most energy?

Bananas! My early morning runs are fueled by bananas because they are tasty, full of simple carbohydrates, quick to eat, and easy on my stomach.

Do you take any supplements?
I supplement with protein powder, vegan glucosamine, BCAAs, and digestive enzymes.

ADVICE

What is your top tip for gaining muscle?
Lift heavy, lift often, and give your muscles the fuel (calories) they need to grow.

What is your top tip for losing weight?
Lift heavy (you may not lose weight, but you'll lose fat!), slight calorie restriction, stay active, and eat clean.

What is your top tip for maintaining weight?
Eat clean, eat by feel, weigh yourself periodically - maybe once a month - to make sure you're on track. After years of over-eating, followed by years of dieting, many of us no longer eat when it feels natural. We rely on the clock and macronutrient intake to tell us what to eat. Macros should be used only when training for an event, looking to lose fat, or looking to gain muscle.

What is your top tip for improving metabolism?
Gain muscle, implement interval training (sprint intervals if you're running), and eat clean.

What is your top tip for toning up?
I'm not a fan of "toning."

How do you promote veganism in your daily life?
I try to be a beaming beacon of all that's good in veganism. I love posting photos of my beautiful, tempting, vegan creations on my social networks. I also have a small selection of vegan message tees that I wear whenever I can.

How would you suggest people get involved with what you do?
If you're interested in running, just get a pair of sneakers and go do it - no fancy equipment required. That's the beauty of running, it's so easy to get started and an ability that we are all born with - some might be faster than others, but we can all do it. If you want to try veganism, I recommend reading "Forks Over Knives" and "Thrive", and getting a few cooking books to help you learn new ways to combine foods.

"I'm sure that there are some vegans that do get a little "preachy," and I get it – we are a passionate lot. If you give me the opportunity, I will talk your ear off, but I only do it when the message is well received. I prefer to concentrate on the positives – the benefits that I experience – and steer clear of negative, condemning language. Sort of the "you catch more flies with (vegan) honey" mentality."

BETSY BAILEY
VEGAN VOLLEYBALLER

USA and France
Vegan since: 2002

veganvolleyballer.com

Betsy Bailey thrives under the philosophy that playing hard improves her work, and working hard improves her play. She enjoys the challenges of discovering simple yet indulgent ways to live mindfully wherever her travels take her. Though she has ambitions of maintaining a beautiful, informative blog, her websites only gets updated about once a year.

WHY VEGAN?

How and why did you decide to become vegan?
My journey was very gradual. When I was 16, I decided to stop eating red meat, mostly because I discovered it wasn't healthy. Then, little by little, I found more and more reasons to cut out all animal products. What started out as a quest to be as healthy as possible, led to discovering all of the other reasons to become vegan - environment, animal rights, human rights, etc.

How long have you been vegan?
I don't have an exact date of the last time I purposely ate something animal-derived, but I would say it was 12 or so years ago.

What has benefited you the most from being vegan?
More variety in what I eat - I discovered so many new fruits and vegetables - and a clear conscious knowing that I don't have to hurt any living being in order to survive and thrive.

What does veganism mean to you?
Being vegan touches so many aspects of my life, because being compassionate towards others (human or animal) is good for my physical, mental and spiritual wellbeing. It's not just about what we eat or wear, but about how we live and view the world around us.

TRAINING

What sort of training do you do?
I play volleyball, so my training consists of practice with my team, plus weights, plyometrics, conditioning and yoga at least once a week.

How often do you (need to) train?
At least 5 days per week, which often includes morning lifting/conditioning and evening volleyball practice. In general, we also have one match per week.

Do you offer your fitness or training services to others?
I don't have any official credentials, but it's something I would like to look into in the future. I do have quite a bit of experience coaching junior volleyball, but it's not something I'm doing presently.

What sports do you play?
Indoor volleyball and beach volleyball. I also love basketball, tennis and soccer, but I don't get the chance to play them that often. I pretty much like any sport or activity that has a competitive element, makes me sweat and requires strategic thinking.

STRENGTHS, WEAKNESSES & OUTSIDE INFLUENCES

What do you think is the biggest misconception about vegans and how do you address this?
There is always the protein question, but if someone who knows me actually thinks about that question before asking, they will quickly understand that it's not an issue.

What are your strengths as a vegan athlete?
I think I recover more quickly than most of my counterparts, even those who are 10 years younger! I tend to have more energy as well, but I think only part of that has to do with what I eat. The other part is my natural competitive drive.

What is your biggest challenge?
Eating on the road. Whenever we have away games, I always have to bring food with me. France is not the most vegan-friendly when it comes to eating out or buying food at rest stops.

Are the non-vegans in your industry supportive or not?
Some are, some aren't. My first year playing in France, my coach, when he found out I was vegan, told me I must eat pasta every day for energy. I told him that if he ever notices I'm lacking in energy, then he can then tell me what to eat. Since then, I've had a few teammates actually go vegan for a few weeks to try it out. Usually, they discover they feel great eating vegan, but aren't necessarily mentally ready to go full-time yet. Baby steps.

Are your family and friends supportive of your vegan lifestyle?
Yes. They are great and all very accommodating and open to trying new recipes. I'm lucky.

What is the most common question/comment that people ask/say when they find out that you are a vegan and how do you respond?
I think the most common is the protein question, but I also get a lot of "I could do vegetarian, but not vegan. I love cheese." My general response is "you can do vegan, you just don't want to right now". I also explain that cheese was the hardest part for me too, and that if you do your research, you'll understand why humans do not need milk products and chances are, you'll feel better without them.

Who or what motivates you?
Fellow vegan athletes, watching any high-level sporting event, busy people who still make time to exercise and eat healthy - for example working parents - listening to music and playing music/singing, people who devote their time to helping others in need, and people who are really good at what they do.

FOOD & SUPPLEMENTS

What do you eat for Breakfast?
Usually fruit or a smoothie.

What do you eat for Lunch?
A big salad with whatever veggies I have on hand and maybe some chickpeas, tofu, nuts or something like that. I love having different kinds of soup in the Winter.

What do you eat for Dinner?
Often rice, quinoa or potatoes with either sautéed or steamed veggies.

What do you eat for Snacks - healthy & not-so healthy?
Smoothies, energy bars (I love Vega stuff and Lärabars), dark chocolate, apple with peanut butter, home-made kombucha, coconut water. I'm "lucky" that in France, a lot of the vegan convenience junk foods aren't readily available, so I stay away from them by default. When I'm in the US, I let myself eat vegan pizza with Daiya cheese and vegan ice cream, once in a while - maybe a little too often...

What is your favourite source of Protein?
Chickpeas, lentils, other beans, tofu, tempeh, nuts, mushrooms, hemp, broccoli - the list is endless.

What is your favourite source of Calcium?
Sesame, greens, beans, nuts and seeds.

What is your favourite source of Iron?
Lentils, greens.

Honestly, I don't pay much attention. As long as I eat a variety of whole fruits and vegetables, I will get enough protein, calcium and iron.

What foods give you the most energy?
Fruit.

Do you take any supplements?
I take B12 and sometimes iron and vitamin D in the winter. I've had borderline low iron levels since my early teenage years - long before being vegetarian or vegan - so I try to keep track of my levels with annual blood tests and supplement when needed.

ADVICE

What is your top tip for gaining muscle?
Hit the weights and eat whole foods.

What is your top tip for losing weight, maintaining weight and improving metabolism?
Get active and eat whole foods.

What is your top tip for toning up?
Get active, hit some weights, and eat whole foods. It's all pretty simple.

How do you promote veganism in your daily life?
I find that I don't usually need to bring up the subject. Others usually want to talk about it when they find out I'm vegan, which then allows me to share my lifestyle without forcing it upon anyone who doesn't want to hear it.

How would you suggest people get involved with what you do?
If you want to try a vegan lifestyle, but aren't sure you're quite ready for it, try replacing some of your daily staples with a plant-based version. For example, if you usually have cow's milk with cereal, swap it out for a rice, soy, almond, coconut, etc. version. It doesn't have to be an overnight change.

If you want to play volleyball, check out your local YMCA or Google "volleyball" in your city. There are tons of recreational leagues out there for any level.

BIANCA PERRY
VEGAN MARATHON RUNNER

Gold Coast, Queensland, Australia
Vegan since: 2009

taonutrition.com.au
SM: *FaceBook, Instagram, Twitter, YouTube*

Over 10 years ago, Bianca Perry decided that life was more than just existing, and that she would consciously make her life about living every moment of every day. As a result, she became a better version of herself, from a person who didn't really think too much about her health, to a person who now loves to run marathons. As a result, she became a better version of herself. From a person who didn't really think too much about their health, to a person who now loves to run marathons.

She decided that she wanted to share the freedom, fun and spirit of being alive and healthy with others, and co-founded a business called Tao Nutrition. Offering an awesome natural plant-based protein superfood to share and inspire health through optimal nutrition. Tao Nutrition is the mantra of how Bianca approaches life and is honoured to be able to share the potential of life, strength, fitness and vitality with others through 100% natural plant-based nutrition.

WHY VEGAN?

How and why did you decide to become vegan?
Like many people, I became vegetarian before becoming vegan. I remember one day eating lunch and it dawned on me what I was actually eating: an animal. I loved animals, yet I was eating one. I couldn't be an animal lover and eat them too, so that was it for me. No more meat. The choice was easy and I never looked back. A few years later my husband and I had a conversation about what being vegetarian actually meant to us. This conversation highlighted to me that I was still causing pain and suffering to animals by eating eggs and dairy. Again this was not something that I wanted to cause to other living creatures, so from that conversation I decided to become vegan. It was one of the best decisions I have ever made.

How long have you been vegan?
Over five years.

What has benefited you the most from being vegan?
My health, fitness and outlook on life has flourished since being a vegetarian, and increased even more after becoming vegan. I feel unstoppable now. I truly feel alive, creative, fit and healthy. Prior to my change, I felt sluggish, unimaginative and uninterested. I love my outlook and approach to life now.

What does veganism mean to you?
It's more than a diet, it's an approach to life and a deep respect for the earth and its creatures. I feel more connected to the earth and the souls around me now.

TRAINING

What sort of training do you do?
I run marathons, so my training involves a lot of running, strength training and stretching.

How often do you (need to) train?
I train specifically for running 4 days a week, however I aim to be active every day of the week.

Do you offer your fitness or training services to others?
My husband and I thought deeply on how we could provide a conscious and meaningful service to others and it clicked that we could do this with something we are both passionate about, nutrition. We had been making our own natural plant-based protein and superfood mixes for about 10 years to fuel our active lives. So, it made huge sense to take something that we were having a huge success with and offer it to the community – Tao Nutrition. We also put a lot of time and effort into writing health and wellbeing articles so that we are educating people on how they can make the changes they want to see.

STRENGTHS, WEAKNESSES & OUTSIDE INFLUENCES

What do you think is the biggest misconception about vegans and how do you address this?
The common questions are concerned with the adequacy of the vegan diet. I address this by being a beacon of health, fitness, vitality and positivity. It's hard to question if the diet is adequate if you are flourishing!

What are your strengths as a vegan athlete?
I recover fast and always feel fit, healthy and strong. I haven't had a cold for as long as I can remember, which means I can train more.

Are your family and friends supportive of your vegan lifestyle?
My friends and family are very supportive now. In the beginning, they were concerned because they didn't know much about a vegan diet - but now they see how healthy I am and they are no longer concerned.

What is the most common question/comment that people ask/say when they find out that you are a vegan and how do you respond?
"Where do you get your protein?" My response is, "Plants, vegetables, seeds, beans and Tao Nutrition of course!"

Who or what motivates you?
My family motivates me to be the healthiest I can be so that I can enjoy our wonderful life together.

FOOD & SUPPLEMENTS

What do you eat for Breakfast?
I love my smoothies and in winter something warm. Two of my favourite breakfasts are Tao Nutrition Smoothie and Tao Nutrition Porridge. Also Tao Nutrition rice milkshake poured over muesli.

What do you eat for Lunch?
A large salad.

What do you eat for Dinner?
Roasted vegetables, homemade pizza, homemade veggie burgers, laksa, curries, stir-fry.

What do you eat for Snacks - healthy & not-so healthy?
Tao power balls, choc mint smoothie, organic vegan fair-trade dark chocolate, fruit salad.

What is your favourite source of Protein?
"Where do you get your protein?" My response is, "Plants, vegetables, seeds, beans and Tao Nutrition of course!"

What is your favourite source of Calcium?
Sesame seeds.

What is your favourite source of Iron?
Leafy greens.

What foods give you the most energy?
I love my smoothies. They are a great and tasty way to get a vast variety of nutrients.

Do you take any supplements?
B12 and Tao Nutrition.

ADVICE

What is your top tip for gaining muscle?
Lift weights, stretch and recover - do this each session, 3 times a week.

What is your top tip for losing weight?
If you are looking to lose weight and generate health, Tao Nutrition is perfect for replacing less healthy snack or meal options such as those containing processed foods in particular sugar and fat. By replacing these 'foods' devoid of nutrients, you are removing a health degrader (often the cause of weight gain) and adding a health builder. Providing your body with high nutrient density ingredients making it completely filling, satisfying and nourishing. The result of nourishing your body will be a generation of health and an improved body composition ie weight loss. To achieve optimum results, combine with a healthy balanced diet, optimal hydration and exercise.

What is your top tip for maintaining weight?
Keep a food diary - it is a great way to ensure you are staying on track for your long-term goals.

What is your top tip for improving metabolism?
Eat the right foods often. Stay away from anything unnatural. If it has a chemical, preservative, added sugar or other nasty - avoid it!

What is your top tip for toning up?
There is no cheating here - nutrition and movement are the answer. A mix of cardio, weights and proper nutrition is the answer.

How do you promote veganism in your daily life?
1) By being a beacon of health, fitness, vitality and positivity

2) Being the co-founder of a plant based premium protein superfood

How would you suggest people get involved with what you do?
Visit our website.

BILL NORTON
VEGAN FITNESS INSTRUCTOR

Perth, Western Australia, Australia
Vegan since: 2013

SM: FaceBook

Bill Norton is an Australian Fitness Instructor, CrossFit Coach and animal rights advocate and activist. Passionate about a vegan lifestyle for ethical, environmental and health benefits, he is enthusiastic about helping people to get the most out of themselves. He believes education and intestinal fortitude are key to staying in great shape and being happy. He's had the privilege to have been educated, coached and trained alongside some of Melbourne and Perth's best and desires to pass on what he's learnt to others.

WHY VEGAN?

How and why did you decide to become vegan?
Ironically I grew up on a hobby farm and we lived primarily off the land - we grew fruits and vegetables and raised sheep, cows and poultry. I also took part in the slaughter of these animals, so I was under no illusion as to where my food came from. It wasn't until I moved in with a vegan in Melbourne did I make the connection and begin to rationalise ethics on an equal level. I started doing some soul searching and was vegetarian for three weeks, watched the documentary "Earthlings" and become vegan overnight. I could no longer participate in a system that exploits the innocent.

How long have you been vegan?
Since August 2013.

What has benefited you the most from being vegan?
Been able to look myself in the mirror with a clear conscience, giving me a sense of purpose, and feeling great in the process.

What does veganism mean to you?
Standing up for what is right. Not condoning the unnecessary imprisonment, torment and murder of other living beings (human and non-human alike). This too takes into consideration the environment, since the main cause of environmental destruction is caused through animal agriculture. Also through our health and wellbeing, there are no known diseases caused from a vegan lifestyle! Veganism encompasses all sentient life and eliminates speciesism, racism, sexism and homophobia, for good.

TRAINING

What sort of training do you do?
I mainly follow the CrossFit methodologies whilst also incorporating strength, gymnastics and Olympic lifting disciplines.

How often do you (need to) train?
I train 5 to 6 days a week.

Do you offer your fitness or training services to others?
I'm a qualified Fitness Instructor and CrossFit Coach, I take classes at CrossFit Artax in Perth, Western Australia.

What sports do you play?
CrossFit, that's my jam! I enter in local competitions and I competed in the 2015 Reebok CrossFit Games Open, a worldwide event where people from all around the world challenge themselves to five workouts over five weeks to test their fitness. Other than that I enjoy going for a run every other weekend.

STRENGTHS, WEAKNESSES & OUTSIDE INFLUENCES

What do you think is the biggest misconception about vegans and how do you address this?
The biggest misconception is that vegans are undernourished and are physically at a disadvantage. However the truth is quite the opposite. I've personally never felt better, I'm stronger, faster, and recover much sooner than I ever used to. I address this by being the exception, breaking the stereotypes and setting a good example.

What are your strengths as a vegan athlete?
I don't get sick. Better recovery time between workouts and I feel lighter.

What is your biggest challenge?
Promoting veganism in a meat, dairy and egg dominant industry that is bombarded with clever, aggressive and misleading marketing that has virtually unlimited resources and funding. The important thing is that I keep true to myself and continually improving in the way of performance and educating others along the way. Other than that, the only challenges I have are the ones I set for myself.

Are the non-vegans in your industry supportive or not?
Some are and some are not, that's the way life is. For every hater, there's someone else who thinks you're a freaking inspiration.

Are your family and friends supportive of your vegan lifestyle?
At first they couldn't understand why and thought it was a phase, but are supportive and respectful of my decision to live a cruelty-free lifestyle.

What is the most common question/comment that people ask/say when they find out that you are a vegan and how do you respond?
"You're a vegan!?" "What do you eat?" and the classic "Where do you get your protein from?" There is a lot of false and misleading information about vegan nutrition and anyone who asks me about the topic, I'm more than happy to inform and educate them in a way that's not forceful or intimidating, and leaves people asking more.

Who or what motivates you?
I'm motivated by doing what is right through a virtuous lifestyle, by trusting myself, breaking the rules (stereotypes), not being afraid to fail, ignoring the naysayers, doing my best and giving back through education and my actions.

In regards to who motivates me, Billy Simmonds, Joel Kirkilis, Ed Bauer, Frank Medrano, Patrik Baboumian, Brendan Brazier, Mike Tyson and the PlantBuilt Team, basically anyone in any form of athletic disciple that promotes a cruelty-free lifestyle. Also people who openly create awareness of speciesism such as, Gary Yourofsky, Dr. Richard Oppenlander, Dr. Melanie Joy, Capt Paul Watson, Philip Wollen, Gary L. Francione, Will Potter, Bill Clinton and Howard Lyman, just to name a few.

FOOD & SUPPLEMENTS

What do you eat for Breakfast?
Rolled oats with mixed berries, seeds and grains, Maple Crunch from Freedom Foods and soy milk. Sometimes peanut butter and vegemite on toast, and occasionally pancakes.

What do you eat for Lunch?
I don't usually eat lunch, if I do it's at a vegan café such as Loving Hut.

What do you eat for Dinner?
This varies, as it's my main meal of the day so I like to get creative at times. This can range from a simple tofu, spinach, tomato, carrot, and avocado wrap; to a stir-fry or a full out mushroom pasta dish filled with beans, fruits and veggies. All depends on what I've got in the kitchen and what I'm in the mood for.

What do you eat for Snacks (healthy & not-so healthy)?
Almonds, fruit, Clif Bars, Pringles and dairy-free ice cream.

What is your favourite source of Protein?
Tofu, peanut butter, beans and almonds.

What is your favourite source of Calcium?
Leafy greens such as kale and spinach, almond milk and almonds.

What is your favourite source of Iron?
Leafy greens, beans, grains and almonds - I like almonds.

What foods give you the most energy?
Fruit and almonds.

Do you take any supplements?
Flaxseed oil with breakfast, Prana ON protein powder (with almond milk), Clean Machine's BCAA's and Cell Block 80 on occasion.

"It wasn't until I moved in with a vegan in Melbourne did I make the connection and begin to rationalise ethics on an equal level. I started doing some soul searching and was vegetarian for three weeks, watched the documentary "Earthlings" and become vegan overnight. I could no longer participate in a system that exploits the innocent."

ADVICE

What is your top tip for gaining muscle?
Lifting big, eating well and sleeping lots.

What is your top tip for losing weight?
The key is high intensity interval training, keep it constant, keep it varied, keep it functional but keep it fun, or you won't keep it up.

What is your top tip for maintaining weight?
Need to find the balance between the training you're doing or not doing and the amount of food you consume.

What is your top tip for improving metabolism & toning up?
Train mean, eat clean and get lean! Sleep and drink plenty of water.

How do you promote veganism in your daily life?

By being the example, the standard you walk by is the standard you accept. By not taking part in any form of animal cruelty and performing well in the gym creates controversy, people are more interested in a topic when they ask the questions themselves.

How would you suggest people get involved with what you do?

Start by questioning everything i.e. Where does my food come from? Why are cows, sheep, pigs, poultry and fish considered edible, and all the other millions of species considered inedible? The Internet is a good resource however not all sites are reliable. There are heaps of documentaries filled with facts and credible sources, some good ones are: "Speciesism The Movie", "Lucent" (Aussie made), "Earthlings" and "Cowspiracy." More importantly why do we never ask ourselves why to begin with? Once you start asking these questions you begin to think logically and your perception on veganism changes. Then education is key, find the answers to these questions. The internet is a good resource however not all sites are reliable. There are heaps of documentaries filled with facts and credible sources, some good ones are: Speciesism The Movie, Lucent (Aussie made), Earthlings and Cowspiracy. Get involved with your local vegan movement group, live by example and when asked about veganism, be patient and coherent. Ignore the naysayers and be the vegan that gives vegans a good name.

"It's challenging to promote veganism in a meat, dairy and egg dominant industry that is bombarded with clever, aggressive and misleading marketing that has virtually unlimited resources and funding. The important thing is that I keep true to myself and continually improving in the way of performance and educating others along the way."

Veganism is Just One Step

Being vegan is a great way of putting compassion into action, living in line with your beliefs, and leading by example to show others how you want our world to be. But it's just one step - an awesome and important step - but still just a step. Find out more about other social justice issues, how they intersect with veganism, and how we can support their causes. Together we can really make some changes!

- Leigh-Chantelle

BILLY SIMMONDS
VEGAN BODYBUILDER

Gold Coast, Queensland, Australia
Vegan since: 2009

billysimmonds.com
pranaon.com
SM: *FaceBook, Instagram, Twitter*

Billy Simmonds is an Australian Professional Natural Bodybuilder, Powerlifter, Martial Artist, CrossFitter and Vegan. He is the founder of Prana ON – a vegan fitness nutrition company. He is the winner of the 2009 Mr. Universe title, holds multiple Black-belts in different Martial Arts, and has set world titles performing feats of strength. He is a passionate advocate of a vegan lifestyle for its health, environmental and ethical benefits.

WHY VEGAN?

How and why did you decide to become vegan?
As a teenager I started to question what was on my plate - where it came from and what it was doing to my body. After learning many of my role models are or were vegetarian or vegan, I followed that path for myself.

How long have you been vegan?
Vegetarian for 10 years then vegan for 5.

What has benefited you the most from being vegan?
A clearer conscience, more energy and a sense of purpose.

What does veganism mean to you?
Each and every person who decides to be vegan makes a massive difference. From literally saving animals from suffering and death, to improving their health and the environmental benefits - being vegan means seeing the bigger picture and saying I'm going to do what I can and take a stand.

TRAINING

What sort of training do you do?
I compete in natural bodybuilding, power lifting and martial arts competitions. Depending on my specific competition goals I will temper the volume of each to accommodate each modality. I also incorporate yoga and other cross training into my schedule.

How often do you (need to) train?
I'll train typically twice a day - weights in the morning and martial arts (Taekwondo, Hapkido, Muay Thai or Brazilian Jiu-Jitsu) in the evening. I'll also surf regularly if the conditions are right.

Do you offer your fitness or training services to others?
I have put my energy into building a company that supports the whole fitness community with the very best vegan nutrition products on the market.

What sports do you play?
Other than my main disciplines - I love surfing and enjoy going for a run or doing sprints, which helps my overall fitness.

STRENGTHS, WEAKNESSES & OUTSIDE INFLUENCES

What do you think is the biggest misconception about vegans and how do you address this?
The biggest misconception is that it's a disadvantage physically and even socially. I have never felt better, been fitter and even many of my non-vegan friends love coming out to eat with me at veg restaurants. I've learnt how to make the nutrition aspect work and also control my environment so there's only upsides.

What are your strengths as a vegan athlete?
Nutritionally I'm eating specific high nutrient, alkaline foods that fuel my body for performance, growth and repair.

What is your biggest challenge?
Only those I set for myself!

Are the non-vegans in your industry supportive or not?
My putting myself out there in competitions and winning I would say that they see my approach as a legitimate alternative to the 'traditional' methods - and many are open to learning more.

Are your family and friends supportive of your vegan lifestyle?
My parents thought it was a phase, but over the years they have become more and more supportive and respectful.

What is the most common question/comment that people ask/say when they find out that you are a vegan and how do you respond?
Of course the cliche "Where do you get your protein?" but also, "What exactly do you eat?" There is still a lot of mystery around vegan nutrition and the idea you can't feel full, let alone get enough protein. I'll always just discuss the sort of foods I eat and why they are more beneficial than animal-based foods.

Who or what motivates you?
I'm motivated by being the best example I can of what can be achieved physically and ethically. I strive to excel in what I love doing and don't believe in the idea that I can't be strong and muscular because I'm vegan, or that I can't be fast or flexible because I'm a bodybuilder, and that one person can't make a difference.

FOOD & SUPPLEMENTS

What do you eat for Breakfast?
Green smoothie with raw Power Plant Protein, banana, berries, avocado and coconut water.

What do you eat for Lunch?
Tofu or tempeh, bean and kale salad.

What do you eat for Dinner?
Bean pasta with seeds and steamed greens, perhaps a yam if needed.

What do you eat for Snacks - healthy & not-so healthy?
Rice cakes with almond butter, raw vegie sticks with hummus, fruit and dark chocolate.

What is your favourite source of Protein?
At the moment it's a toss between mung bean pasta, tempeh, and Prana ON Power Plant or Phyto Fire Protein Powder.

What is your favourite source of Calcium?
Greens like kale, and nuts like almonds.

What is your favourite source of Iron?
The gym! - and of course dark leafy greens, lentils and broccoli.

What foods give you the most energy?
Kale, bananas, fresh dates and yams.

Do you take any supplements?
Yes – I've designed the Prana ON range to support high levels of activity to support recovery, growth, repair and immunity.

ADVICE

What is your top tip for gaining muscle?
Lift heavy weights, eat protein-rich plant foods, be patient and do it naturally.

What is your top tip for losing weight?
Reduce your portion sizes, do more cardio, cycle starchy or sugar carbohydrates and take your time.

What is your top tip for maintaining weight?
Find your baseline Basal Metabolic Rate (BMR) and get the ratio of protein, fats and carbohydrates right.

What is your top tip for improving metabolism and toning up?
Do more High-intensity interval training cardio, or CrossFit.

How do you promote veganism in your daily life?
By trying to create the most compelling contradiction of what a 'typical vegan' is so that others just simply have to ask. People are much more receptive when they are asking the questions. If you wear the vegan badge, then wear it proudly, and know that people will make a judgement if it's right for them based on how well you articulate and demonstrate its benefits.

How would you suggest people get involved with what you do?
People can read my personal blog, try Prana ON's amazing range of vegan fitness nutrition, and of course both of these have great Social Media channels to connect with as well!

"I'm motivated by being the best example I can of what can be achieved physically and ethically. I strive to excel in what I love doing and don't believe in the idea that I can't be strong and muscular because I'm vegan, or that I can't be fast or flexible because I'm a bodybuilder, and that one person can't make a difference."

BRENDAN BAILEY
VEGAN CYCLIST

Melbourne, Victoria, Australia
Vegan since: 2001

thenewtimer.blogspot.com

Brendan Bailey has been vegan since 2001 and has been cycling competitively since 2008. In that time, he has risen through the ranks to become an elite level cyclist on the velodrome, specializing in endurance events such as the points race and the Madison. He also races on the road and in 2010 became Brunswick Cycling Club's Road Race Champion. His thoughts on cycling, veganism and everything in between can be found on his website.

WHY VEGAN?

How and why did you decide to become vegan?
I'd been vegetarian since 1993, and when you're vegetarian, you're always aware that you're a little pissweak. It's more of an effort to continually justify consuming animal excretions than it is to actually turn vegan. Therefore, I made the jump on the occasion of moving to another country. The shock to the system made it easier in the long run.

What has benefited you the most from being vegan?
Strange question. I'm not vegan because it benefits me. I'm vegan because it benefits animals.

What does veganism mean to you?
It means that every day I'm doing something to combat oppression and help lessen suffering. It also means I get to annoy waiters in non-vegan restaurants.

TRAINING

What sort of training do you do?
Cycling is tough in that you need to spend a lot of time on the bike in order to reach your peak, but you also need to back it off at times to avoid overtraining. Right now I'm on a break, but on heavy weeks in the past I've been doing about 20 hours of training, including 4 or 5 hours in the gym doing weight training, a couple of ergo sessions on the stationary bike, a training session or two on the track, racing, and a whole lot of road miles.

STRENGTHS, WEAKNESSES & OUTSIDE INFLUENCES

What do you think is the biggest misconception about vegans and how do you address this?
I think the biggest misconception is that we won't be able to do it. The best way to answer this is by winning, and fortunately, I've been able to do that enough to shut people up. The next biggest misconception, however, is that we're doing it to achieve some kind of advantage in our performance. While we might gain some advantage,

that's an added bonus, not the reason itself. It's about the animals, remember?

What are your strengths as a vegan athlete?
Tenacity, Moral Strength and Discipline.

What is your biggest challenge?
It is difficult to get enough calories, but there is an awesome answer to that – eat more food! Being vegan you also need to be more careful than the average person about receiving all the necessary nutrients, both macro and micro. I keep a daily food and training journal to make sure I'm getting enough, and also to document how certain foods make me feel. That's kind of a pain in the ass at the end of a tough day.

Are the non-vegans in your industry supportive or not?
As long as I keep winning, sure!

Are your family and friends supportive of your vegan lifestyle?
See above.

What is the most common question/comment that people ask/say when they find out that you are a vegan and how do you respond?
Where do you get your protein? Where do you get your iron? Where do you get your calcium? I tell them I get it all from plants.

Who or what motivates you?
I like winning.

FOOD & SUPPLEMENTS

What do you eat for Breakfast?
Big bowl of fruit with a seed mix or protein shake.

What do you eat for Lunch?
Usually a big salad of some description, but if it's cold I'll hit up some baked beans, mix in some pumpkin seeds and eat it all on Turkish bread.

What do you eat for Dinner?
Whatever's going on. Like every other trendsetter, I'm crazy about Mexican food right now, so I'm making a lot of quesadillas with salad on the side lately.

What do you eat for Snacks - healthy & not-so healthy?
Usually fruit and nuts, but occasionally I'll hit up some chocolate. Man's not a camel.

What is your favourite source of Protein?
Sunwarrior protein powder.

What is your favourite source of Calcium?
Leafy greens.

What is your favourite source of Iron?
Leafy greens, with a little vitamin C to help absorption.

What foods give you the most energy?
I'm quite fond of dates when I'm on the bike – they're sweet and pack in a bunch of calories, which is pretty much exactly what you want in the second hour of a three hour bike race.

Do you take any supplements?
Yeah, a bunch. Protein powder, iron supplements, vitamin D, a B complex and a magnesium mix. Mostly for muscle repair, but some of them are basic vegan nutrition, which I'd be taking regardless.

ADVICE

What is your top tip for gaining muscle?
Go to a weightlifting gym, smash the protein.

What is your top tip for losing weight?
Do more time on the bike, eat less food.

What is your top tip for maintaining weight?
The more exercise you do, the more food you should eat.

What is your top tip for improving metabolism?
Don't eat shit food.

What is your top tip for toning up?
I don't ever know what this means. It's a misconception. If you want your muscles to show, you're either gaining muscle or losing fat. See above for my advice on those matters.

How do you promote veganism in your daily life?
By living it.

How would you suggest people get involved with what you do?
If they're interested in competitive cycling, they should contact Cycling Australia and find out who some of their local cycling clubs are. If you think beating someone in the bike lane on your way to work is satisfying, you should try beating someone on the velodrome.

If they're interested in veganism, they should probably continue reading this book and check out the website that this interview is a part of.

"When you're vegetarian, you're always aware that you're a little pissweak. It's more of an effort to continually justify consuming animal excretions than it is to actually turn vegan. Therefore, I made the jump on the occasion of moving to another country. The shock to the system made it easier in the long run."

BRETT BLANKNER
VEGAN ULTRA-ENDURANCE ATHLETE

College Station, Texas, US
Vegan since: 2011

zentriathlon.com

Brett Blankner is an ultra-endurance athlete, coach, and host of the Zen and the Art of Triathlon Podcast. In less than one year, he ran 100 miles (160km) non-stop, swam the length of Lake Tahoe (22 miles/35km) in 13 hours, completed two Ironman triathlons (2.4 mile swim, 112 mile bike, 26.2 mile run) and also swam from Alcatraz Island to San Francisco. He powers all this on a vegan diet while also working full-time and raising his seven year-old with his wife, Emily. You can find out more about Brett on his website.

WHY VEGAN?

How long have you been vegan?
Over 3 years.

What has benefited you the most from being vegan?
My energy levels are much higher and more consistent.

What does veganism mean to you?
Using great nutrition to open up so many more doors in life. It's amazing what you can do with your body and mind!

TRAINING

How often do you (need to) train?
Twice a day. Two hours a day on weekdays, four hours a day on weekends.

Do you offer your fitness or training services to others?
Yes! I am a certified triathlon coach and you can find out more about my coaching online.

What sports do you play?
I am an Ironman triathlete, ultra runner, and adventure swimmer.

STRENGTHS, WEAKNESSES & OUTSIDE INFLUENCES

What do you think is the biggest misconception about vegans and how do you address this?
That being vegan makes you physically weaker. I show them my race results before and after going vegan and the difference is huge.

What are your strengths as a vegan athlete?
I have a much faster recovery time after a race or hard workout because the nutrition is so much better. This allows me to get back to training sooner, so I am able to keep improving while others are still recovering.

What is your biggest challenge?

I have to travel to most races, so finding healthy food on the road or at the airport is sometimes difficult. I can do it, but what is most heartbreaking is how our food system is set up to make everybody fail. It should be harder to eat bad food than good food, and the opposite is true.

Are the non-vegans in your industry supportive or not?

Vegans are definitely becoming a known force in endurance sports. It really works and this sport is basically about pushing your body to the limit for hours or days. If anything is going to help, people will do it. Being vegan has proven to be a competitive advantage for those of us that give it a try. I recommend it, unless you're my competition. If you're racing against me, then by all means, eat all the meat you can find. Just kidding. Mostly.

Are your family and friends supportive of your vegan lifestyle?

Some friends are, others laugh at it. It is not something I worry too much about it because the results speak for themselves and are pretty obvious. When you take over an hour off of a twelve-hour race simply by going vegan, you don't worry about what somebody that is very overweight and out of shape says. My wife is vegetarian and definitely gets a kick out of watching me try to take it all to the next level.

What is the most common question/comment that people ask/say when they find out that you are a vegan and how do you respond?

"Where do you get your protein from?" Honestly, I thought this was a big issue as well until I learned that plants have tons of protein in them. Oatmeal has more protein than eggs!

Who or what motivates you?

Rich Roll is a prominent vegan endurance athlete and he opened my eyes to what this eating style can do for us. It was amazing how it turned his health around and since he's a public figure, it was easy to follow suit. He's even got a cookbook on his website that you can order to eat like he does.

FOOD & SUPPLEMENTS

What do you eat for Breakfast?

Ezekiel cinnamon and raisin cereal with coconut milk and some coffee.

What do you eat for Lunch?

I go to a local burrito shop called "Freebirds" and get a hand-made burrito. I have them put in beans, greens, corn, salsa, guacamole, and roasted peppers and onions. It's awesome!

What do you eat for Dinner?

Peanut butter and jelly sandwiches, greens, Indian food, lots of great stuff that's pretty random.

What do you eat for Snacks - healthy & not-so healthy?

I make a green smoothie every day with kale, fruit, and carrots in it. It's fantastic! I also like to snack on Lara Bars.

What is your favourite source of Protein?

I don't worry about it too much. Protein is in nearly everything.

What is your favourite source of Calcium?

Kale and other greens.

What is your favourite source of Iron?
Beans and greens are very high in iron, so I'm doing really well.

What foods give you the most energy?
Simple carbs like dates or bread pick me up the fastest, but they also fade quickly. I add in nuts and seeds if I need more staying power and that works very well.

Do you take any supplements?
Not really. A little B12 here and there, but that's about it.

"I have a much faster recovery time after a race or hard workout because the nutrition is so much better. This allows me to get back to training sooner, so I am able to keep improving while others are still recovering."

ADVICE

What is your top tip for gaining muscle?
Definitely lifting weights. It puts on muscle really fast.

What is your top tip for losing weight?
Eat whole foods and stop eating a little before feeling full.

What is your top tip for maintaining weight?
Nuts and oils have all the calories you could want and can help put on weight fast.

What is your top tip for improving metabolism?
Weight lifting and running.

What is your top tip for toning up ?
Swimming HARD and weight lifting.

How do you promote veganism in your daily life?
I post pictures on Twitter of what I eat, then turn around and post the results of my workouts. Showing how I do a 60 mile bike ride at 20 MPH after eating vegan all week really makes people start considering eating more healthy food. I also host a popular triathlon podcast called Zen and the Art of Triathlon and talk about it there. I never tell people they have to eat this way. Rather I lead by example.

How would you suggest people get involved with what you do?
Triathlons come in all sizes and distances. Most are quite short and fun. You can easily find one in your area on Active.com. Once you start training for one, you'll notice you don't need anywhere near the energy it takes to get all of the work done without cleaning up your diet. That's where I show up with a big bag of kale and a smile.

"I have to travel to most races, so finding healthy food on the road or at the airport is sometimes difficult. I can do it, but what is most heartbreaking is how our food system is set up to make everybody fail. It should be harder to eat bad food than good food, and the opposite is true."

Brian Evans
VEGAN EXERCISE ENTHUSIAST

New York City, New York, USA
Vegan since: 1993

E: bevans628@yahoo.com

Brian Evans is a university professor at Pace University in New York City. He primarily prepares students to teach mathematics. He has traveled extensively and has been to all 50 U.S. states, nearly 100 countries, and all seven continents. He also enjoys hiking, cycling, martial arts, and exercise.

WHY VEGAN?

How and why did you decide to become vegan?
I adopted the vegan lifestyle primarily for ethical reasons. I soon learned about the health, environmental, and human welfare implications and consider all of these good reasons for being vegan. Peter Singer's "Animal Liberation" was a book I read soon after becoming a vegetarian and this gave me a solid philosophical grounding for my new lifestyle. I also became involved in the straight edge hardcore music scene, which also had strong vegan influence and highly assisted in my move from vegetarian to vegan.

How long have you been vegan?
I have been vegan since 1993, which means I've been vegan for over 20 years. I was vegetarian for one year before I decided to adopt the vegan lifestyle.

What has benefited you the most from being vegan?
Personal benefits have primarily been the physical health and psychological benefits of a vegan lifestyle. I was born in 1976, and I'm often told I look much younger than my physical age and that I'm in great physical shape. While I do not know the extent my diet has contributed as compared to genetics and exercise, I would like to think diet has a significant impact. I add psychological benefits because being a vegan means reducing the harm to other sentient beings, which has significant personal psychological implications.

What does veganism mean to you?
My primarily motivation is the ethical consequences of a vegan lifestyle, which is the process of reducing animal suffering to the greatest degree possible. It also means reducing environmental degradation and improving human health to the greatest degree possible.

TRAINING

What sort of training do you do?
The primary interest to the reader is likely to be the quantity of pushups I do each day. My usual morning involves 500 one-arm pushups on each arm along with 500 regular two-arm pushups in sets of 100 to 125. If I'm not overly busy, I do it again

in the evening before dinner. This means my typical day involves 3000 pushups. I recently found out that I'm not terribly far away from several world records. I've been encouraged to attempt to break a record or two by many friends, and I have been considering working on it.

In between sets of pushups I practice martial arts, stretch, and do squats. I have a black belt in Shotokan and have practiced Aikido, and I frequently teach self-defense classes to my students at my university. While probably not as impressive, I do 3000 squats a day in addition to the pushups. Several days a week, I run three to four miles and do pull ups, and I also frequently cycle. I enjoy getting outdoors to hike and the picture I used for this interview online is on a hike in the Annapurna region of the Himalaya Mountains in Nepal.

How often do you (need to) train?
I know I'll receive some criticism for this but I usually train every day. I enjoy training very much and my day does not feel right without it. When extraordinarily busy I will skip the evening workout. However, it's extremely rare for me to skip the morning workout.

Do you offer your fitness or training services to others?
Yes, I frequently give talks to college students at my university on exercise, healthy lifestyle, and veganism. Friends often solicit advice as well.

What sports do you play?
Most of my physical interests are exercise, martial arts, cycling, and hiking. I do not have the opportunity to play team sports very often, but I do enjoy playing basketball, soccer, and volleyball. Quite a few years ago a friend and I were affectionately called the "vegan power houses" by some non-vegan friends who often played basketball with us.

STRENGTHS, WEAKNESSES & OUTSIDE INFLUENCES

What do you think is the biggest misconception about vegans and how do you address this?
In the 20 years I've been vegan I've seen much improvement in the way in which people perceive veganism. In fact, 20 years ago most people didn't know what a "vegan" was. I rarely encounter that today. The biggest misconceptions I encounter are around the nutritional adequacies of the vegan diet. I am not formally educated in nutrition, but have learned much about it on my own. I do my best to address concerns presented to me. I find that presenting myself to people as a friendly, smart, and physically fit example of a vegan has been helpful.

What are your strengths as a vegan athlete?
Since readers will likely be most interested in the quantity of pushups I do, I would say my upper body strength, while remaining slim and athletic, is my great physical attribute. I'm well suited for performing large numbers of pushups because I'm strong but have a slim and athletic build. Being too muscular is good for weightlifting, but probably would not help as much with pushups. Not surprisingly, I won a pushup competition in college and had no problem beating much larger athletes.

What is your biggest challenge?
Probably like most people, finding the time to remain active is a challenge. I have a very busy schedule, but I prioritize my exercise. Motivation was never a problem for me, but I acknowledge lack of motivation is probably the other major factor for most people.

Are the non-vegans in your industry supportive or not?

When I encounter non-vegan athletes, I sometimes receive negative comments about how introducing some animal products into my diet would likely benefit my physical performance. I politely disagree. However, most non-vegan athletes are more interested in my lifestyle and have many questions. Most people I've encountered seem supportive.

Are your family and friends supportive of your vegan lifestyle?

Yes, my parents now know that after 20 years my diet is not a teenage fad.

What is the most common question/comment that people ask/say when they find out that you are a vegan and how do you respond?

Usually the most common questions revolve around nutrition. I do my best to present what I know about vegan nutrition to those who will listen.

Who or what motivates you?

In terms of vegan athleticism, the great vegan athletes, such as many being profiled here in this book, are quite inspirational. I feel very honored and humbled that my story is included in the same work as theirs. In terms of what motivates me, I have been fortunate that most of my life I've had a strong intrinsic motivation for success.

FOOD & SUPPLEMENTS

What do you eat for Breakfast?

My breakfast and my dinner are nearly identical. I usually eat about a pound of leafy greens (collards or kale) and about a third of a pound of legumes (lentils or beans) with crushed flax seeds and salt for breakfast and again for dinner.

What do you eat for Lunch?

I mostly eat fruit and nuts or seeds for lunch.

What do you eat for Dinner?

Dinner is the same as breakfast on most days. This means I'm eating about two pounds of leafy greens and two-thirds of a pound of legumes each day. I've done a nutritional analysis of my typical diet to be certain I was receiving adequate quantities of the nutrients I need. I understand that most people would find my diet a bit repetitive and boring, but I like it. I also think the most nutritious of all vegan foods are leafy greens and legumes. I do my best to stay away from processed foods and I promote a healthy plant-based diet based around whole vegan foods.

What do you eat for Snacks - healthy & not-so healthy?

Like my lunch, if I snack it's going to be mostly fruit and nuts or seeds.

What is your favourite source of Protein?

Legumes (lentils or beans.)

What is your favourite source of Calcium?

Leafy greens (collards or kale.)

What is your favourite source of Iron?

Legumes (lentils or beans.)

For all three I would advocate for leafy greens and legumes. I get more protein, calcium, and iron than I need particularly as a very active person.

What foods give you the most energy?
I really like raisins and peanuts on long hikes. Dried fruit, while being high in calories, can be quite good for instant energy.

Do you take any supplements?
I take a B-12 and vitamin D supplement every day. I sometimes take a pill for additional omega 3's in addition to the crushed flax seed in my breakfast and dinner.

ADVICE

What is your top tip for gaining muscle?
There is much to say about the science of muscle gain, but I would say legumes are my favorite source of protein for those concerned about protein intake. Many believe fewer repetitions with heavier weights are more effective than many repetitions with lighter weights. This knowledge motivated me to add the one-arm pushups to my routine.

What is your top tip for losing weight?
Reducing processed foods, even vegan processed foods, and eating mostly unrefined whole vegan foods is the best tip I have. I would add that in addition to diet and exercise, sufficient amount of sleep and stress-reduction are two other important variables in promoting overall health. I advocate drinking large quantities of water and avoiding any other drinks except green tea.

What is your top tip for maintaining weight?
Balancing a healthy diet with the amount of physical activity is the best tip I have.

What is your top tip for improving metabolism?
I have a simple general answer to offer. A balanced diet with exercise is the best one can do. I recommend gaining some muscle mass since muscle uses more energy than fat.

What is your top tip for toning up?
I recommend pushups and squats for general toning. Body weight exercises are highly effective and can be done anywhere. I travel frequently and I can do these exercises anywhere. Pushups involve many of the upper body muscles and have the advantage of engaging stabilizing muscles. Pushups, like planks, are great for abdominal muscle strengthening. When I realized this I stopped doing crunches and sit ups, and I don't think my abdominal region suffered at all by doing this.

How do you promote veganism in your daily life?
As mentioned earlier, on a daily basis I promote veganism through example. I present myself as a friendly, smart, physically fit example of a vegan. I think unless one is a full time activist, this is the best approach a regular person can take.

How would you suggest people get involved with what you do?
People are consistently amazed that I do 2000 one-arm pushups and 1000 regular pushups every day. However, it took many years to build to this. I began with 50 pushups in five sets of 10 the mid 1990s. Over the years I've slowly improved and that is how I am reached the quantity I've reached today. Similar advice could be given for switching to a vegan diet. While I would like to see people quickly adopt a vegan diet, I understand that a slower transition is probably more sustainable rather than radically altering one's diet in a very short period of time.

BRIDGET FLYNN
VEGAN EXERCISE ENTHUSIAST

Oberlin, Ohio, USA
Vegan since: 2007

hardfemmephysique.wordpress.com
SM: *FaceBook, Instagram, Twitter*

Bridget Flynn is a vegan athlete from the Midwest, USA who loves her job as the Sustainability Coordinator at Oberlin College. She graduated cum laude from Indiana University with degrees in Environmental Ethics and Religious Studies. She lives with her best friend, Buddy (who is a majestic cat), enjoys being active, reading, spending time with and adventuring with family and friends.

WHY VEGAN?

How and why did you decide to become vegan?
I received a DVD at Warped Tour that portrayed the brutal realities of slaughterhouses, the environmental impact of factory farming, and the health benefits of vegetarian and vegan diets – as well as interviews with bands that have vegetarian and vegan members. This video was the first time I had seriously thought of – or seen – how animals were killed for my food. I was devastated, cried my eyes out and went vegetarian immediately. Over the next few months, I read more and more about being vegan and began to cut out most animal products until deciding to jump into veganism for life. As a deeply empathetic person and a total nerd, I learned as much as I could about veganism and related issues (human nutrition and health, environmental impact, advocacy, etc.) and developed immense passion for the subject.

How long have you been vegan?
Vegetarian since August 2006, Vegan since May 2007.

What has benefited you the most from being vegan?
Becoming vegan has allowed me to be who I am and live at peace with the world in a new way. Prior to going vegan, I didn't know that this was even possible. I feel immense reward from living compassionately and advocating for the animals.

Becoming vegan also opened me up to a whole new world of foods and ushered me into the vegan community! It's so much fun to go to new cities to check out their vegan scene, find new products, meet like-minded individuals, and most importantly feel like I'm living in line with my ethics and making a difference for the animals.

What does veganism mean to you?
Veganism to me is about living in the world with respect to all life and with the desire to minimize suffering. This includes extending our circle of compassion and care to our human and non-human counterparts and the natural world.

TRAINING

What sort of training do you do?
I have been a life-long athlete; more recent accomplishments include running two half-marathons, dozens (if not closer to 100) 5ks, competing in a rock climbing competition, receiving my purple-belt in taekwondo, and completing a Tough Mudder. My current sport of focus is bodybuilding. I competed in my first figure competition in August 2014.

How often do you (need to) train?
I lift weights five times a week, pose once a week, and when in the cutting phase do cardio quite a few times a week.

Do you offer your fitness or training services to others?
Not in any formal capacity. As someone into fitness and nutrition, I am often asked for advice from co-workers, friends, family, and random folks at the gym. More recently, I've led orientation trainings to the weight room and lifting. It's been a lot of fun to encourage and empower people to find and express their strength. Because I was getting so many questions, I also started my blog.

What sports do you play?
I have competed in: basketball, volleyball, track, softball, snowboarding, cross-country, kickboxing, taekwondo, swimming, rock-climbing, running, and now bodybuilding. I also bike recreationally.

"Eat healthy, exercise hard and often, and learn to love your body no matter your size. Lastly, enjoy the journey. Particularly when you are striving for a certain goal, remember that you must enjoy the journey toward the goal, too. Happiness doesn't just arrive and stick around once you've achieved your goal. Enjoy the process and keep striving for more."

STRENGTHS, WEAKNESSES & OUTSIDE INFLUENCES

What do you think is the biggest misconception about vegans and how do you address this?
The biggest misconception or stereotype of vegans is that they are white, pale, scrawny, and need to worry about their protein intake. I combat this misconception by referring people to diverse vegan athletes, like the PlantBuilt team; as well as being an active and informed vegan myself.

What are your strengths as a vegan athlete?
I love to shatter the myths people have about vegans – in particular vegans in athletic arenas. Knowing I'm an ambassador to the animals pushes me to work hard. I want to dispel the myth that in order to be competitive you need animal products. My other strength is empathy and understanding. I love to encourage people to make more vegan choices; it doesn't have to be all or nothing. Do your best!

What is your biggest challenge?
Right now, dieting is hard, but that doesn't have much to do with veganism. It can be difficult to be an ambassador for the animals, because people will always look to your for answers, critique everything you do from your achievements to your purchases. However, that's a small price to pay.

Are the non-vegans in your industry supportive or not?
Some are; some aren't. There are certainly some people that are in awe of vegans with muscle and respect it very much, but there are others that say "Well, just imagine what you could do if you ate animal products." As a whole, I think the athletic community is becoming more and more accepting – and even excited about – veganism.

Are your family and friends supportive of your vegan lifestyle?
The vast majority of my friends and family are now. When I first went vegetarian and then vegan, my family was hesitant and didn't understand it exactly. Now my family sees that I'm healthy, happy, and that veganism has been a positive, affirming choice for me.

What is the most common question/comment that people ask/say when they find out that you are a vegan and how do you respond?
Haha! There's so many. Certainly the top one is "Where do you get your protein?" to which I usually respond by telling them all the foods I eat in a day, and reference the myriad of ways to get plant protein from beans and lentils to whole grains to tempeh and seitan. I also love to mention that dark leafy greens like kale and Brussels sprouts have more protein per calorie than steak.

Who or what motivates you?
Motivation comes from within, but is reinforced by family, friends, fellow athletes, and the "haters." I faced a lot of sexism in athletics growing up which made me develop an underdog-type of prove-them-wrong attitude. As a vegan, too, I am motivated to show that a compassionate lifestyle and fitness are not incompatible. Because I'm from the Midwest, there are a lot of minds to change; I constantly have fruitful conversations with folks about veganism, which is really rewarding. These kinds of conversations further reinforce the impetus to change hearts and minds, which is really motivating for me.

Ultimately, you're the only one there to make those reps count or to stop you from gorging on Oreos. Especially with dieting, it's a mental game and you have to keep yourself in check. Of course, it is extremely helpful to have supportive friends, family, roommates, partners, and coaches.

"Because I'm from the Midwest, there are a lot of minds to change; I constantly have fruitful conversations with folks about veganism, which is really rewarding. These kinds of conversations further reinforce the impetus to change hearts and minds, which is really motivating for me."

FOOD & SUPPLEMENTS

What do you eat for Breakfast?
Nowadays oatmeal with protein powder and strawberries; I also love really hardy green smoothies with fruit and peanut butter for breakfast. I also love healthy pancakes, waffles, tempeh bacon, and other breakfast foods.

What do you eat for Lunch?
High-protein tofu, steamed broccoli, and nutritional yeast with salsa or spices; sweet potato with seitan and a huge salad with dark greens and veggies. I am also a fan of burritos, wraps, sandwiches, and more.

What do you eat for Dinner?

Homemade seitan, brown rice, and steamed veggies like Brussels sprouts, peppers, or spinach with lemon. In the off-season, I like the Vegan Stoner's mac-and-peas, pasta with marinara and nutritional yeast, couscous, quinoa, and more.

What do you eat for Snacks - healthy & not-so healthy?

Veggies and hummus, snap peas, steamed veggies, zucchini, green beans, protein pudding (made with tofu and cocoa powder or protein powder and almond milk), kale chips, and in the off-season Clif bars, trail mix, pretzels. I am a huge fan of baked goods and enjoy making semi-healthy ones like my famous oatmeal raisin cookies, zucchini bread, carrot spice muffins, or cupcakes!

What is your favourite source of Protein?

RawFusion Peanut Butter Chocolate Fudge protein powder, tempeh, tofu, whole grains, quinoa - oh, it's so hard to choose!

What is your favourite source of Calcium?

Broccoli, kale, almond milk, kimchi (fermented cabbage).

What is your favourite source of Iron?

Lentils, spinach, beans, edamame, tofu, tempeh, kale, nuts and seeds (trail mix – yum!)

What foods give you the most energy?

Simply eating healthy foods in the right portions keep me energized – as well as coffee and tea. Sweets give me energy boosts, too.

Do you take any supplements?

Right now, I take quite a few. In general, just an occasional multi-vitamin containing B12 is all I take. For bodybuilding, I also regularly take CLA, Glucosamine, BCAAs post-workout; as well as creatine during the bulking phase.

"Becoming vegan has allowed me to be who I am and live at peace with the world in a new way. Prior to going vegan, I didn't know that this was even possible. I feel immense reward from living compassionately and advocating for the animals."

ADVICE

What is your top tip for gaining muscle?

Lift weights! Bodybuilding.com is a terrific resource.

What is your top tip for losing weight?

This can be hard. Eat right and exercise regularly. I think too many people focus on losing weight instead of gaining health and fitness and simply feeling good. The number on the scale or even your BMI doesn't determine your worth, your fitness, or your health. In the US, too many people rely entirely on the scale. Eat healthy, exercise hard and often, and learn to love your body no matter your size. Lastly, enjoy the journey. Particularly when you are striving for a certain goal, remember that you must enjoy the journey toward the goal, too. Happiness doesn't just arrive and stick around once you've achieved your goal. Enjoy the process and keep striving for more.

What is your top tip for maintaining weight?

Keep doing what you're doing.

What is your top tip for improving metabolism?

Eat smaller meals more often. I find that eating five to seven times a day is a great way to boost your metabolism and maintain a more consistent energy level throughout the day.

What is your top tip for toning up?

Again, lift weights and/or do circuit-training exercises – even with your body-weight. There are so many ways to do this. Find activities that you find fun and stick to it.

How do you promote veganism in your daily life?

There are many ways I promote veganism in my personal and professional life. I talk to people intelligently and enthusiastically about veganism often – even simple acts like wearing a t-shirt that says "Vegan" on it at the gym have inspired many conversations. Just about everyone who knows me knows that I am vegan and respects my veganism. I have had conversations about veganism with nearly everyone I know at this point. I love when months, or even years, later people will contact me and tell me they are trying vegan foods or went vegetarian or vegan and that I inspired them. How exciting!

I have worked with Mercy for Animals and Indy (Indianapolis) Vegans. In my current role at work, I have advocated for a Meatless Monday-type campaign, and ensure events we host are vegetarian or vegan, which can mean hundreds of people eating vegan cookies! I am the advisor to the Animal Rights Club, and initiated an intersectional animal rights book club where we discuss how issues of gender, race, class, sexual orientation, and sustainability relate to veganism and animal rights. Occasionally I post pro-vegan messages on my social media pages, volunteer for or contribute to vegan organizations, leaflet, support ethical and innovative vegan/-friendly businesses, and shop strategically among other things.

How would you suggest people get involved with what you do?

Feel free to find or contact me on FaceBook, Instagram and Twitter. Preferably follow my FaceBook page and Instagram, as that's where I post most of my journey. Send me good vibes for my competitions!

"I love to shatter the myths people have about vegans – in particular vegans in athletic arenas. Knowing I'm an ambassador to the animals pushes me to work hard. I want to dispel the myth that in order to be competitive you need animal products. My other strength is empathy and understanding. I love to encourage people to make more vegan choices; it doesn't have to be all or nothing. Do your best!"

CAM F AWESOME
VEGAN PROFESSIONAL BOXER

Kansas City, Missouri, USA
Vegan since: 2013

camfawesome.com
SM: *FaceBook, Twitter*

Cam F Awesome is currently the captain of the USA National boxing team. He aims to win a gold medal in the 2016 Olympics. Cam is originally from Long Island, New York, but currently resides in Kansas City, Missouri, which he considers home. He has been vegan for almost 3 years and loves it. There are sometimes challenges but nothing that Cam can't overcome to maintain his plant-based diet. In between boxing and working out, Cam gives motivational speeches to young adults. He is also pursuing a career in standup comedy.

WHY VEGAN?

How and why did you decide to become vegan?
I became vegan after trying the Engine 2 28-day vegan challenge.

How long have you been vegan?
I have been vegan coming up on 3 years.

What has benefited you the most from being vegan?
My recovery time is better and it's taught me to pack my meals beforehand.

What does veganism mean to you?
It has changed my life and the way I've looked at other lives.

TRAINING

What sort of training do you do?
I do boxing training and strength and conditioning.

How often do you (need to) train?
I train about 6 days a week.

Do you offer your fitness or training services to others?
I coach boxers in Kansas City when I am in town.

What sports do you play?
I'm a boxer.

STRENGTHS, WEAKNESSES & OUTSIDE INFLUENCES

What do you think is the biggest misconception about vegans and how do you address this?
The biggest misconception is that many people don't think tough fighters can be successful without meat.

What are your strengths as a vegan athlete?
My strength in the ring is my defence and agility.

What is your biggest challenge?
My biggest challenge is keeping my nutrients up when I leave the country.

Are the non-vegans in your industry supportive or not?
They are supportive but give me a tough time with jokes. We are a close team. I can take it!

Are your family and friends supportive of your vegan lifestyle?
My friends and family are very supportive of my team.

What is the most common question/comment that people ask/say when they find out that you are a vegan and how do you respond?
"Where do you get your protein?" I let my accomplishments speak for themself.

Who or what motivates you?
Hearing my country's national anthem on the podium.

FOOD & SUPPLEMENTS

What do you eat for Breakfast?
Oatmeal.

What do you eat for Lunch?
I love tofu blend and salads.

What do you eat for Dinner?
Brown rice, lots of greens and veggies.

What do you eat for Snacks - healthy & not-so healthy?
I love Field Roast Italian sausages.

What is your favourite source of Protein?
Garden of Life Marley Coffee.

What is your favourite source of Calcium?
Vanilla almond milk.

What is your favourite source of Iron?
Garden of Life supplement.

What foods give you the most energy?
I love carbing up before a fight.

Do you take any supplements?
I only take Garden of Life supplements.

ADVICE

What is your top tip for gaining muscle?
Strength and conditioning with the proper diet.

What is your top tip for losing weight?
Simple: burn more calories than you take in.

What is your top tip for maintaining weight?
Burning the amount of you take it.

What is your top tip for improving metabolism?
More smaller meals and not eating late meals.

How do you promote veganism in your daily life?
I talk about my diet to those who are curious.

How would you suggest people get involved with what you do?
I suggest watching "Forks Over Knives" to find out more about being vegan.

Get outside of your comfort zone.

"There are three classes of people: those who see, those who see when they're shown and those who do not see."

- Leonardo da Vinci

Permanent Changes Not Quick Fixes.

CHERYL PANNONE
VEGAN MARATHON RUNNER

Warwick, Rhode Island, USA
Vegan since: 2008

plantsrunwild.com
SM: *FaceBook, Pinterest, Twitter*

Cheryl Pannone changed her life forever with a resolution on New Year's Eve 2008. She wanted to become healthier, so trained for a 5km marathon and was instantly hooked. Then, she decided to go back to school and earn her Bachelor's in Health & Wellness and personal trainer certificate. Cheryl eventually went further and earned her certificate in plant-based nutrition at Cornell University. Today 7 years after her resolution, she now runs marathons, cycles, lifts weights, does yoga and has been featured in Vegan Health & Fitness magazine, writes weekly blogs for Happycow.com, and is developing her own vegan website.

Cheryl and her husband are both vegan. They met at a half marathon, he proposed at the finish line of a full marathon, and they recently got married in Las Vegas where they exchanged vows at the start of a half marathon.

WHY VEGAN?

How and why did you decide to become vegan?
After watching the movie "Food Inc.", I decided to become vegetarian, which then led to reading, researching and watching everything I could to learn about the food industry eg Forks Over Knives, Slaughterhouse, China Study, Whole and many others that converted me to becoming a whole foods vegan shortly after. I was devastated on how factory farms treat the animals and how foods end up in our supermarket shelves. I learned that ordering a cheeseburger in the drive through window for a buck, impacts the health epidemic, welfare of our animals, oceans, lakes, land and air. I became vegan to become healthier, save animals and our earth.

How long have you been vegan?
Over 6 years.

What has benefited you the most from being vegan?
I am now in my 40s and I have never felt better. I have more energy, my endurance for races has increased and my recovery is much quicker, allowing me to get back out there sooner. My hair, skin, nails and body feels and looks younger. Most of all, I know that I am not contributing to the horrible treatment of animals, supporting big business, or wasting our resources.

"People are so brainwashed with what the food industry tells us with commercials, news reports, product labels, and government agencies, that they simply don't realize that whole foods such as kale and other leafy greens have more protein than meat."

What does veganism mean to you?
Veganism to me means a lifestyle where I know that I am consuming foods that have not come from sick, mistreated, angry, and drugged animals. I know I am not contributing in using our most precious natural resources to feed, water, and process these animals and other processed foods. I am living a lifestyle that I know is healthy for my body, mind and soul.

TRAINING

What sort of training do you do?
During the off season I run on my treadmill on average 10-15 miles (16-24km) in the morning or I mix it up and ride the stationary bike or elliptical. During the nicer weather, I run outside in the morning and my long run days are Sundays running usually around 20 miles. I average 50-60 miles a week. I also, go to the gym 4 nights a week to lift weights, participate in kick boxing classes or yoga.

How often do you (need to) train?
I train 7 days a week, with Saturdays being my light easy days.

Do you offer your fitness or training services to others?
Although I don't have a regular clientele right now, I do have my Personal Trainer certificate and I do offer my services to family and friends whenever they need it. I am building up my website to offer my wellness services that includes educating, recipes, fitness and resources to turn to.

What sports do you play?
I run long distance, bike long distance and lift weights.

STRENGTHS, WEAKNESSES & OUTSIDE INFLUENCES

What do you think is the biggest misconception about vegans and how do you address this?
If I had a dime for every person who thinks I don't get enough protein, I would be rich. People are so brainwashed with what the food industry tells us with commercials, news reports, product labels, and government agencies, that they simply don't realize that whole foods such as kale and other leafy greens have more protein than meat. They believe that because meat is a complete protein in amino acids and that veggies are not, therefore are inferior and do not provide essential nutrients when in fact the opposite is true. I am always asked the same question, "Well what is it that you eat then?" I simply explain to them what I eat and that I am getting all of the nutrients my body needs to keep me healthy through whole foods.

What are your strengths as a vegan athlete?
My biggest strengths is being able to increase my endurance and having enough energy to do so. I am increasing in muscle mass and decreasing body fat. I recover much quicker after an endurance event. My last marathon I was at the gym the next day and felt great.

What is your biggest challenge?
I have faced many challenges over the years being a vegan. Since I am the only vegan in my family, I think the hardest challenge was my family and friends, and convincing them that this is my lifestyle and trying to explain to them why. Family gatherings, holidays, going out to eat, and travel were all challenging but, I have overcome them

and plan ahead meals, call restaurants to see if they can accommodate, and make dishes I can eat for holidays.

Are the non-vegans in your industry supportive or not?
The people who I work with simply do not understand what it is to be a vegan. They will ask me if I can eat fish or eggs and can't understand why I do not. I am often asked exactly what it is that I eat and if I only eat salads. They will make comments saying that healthy food is expensive, doesn't taste good and is boring which also leads to another misconception. Vegan foods made from whole foods are the most delicious and nutritious, and can be easy, fun and inexpensive to cook.

Are your family and friends supportive of your vegan lifestyle?
It took my family and friends a very long time to accept my lifestyle, simply because they didn't know anything about it. I had always grown up in a meat and potatoes household. Both of my children are not vegan, although they do enjoy vegan dishes that I cook, they will not give up animals products. My son loves bacon so much that he has a bacon air fresher in his car. I still get the occasional joke or comment, like someone offering me a hot dog or burger at gatherings. I mostly laugh and brush it off, knowing that I am putting healthy food in my body and saving animals.

What is the most common question/comment that people ask/say when they find out that you are a vegan and how do you respond?
"Where do you get your protein?" "How can you run marathons eating no meat?" "You are not getting enough nutrients, you are going to become anemic", and "You need calcium from milk and protein from meat." I respond by telling them that I eat a very healthy well-balanced diet and foods such as, leafy greens, other vegetables, fruits, whole grains, nuts and seeds all contain the required nutrients that my body needs to keep me healthy and strong. Animal products often lack essential nutrients such as fiber and phyto-chemicals that have been proven to fight cancer and other chronic illnesses. Animal proteins have saturated fats and high cholesterol, which contributes to many illnesses.

Who or what motivates you?
I have a few favorite vegan athletes who I deeply admire and inspire me to keep me motivated and help me to improve in my athletic goals, runners such as Richard Roll, Scott Jurek, Brendan Brazier (I have read their books), Matt Frazier, Ruth Heidrich and Catra Corbett. I follow their websites for great inspiration, articles and recipes.

FOOD & SUPPLEMENTS

First I just want to mention that 90% of what I eat is made from scratch. I make meals in bulk and plan ahead of time. My husband (who is also vegan) and I like to eat out at our favorite vegan restaurants once in a while.

What do you eat for Breakfast?
Every morning I have my favorite breakfast, which is organic peanut butter or almond butter on spouted whole grain bread - sometimes I make my own waffles for this - with banana and a glass of fresh squeezed orange juice.

What do you eat for Lunch?
I have a smoothie that usually consists of kale, spinach, little bit of fresh cilantro and parsley, blueberries, banana, pumpkin, sweet potato, avocado, celery, nuts, chocolate protein, wheat grass, spirulina, chia seeds and a splash of agave. I like to mix it up and put other great veggies in them.

What do you eat for Dinner?

We always have a garden salad with homemade dressings. My favorite is a miso ginger dressing, topped with crunchy lentils, homemade pickled beets and other veggies. With the salad, I will sometimes make a soup such as tomato or cream of broccoli, or dishes such as Soba noodle pasta with sauces, black bean burgers, rice or quinoa casseroles, and the list goes on.

What do you eat for Snacks - healthy & not-so healthy?

My favorite snack is crunchy chickpeas with lots of seasoning. I also make granola, energy bars and crackers. I snack on fresh fruits sometimes dipped in peanut butter. I will bake once in a while making healthy treats such as brownies, cupcakes and breads. My one bad not-so healthy snack that we both have a weakness for is tortilla chips usually the Whole Foods brand. We don't buy them that often because we simply don't have control over eating the whole bag. We usually save them for holidays. Oh and lots of water throughout the day.

What is your favourite source of Protein?

Sunwarrior chocolate protein blend.

What is your favourite source of Calcium?

Kale, kale and more kale, broccoli, tahini, oranges, dates and fennel - just to name a few.

What is your favourite source of Iron?

Pumpkin seeds, lentils, beans, collard greens, and of course more kale - just to name a few.

What foods give you the most energy?

Since most of what I eat is whole foods, I have to say all of it. But if I have to choose I would say fruits such as dates, which are an athlete's favorite, Also, bananas, kiwi, lemons - all of which provides a natural source of fructose, and chia seeds or sprouted barley.

Do you take any supplements?

The only supplement I do take is a vegan B12, Sunwarrior protein in my smoothies and spirulina.

"I was devastated on how factory farms treat the animals and how foods end up in our supermarket shelves. I learned that ordering a cheeseburger in the drive through window for a buck, impacts the health epidemic, welfare of our animals, oceans, lakes, land and air. I became vegan to become healthier, save animals and our earth."

ADVICE

What is your top tip for gaining muscle?

Eat lots of foods that contain natural fats and proteins such as, quinoa, millet, avocados, sweet potatoes, peanuts or other nut butters. Do less cardio and lift heavier weights with less repetition.

What is your top tip for losing weight?

Although the above are essential sources of proteins, to lose weight I would recommend limiting some of these and eating more foods that will provide healthy fibers and carbohydrates for energy such as leafy greens, and some fruits. Exercise with more cardio and light weights and more repetitions to build tone in the muscles that will burn fat calories faster.

What is your top tip for maintaining weight?

Eat a well-balanced diet consisting of mostly vegetables, fruits, some nuts and seeds and whole grains. With a balance of exercise consisting of light weights and cardio.

What is your top tip for improving metabolism?

Eat foods that are high in calcium and omega 3s. Citrus fruits, spices, green teas, whole grains and broccoli. Also, eat at least 6 smaller meals throughout the day and have an exercise plan that includes weights. Muscle will increase metabolism.

What is your top tip for toning up?

Eat foods that are not processed and in their whole form in small meals throughout the day, while maintaining an exercise program that includes cardio, circuit training and light weights with more repetitions to tone the muscles.

Timing is also important when it comes to eating foods. Eat healthy carbohydrates - such as fruits and not refined white processed carbohydrates - before a work out and earlier in the day to give your body energy. Eat protein-rich foods after a workout - smoothies are best because it gets absorbed quicker replacing nutrients lost during workouts. Protein meals should be eaten more at night.

How do you promote veganism in your daily life?

I always answer anyone's questions if they're interested in the vegan lifestyle. I offer recipe samples, books to read or movies ideas to watch. If I make a dish, I will offer some of it to others to try or give them the recipe. If they want to learn how to workout, I put a suggested plan together for them that meets their needs and lifestyle. I am proud of living this lifestyle and try to promote it when I can.

How would you suggest people get involved with what you do?

I first give them websites (starting with my own) to look at, give them very simple and easy recipes that tastes great. Suggest books or documentaries to watch, and vegan groups to join in their area. I have even taken friends and family on field trips to Whole Foods to teach them how to shop and what to look for. I invite them to the gym with me to give them some ideas and tips for working out either there or at home.

"Veganism to me means a lifestyle where I know that I am consuming foods that have not come from sick, mistreated, angry, and drugged animals. I know I am not contributing in using our most precious natural resources to feed, water, and process these animals and other processed foods. I am living a lifestyle that I know is healthy for my body, mind and soul."

CHRISTINE HO
VEGAN GYMNAST

Markham, Ontario, Canada
Vegan since: 2011

instagram.com/christinehsj

Christine Ho is a vegan fitness junkie based in Markham, Ontario, Canada who used to eat at McDonald's and KFC everyday. Her favorite things to do are working out, reading fitness magazines, reading recipes and "veganizing" them and coming up with new ones! Christine hopes to have her own fitness centre with a raw/vegan restaurant/cafe and also to perform in the circus one day! May sound a bit crazy, but after looking back and seeing how much her life has changed and that she's still here enjoying the things that she loves to do, Christine really believes that nothing is impossible.

WHY VEGAN?

How and why did you decide to become vegan?
Becoming a vegan was a very gradual transition for me. I used to eat McDonald's almost everyday! One day, I read a book by Kevin Trudeau on the truth about the meat industry, which prompted me to cut out poultry from my diet. Seafood was the next to be eliminated from my diet, then eggs, and lastly dairy. I went vegan in January 2011 after suffering from a terrible cold over the Christmas break because I assumed that dairy had something to do with it. I barely get sick ever since then.

How long have you been vegan?
I have been vegan since 2011, and loving it!

What has benefited you the most from being vegan?
After becoming a vegan, I rarely get sick, I became leaner and stronger, I recover quicker, and I'm getting better grades because I can think clearer and memorize better!

What does veganism mean to you?
To me, veganism is not just a diet. It's a lifestyle. It is so much more than just food. I feel great knowing that my choice to go vegan has spared the lives of many innocent animals, be it for food or for fur. In addition, when I think of veganism, I conjure up images of peace, nature, and a green, environmental friendly lifestyle.

TRAINING

What sort of training do you do?
I do a variety of exercises, which includes strength/weight training, plyometrics, kickboxing, endurance training, yoga, Pilates, and dance. I also train for competitive gymnastics and I will start to train for a 10k soon.

How often do you (need to) train?
I workout six days a week and do gymnastics twice a week.

Do you offer your fitness or training services to others?
Yes. I used to be a competitive cross country and track and field distance runner in high school. Now I train my high school team.

What sports do you play?
Gymnastics and running.

STRENGTHS, WEAKNESSES & OUTSIDE INFLUENCES

What do you think is the biggest misconception about vegans and how do you address this?
I think the biggest misconception about vegans is that we don't get enough protein or that we will never be as strong as meat eaters. I often prove them wrong by telling them that I'm vegan every time I do very well in my competitions. I have gotten first place in my age category in the 5k event for Scotiabank Toronto Waterfront marathon, and I have won fitness challenges held in school. I even beat the guys!

What are your strengths as a vegan athlete?
Others often say that I am a tough person, which I agree. I've learned to persevere, work harder than everyone else, and never give up through distance running because I was not born naturally good at running. I have to work extremely hard just to achieve a time that natural born runners can achieve. I've been able to transfer everything that I've gained from sports into my life. No matter what I do, I know that hard work will always payoff. Because I want to show others that vegans can be just as strong or stronger than meat eaters, my intrinsic motivation to excel is very strong.

What is your biggest challenge?
My biggest challenge is to eat out with friends and family.

Are the non-vegans in your industry supportive or not?
Some of them are, some are not.

Are your family and friends supportive of your vegan lifestyle?
My parents are not, but my friends are.

What is the most common question/comment that people ask/say when they find out that you are a vegan and how do you respond?
The most common question is the most popular one: "Where do you get your protein?" I simply list all the plant-based protein sources to them and they are usually left speechless.

Who or what motivates you?
Other vegan athletes (i.e. Ironman triathlete Brendan Brazier) and food motivates me.

FOOD & SUPPLEMENTS

What do you eat for Breakfast?
Large green smoothie made with green leafy veggies, berries, bananas, flaxseeds, nuts, sprouts everyday. Also sprouted bread with jam, nut butter or coconut oil, oatmeal, homemade muffins, raw crackers, sprouted grain cereal etc.

What do you eat for Lunch?
Big salad, with a sandwich, wrap or noodles, etc (whole grain, most are raw and made with raw sprouted grains, nuts and seeds and veggies).

What do you eat for Dinner?
Big salad with stir-fries, curries, stews, soups with veggies, tofu or beans and lentils or tempeh etc.

What do you eat for Snacks - healthy & not-so healthy?
All sorts of fruits, dried fruits, nuts and seeds, coconut water etc.

What is your favourite source of Protein?
Vega Whole Food Optimizer or Vega smoothie.

What is your favourite source of Calcium?
Sesame seeds.

What is your favourite source of Iron?
Spinach.

What foods give you the most energy?
Sprouts, fresh and dried fruits.

Do you take any supplements?
Daily multivitamin and Vitamin D.

"To me, veganism is not just a diet. It's a lifestyle. It is so much more than just food. I feel great knowing that my choice to go vegan has spared the lives of many innocent animals, be it for food or for fur. In addition, when I think of veganism, I conjure up images of peace, nature, and a green, environmental friendly lifestyle."

ADVICE

What is your top tip for gaining muscle?
Strength training and consuming complete protein sources such as quinoa, hemp seeds, and by combining legumes and grains. Enough sleep and reducing stress is also essential to repair and rebuild the body. Daily workout, food or sleep journal is also helpful.

What is your top tip for losing weight?
A mix of steady state and interval cardio training, strength training to reduce loss of muscle mass, and watch what you eat. Many people assume that vegan foods are healthy, but that's not the case. Just because something is vegan doesn't mean that they are low calories or good for you. Again, get enough sleep and try to reduce your stress level as much as possible! Daily workout, food or sleep journal is very helpful.

What is your top tip for maintaining weight?
Workout most days of the week doing a variety of cardio, strength, and flexibility training that you enjoy to prevent boredom. Eat healthy food that gives you energy and makes you feel good, and don't count calories because that stresses people out. Cookies and cakes are not going to make you fat and unhealthy as long as they are eaten in moderation. Always think of food as fuel and take time to enjoy everything that you eat. This tends to help people make smarter food choices.

What is your top tip for improving metabolism?
Cardio intervals and strength training.

What is your top tip for toning up?
The best way to tone up is to do a combination of cardio, strength, and flexibility training and of course, eating a clean, whole and natural food-based diet with adequate

protein, carbohydrates, and healthy fats.

How do you promote veganism in your daily life?

I bring interesting lunches to school and work so that others will want to know what I'm eating. I wear T-shirts that say something about veganism. Once a conversation about veganism is started, I tell the story about my journey towards becoming vegan. Many of my friends started to eat less meat and more plants under my influence. I also volunteer for the Toronto Vegetarian Association as an outreach specialist at different events.

How would you suggest people get involved with what you do?

The best way to get involved is through volunteering for various vegetarian/vegan associations and humane societies in the city. You'll learn a lot when chatting with others who have the same interests. Also, search for vegetarian/vegan social or meet up groups who meet up on a regular basis for potlucks and to visit vegetarian/vegan restaurants. It's a great way to meet more people and try different food.

"I've learned to persevere, work harder than everyone else, and never give up through distance running because I was not born naturally good at running. I have to work extremely hard just to achieve a time that natural born runners can achieve. I've been able to transfer everything that I've gained from sports into my life. No matter what I do, I know that hard work will always payoff".

Strive for Progress
Not Perfection

CHRISTINE VARDAROS
VEGAN PROFESSIONAL CYCLIST

Everberg, Belgium, EU
Vegan since: 2000

christinevardaros.blogspot.com
SM: *FaceBook, Twitter*

Christine Vardaros is a world-class vegan cyclist who has been both vegan and racing professionally since 2000. She currently races for STEVENS Pro Cycling Team. Christine is a professional road, mountain and cyclocross racer who has competed at top-level events like World Cups and World Championships. Since 2002, she has been one of the best cyclocross racers in the world. Christine is an athlete spokesperson for In Defence of Animals (IDA), Physicians Committee for Responsible Medicine (PCRM) and The Vegan Society (UK). In addition, she is a founding member of the Marin County Bicycle Coalition, and is a member of the athlete's advisory board for the Stone Foundation for Sports Medicine and Arthritis Research. Christine has never owned a car. Originally, from California, Christine now resides in Belgium with her husband Jonas, their seventeen bikes and an organic garden in the backyard.

WHY VEGAN?

On a vegan diet, I feel clean – as if I am able to magically hold onto that freshly showered feeling all day, every day no matter how dirty I get while riding my bike. This sensation partly originates from eating an incredibly healthful plant diet but it also stems from living with a clear conscience, knowing that my lifestyle allows me to be clean of all moral shame.

How and why did you decide to become vegan?
I originally became vegan to benefit from its sporting advantage, as I had just become a professional cyclist. Once I changed my diet, I quickly realized the ethical ramifications of my choices and this is what keeps me 100% strict with how I eat and how I live. I want to be able to say that nobody was hurt for me to achieve my successes on the bike. Thanks to my vegan diet, I am still racing at the top professional level well into my mid-forties.

How long have you been vegan?
Since 2000.

What has benefited you the most from being vegan?
My breathing is much better. When I was only vegetarian, I had to quit races because I thought I was going to die. My breathing was so bad that other athletes were asking me if I was okay – even during World Cups! The moment I cut animal milk from my diet, my breathing significantly improved. I also found that I wasn't spitting and coughing every few seconds on training rides as well.

What does veganism mean to you?
It is a lifestyle – a way of being.

TRAINING

What sort of training do you do?

I am mainly considered a cyclocross specialist. It is a Winter cycling sport that runs from September to February where you race for under an hour, jump over barriers, ride through sand and mud and run up steep hills while shouldering the bike. My winter training includes mainly rides of under three hours to include short intervals and some running workouts. Over the Summer, I do longer rides, mainly on the road, to work on my base training so that my fitness platform can support the short hard efforts in the Winter. I also add some road races to keep in touch with my top end speed in the "offseason."

How often do you (need to) train?

I train almost every day, especially in the winter because our cyclocross racing schedule is as intense as the training needed to compete in this sport where we're racing in upwards of five times per week. While others are celebrating Christmas and New Year's, we are racing on those days.

Do you offer your fitness or training services to others?

I currently coach a few kids ages 13 to 16 for road and cyclocross racing. I also privately consult many athletes on both fitness and pre-event training. In addition, I've written many articles on these topics for newspapers and magazines such as VegNews Magazine and one of San Francisco's newspapers the Marin Independent Journal. I will also begin writing on fitness and training for Vegan Health & Fitness Magazine.

What sports do you play?

I am a professional road, cyclocross and mountain bike racer. I also like to think of myself as a runner but I am not particularly good at it. Before that, I fenced.

STRENGTHS, WEAKNESSES & OUTSIDE INFLUENCES

What do you think is the biggest misconception about vegans and how do you address this?

The biggest misconception nowadays is that people think we all own yoga mats and wear tie-dyed tees and camp everywhere. Just last week I was accused of this– oddly enough by someone who knows me well, which proves just how powerful stereotypes can be. I address this with my unwavering behavior. I have found that by example I can personally have the greatest impact on others.

What are your strengths as a vegan athlete?

I can recover much faster than my fellow competitors after hard trainings and races. I am also rarely sick which gives me extra days to train.

What is your biggest challenge?

When traveling throughout Europe, the food options can sometimes get a bit boring. I once raced the women's Tour de France and had to subside on string beans and French bread because to many French chefs thought those two foods define a vegan diet. I survived.

Are the non-vegans in your industry supportive or not?

In the past, I found that my diet was put on the chopping block any time I had a bad race. But now people who have personal experience with me know that the diet works and that it is natural to have good and bad days when you race drug-free. Many of them have actually lowered or eliminated their animal consumption altogether based on my example.

I have also won many over through my baking. For the last few years at the final event of the season, I have held a cookie party where I'd serve ten varieties of vegan cookies – all baked by me. It has become so popular that my supporters and fellow cyclists talk about it year round. It has changed how many of them view my "funny" diet. They now see that it can be not only as normal as theirs but much more flavorful. Attendees at my cookie parties are usually so blown away that, at its conclusion, I am left with a bunch of email addresses from spectators as well as fellow racers attached to requests for recipes…and information on how to transition to a plant-based diet.

Are your family and friends supportive of your vegan lifestyle?
My family and friends are very supportive of my lifestyle. Although my Dad doesn't quite understand it all, he is very accepting of it. My Mom was vegan for six months and is still mainly vegan. My husband Jonas' mom makes us vegan meals every time we visit. She now owns about ten vegan cookbooks. Heck, I didn't even know there were that many vegan cookbooks written in Dutch! As for our friends, they too are very accommodating. We have even attended barbeques where we had our own grill and cooking tools with a variety of plant-based items to choose from.

What is the most common question/comment that people ask/say when they find out that you are a vegan and how do you respond?
They ask if I can really compete at the top level eating only plants. Shortly after the question comes out, they quickly realize that my results and many wins over the years, speaks for itself and they usually retract the question.

Who or what motivates you?
I went vegan at the same time as "Elmo", my coach. Watching him to see if he dropped dead helped a lot. When he not only didn't drop dead but progressively got faster on the bike and was also able to recover almost instantly from hard trainings just as I had, it gave me a bit of feedback needed when at that time I was surrounded by the naysayers who thought I was crazy.

As for direct motivation to race my bike hard, I do it as a "thanks" to all my supporters, friends and family who have believed in me from the beginning. Since the winter of 2007, my husband Jonas has helped immensely with my motivation. He has become the ideal teammate I never knew existed. He has made it more enjoyable to be a bike racer. We work incredibly well together to prepare for races and to compete in them. He handles all the driving, bikes, and other logistics while I just focus on riding my bike, eating, and recovering. It is also nice to have someone to celebrate the great results with as well as someone who will let me cry in his arms when it doesn't work out.

Additionally, I dig that little bit deeper for my sister who died many years ago. If you look under my saddles, you will see a little ribbon that I placed there that reminds me of my little sister. And lastly, I am motivated by the animals. When I succeed, it is a success for them too as I prove that their suffering and death is not needed to fuel a body for top level sports. I am now at the point in my career where I can hand pick the sponsors that go on my jersey. Each one of them parallel my beliefs on living an animal-friendly, earth-friendly lifestyle. This upcoming season my new race clothing sponsor, NoDrugs, has added a plethora of fruits and vegetables to my race clothing where it encompasses my sponsors like T. Strong Transportation – a green transport company, HempAge – maker of my casual clothing, BOOOM Energy products – creater of one of the first vegan recovery drinks to make it to Belgium, and STEVENS Bikes, 3T and Challenge that master the art of recycling. On my butt and collar of my clothing is The Vegan Society (UK) logo which gets lots of attention. NoDrugs has also just created a friend and family and supporter clothing line based on my race clothing for purchase by those who want to wear their animal, earth, health-friendly support literally on their sleeves.

FOOD & SUPPLEMENTS

What do you eat for Breakfast?
Oats and muesli with an apple and banana with tepid water.

What do you eat for Lunch?
Usually eaten on the bike: BOOOM bars and gels, washed down with their energy drink. On occasion, I will supplement it with dried mangos, papaya, figs, dates or the periodic steamed sweet potato.

What do you eat for Dinner?
Pasta with homemade pesto, mixed salad with a balsamic vinaigrette and soup. Last night it was lentil soup, rucola salad and Vegetable Green Curry.

What do you eat for Snacks - healthy & not-so healthy?
I am addicted to dark chocolate as I live mainly in Belgium. I also love my own home-baked cookies, which is why I cannot make them very often. My new addiction is well-blended frozen bananas with some shredded coconut, a squeeze of lemon, and chopped dark chocolate bits. It actually tastes like real ice cream but without that heavy mucous aftertaste.

What is your favourite source of Protein?
I keep my protein very low - never more than 6-10% for health reasons. I never ever go out of my way for protein. I once broke my leg and after three weeks, I went back to the doctor for a checkup. He viewed the x-ray and immediately pulled my coach aside to ask what I did because he just witnessed a miracle. A break that should have taken a minimum of six weeks was completely healed in three. My coach responded that I am on a strict low-protein plant-based diet. When I am in a heavy training or racing period, I am very careful to keep my protein low as well for added performance benefits. Even if I weren't a strict vegan, I would still never go back to eating animal protein as it comes in a very complex form which zaps your body of energy, robs it of amino acids, creates toxins and leaves you dehydrated just to break it down.

What is your favourite source of Calcium?
I just had my calcium and bones checked and was told that everything is perfectly in order. I suppose it is due to the leafy green veggies that I eat mostly every day – and of course also due to my low protein diet.

What is your favourite source of Iron?
I eat a lot of parsley sprinkled on my foods with a squeeze of lemon for its vitamin C which helps iron uptake.

What foods give you the most energy?
Apples are one of my favorite foods for energy. I keep to the sour green ones whenever possible as that is closest to how nature intended them to be. I also drink lots of green tea for its sustained energy...and fat-burning benefits.

Do you take any supplements?
Iron once a month, 2 grams of vitamin C per day. Every month or so, I also take a B12 pill since I don't really eat any supplemented foods. According to my blood tests that I have done for my sport, everything is perfectly in order every time. In fact, newest studies are proving that animal-eaters are having more of a tough time getting in their B12 than plant-eaters as everything nowadays is overly sanitized.

ADVICE

What is your top tip for gaining muscle?

That is mainly genetic. The rest has to do with how you train that specific muscle you want to grow. DO skip protein shakes, as they certainly do not help to make your muscle any bigger or more optimally recovered. Your muscles need very little protein to get the job done. Anything above that level is simply wasted – and will do damage on your body as it's processed on its way out the other end.

What is your top tip for losing weight?

Increase your raw vegetable intake. Cutting sugar from a diet really helps if you have a sweet tooth. Cut meal portions down a bit. Eat according to your body demands. If you need your body to do "big work", then eat a big meal beforehand. If all you will do that day is sit at your desk, then eat a light meal. Add green tea or better yet oolong tea to your daily routine. They also sell green tea in pill form called EGCG for those who aren't tea drinkers. Three of those pills can burn up to 225 calories per day.

What is your top tip for maintaining weight?

Eat only when you are hungry, unless you need your body for something strenuous.

What is your top tip for improving metabolism?

Ginger, cinnamon, spicy food, green tea and oolong tea. Exercise is the best for this!

What is your top tip for toning up?

Exercise a bit each day. Start the day with a walk around the block or to the bakery for a loaf of bread. Buy yourself mini weights and do them every other day. Buy a simple exercise video and do it as often as possible.

How do you promote veganism in your daily life?

Mainly by example which seems to work very, very well, especially now that we have social media like FaceBook and Twitter at our disposal. I cannot even begin to tell you how many emails, calls and comments I have steadily received over the years from people who thanked me for their conversion to a plant-based diet. Many of them also said that they were initially turned off by the "crazies" who were shoving the animal rights stuff down their throat and beating them down for their choices. When they saw my example, they realized that there were all sorts of folks who live vegan. I also periodically mention or share tidbits here and there through social media about veganism for health and about the animal abuse. I spend a lot of time giving interviews for publications as well as answer many private emails inquiring about a vegan diet.

In addition, I spread the word as a spokesperson for In Defence of Animals (IDA), Physicians Committee for Responsible Medicine (PCRM) and The Vegan Society (UK). I have spoken at many events such as Paris Vegan Day, World Veggie Day in San Francisco, Veggie Pride Parade in NYC, International Animal Rights Conference in Luxembourg, VegFest UK London, ECOPOP (Ecological conference in Belgium) and for EVA (Belgium's Vegetarian Society.) At these events, I talk mainly about a plant-based diet for active lives. Considering my choice to be vegan is also a moral one, I am thankful for all those who work hard to promote a cruelty-free world as it takes many approaches towards the common goal to reach all people.

How would you suggest people get involved with what you do?

Contact a local bike shop and ask about cyclocross or bike racing. They will usually be able to steer you in the right direction.

CHRISTY MORGAN
VEGAN PERSONAL TRAINER

Dallas, Texas, USA
Vegan since: 2002

blissfulandfit.com
SM: *Facebook, Instagram, Twitter, Pinterest*

Christy Morgan, known as The Blissful (& Fit) Chef, has been tantalizing taste buds for years as a vegan chef, cooking instructor, food writer, and cookbook author; now athlete and NASM certified personal trainer. She is the author of "Blissful Bites: Plant-based Meals That Nourish Mind, Body, and Planet", and the Editor-in-Chief and creator of "Definition Magazine".

WHY VEGAN?

How and why did you decide to become vegan?
I decided to try being vegetarian as an experiment because one of my close college friends was vegetarian. I moved to Los Angeles after college and made another friend who had been vegetarian since she was 15. She showed me the Meet Your Meat video on PETA's website and we went vegan together overnight. There was no way I could contribute to the death and violence of the meat and dairy industry. We connected with other vegans in our community, attended potlucks and that's when I started teaching myself how to cook. I fell in love with feeding people and decided to change careers and go to a natural foods culinary school.

How long have you been vegan?
Since 2002.

What has benefited you the most from being vegan?
It's hard to pinpoint the best benefit because my whole life encompasses my veganism - it's almost like a spiritual practice for me. Being vegan is about the big picture and affects my life physically, emotionally, socially, economically. The benefits are endless and numerous! But to name a few; better health (skin, weight maintenance, sex life, strong immune system), more energy, faster recovery from workouts, discovering amazing foods, building communities and connecting with other like-minded people, and having a greater purpose in life.

What does veganism mean to you?
Creating a life that inflicts the least amount of harm possible, while being the most compassionate and conscious person I am able.

TRAINING

What sort of training do you do?
I'm a diverse athlete and do a lot of cross-training. That includes High-intensity interval training (HIIT), weight lifting, swimming, biking, running, Zumba, kickboxing, yoga, Body Combat, dancing, racquetball, TRX suspension training and more. I don't like to limit myself and I tend to get bored easily.

How often do you (need to) train?
I move my body every day generally. Even on my "rest" days, I take a yoga class.

Do you offer your fitness or training services to others?
I've been the gal you go to when you need help transitioning to a vegan diet, but now that I've become obsessed with fitness, I became a certified personal trainer.

What sports do you play?
I don't play any traditional competitive sports and never have - save for one year on the swim team in high school.

"Being vegan is about the big picture and affects my life physically, emotionally, socially, economically. The benefits are endless and numerous!"

STRENGTHS, WEAKNESSES & OUTSIDE INFLUENCES

What do you think is the biggest misconception about vegans and how do you address this?
The biggest misconception of vegans is that we are sick, pale and weak. This is so far from the truth in most instances! The majority of vegans I know are healthy, vibrant and rarely get sick if they take care of themselves. And those into fitness are far from weak. To address this I keep walking the talk, training hard and showing others how strong I can be on a vegan diet. It's always fun running circles around people at the gym who I know are omnivore.

What are your strengths as a vegan athlete?
When you eat a whole foods vegan diet, you are giving your body the best fuel possible. That makes you stronger, more energetic, and you have quicker recovery times than those who are putting death and violence in their body. Plant foods are alkaline - as opposed to the acid nature of animal foods.

What is your biggest challenge?
Wanting to work out all the time and not giving myself rest periods. Working out, pushing harder, becoming more, transforming my body, all of these things have become almost an addiction. At least it's a healthy one.

Are the non-vegans in your industry supportive or not?
Thankfully, I haven't gotten a lot of pushback from non-vegans. My actions speak for themselves and when they see what I'm capable of in the gym, it gives them something to think about. Those who follow a "paleo" diet tend to be the most closed-minded, but everyone else is pretty laid back.

Are your family and friends supportive of your vegan lifestyle?
At this point in my veganism, almost all of my friends are vegetarian or vegan, so I'm sort of in a bubble. And my family is used to it by now. At first they thought it was interesting at family gatherings. The first Thanksgiving I made all my own food and no one touched it. The second one my grandmother made a separate stuffing for me and I brought a few dishes. By the third one, I was bringing Thai food with me and the fourth one I just stopped going to family gatherings that involved food. It wasn't worth it to me to deal with the stress, and also to continually see their health decline as they stuffed their faces with the most heart-clogging, unhealthy foods. It was heart breaking actually. I haven't been to a Thanksgiving or Christmas with my extended family in 7 years.

What is the most common question/comment that people ask/say when they find out that you are a vegan and how do you respond?
Most people say it's too difficult or that they really love the taste of meat. Since it's my job to help people transition, I offer them advice if they want it. And now that I have created an online wellness program, that gives them all the tools they need to make a successful transition, I usually hand them my card. I encourage them to take baby steps if they aren't ready to go full on - and to incorporate more veggies and greens into their diet while cutting out some processed food. I truly believe that cooking your own food is the best way to health and by learning to cook, you make everything easier for your transition. So my mission in life is to show people how to make quick and tasty meals, how to meal plan, and make it all doable for themselves and their families.

Who or what motivates you?
Reaching the next goal, setting a Personal Record, lifting heavier, running further than I did the day before pushes me. Finding a love of fitness has given me a new outlet for my activism, so being able to share my experiences with others through my blog and social media motivates and drives me. It warms my heart to know that I'm inspiring people every day to get out there and see what they are made of (hopefully plants.) And showing the world that you can be vegan and strong and do anything your heart desires.

FOOD&SUPPLEMENTS

What do you eat for Breakfast?
Protein oats or polenta porridge, topped with fruit and hemp seeds.

What do you eat for Lunch?
Usually a really large mixed green salad with tons of chopped veggies, tofu and homemade dressing.

What do you eat for Dinner?
Depends on what I'm training for, but I usually have my plate divided into three sections with a protein, starchy carbohydrate and greens filling the plate.

What do you eat for Snacks - healthy & not-so healthy?
Green smoothies, rice cake with nut butter, protein shake, fruit, sometimes a raw bar, veggies or rice crackers with hummus, corn chips and salsa, homemade protein treats.

What is your favourite source of Protein?
Tofu, it's so versatile.

What is your favourite source of Calcium?
Greens and beans.

What is your favourite source of Iron?
Collard greens.

What foods give you the most energy?
Complex carbohydrates and fruit.

Do you take any supplements?
B12, Glucosamine, MSM, and protein powder.

"When you eat a whole foods vegan diet, you are giving your body the best fuel possible. That makes you stronger, more energetic, and you have quicker recovery times

than those who are putting death and violence in their body."

ADVICE

What is your top tip for gaining muscle?
Eat! Lift heavy, do a 4 or 5 day split focusing on a small group of different muscles in each session.

What is your top tip for losing weight?
Give up all processed foods, keep sodium low and eat whole, unprocessed foods. Cut out pastries, sugar and alcohol.

What is your top tip for maintaining weight?
Same as above, but enjoy a "cheat" meal once a week.

What is your top tip for improving metabolism?
Don't calorie restrict! Eat 5-6 smaller meals throughout the day.

What is your top tip for toning up?
High-intensity interval training (HIIT) combined with weight training will get you nice and toned with a good diet.

How do you promote veganism in your daily life?
It is my life and my profession to promote veganism and teach others how to make delicious food through my website, cooking classes and online wellness program.

How would you suggest people get involved with what you do?
Check out my website and you can also follow me on Twitter, Instagram and Facebook.

"Finding a love of fitness has given me a new outlet for my activism, so being able to share my experiences with others through my blog and social media motivates and drives me. It warms my heart to know that I'm inspiring people every day to get out there and see what they are made of (hopefully plants.) And showing the world that you can be vegan and strong and do anything your heart desires."

It's a Slow Process
Keep Going

Claire Desroches
VEGAN KICKBOXER & PERSONAL TRAINER

West London, UK
Vegan since: 2010

greatveganexpectations.wordpress.com
greatexpectationsfitness.com
SM: *FaceBook, Twitter*

Claire Desroches is a personal trainer who trains in Brazilian jiu jitsu, although she has previously competed in Thai boxing and kickboxing. She writes about veganism, health and fitness at Great Vegan Expectations, and runs her own training company, Great Expectations Fitness.

WHY VEGAN?

How and why did you decide to become vegan?
There was a very clear moment around the age of 15 when I couldn't face eating dairy – it just seemed wrong to be putting it into my body. It was only later that I understood that we have no right to mass farm animals of other species, and that we have no need to consume so many animal products. I would class myself as an ethical vegan, but my views lean slightly towards the philosophical side of things.

How long have you been vegan?
Over 4 years. I did first go vegan at that moment when I was 15, but I only kept it up for about a year because of the social pressure of constantly having to explain myself to other people. In between that time I did follow a heavily plant-based diet, but I count myself as being vegan from the age of 19.

What has benefited you the most from being vegan?
I have learnt so much about health, cooking and nutrition, and about my own body. It has probably saved me a lot of money too.

What does veganism mean to you?
Taking responsibility for my own health and for leading a compassionate and sustainable lifestyle.

TRAINING

What sort of training do you do?
I take part in Brazilian jiu-jitsu classes (gi and no-gi), which involve drills, techniques, and sparring. I supplement that training with weight lifting, various forms of cardiovascular work, and conditioning sessions.

How often do you (need to) train?
I generally train five or six days a week – usually four days of martial arts classes, and one or two days dedicated to conditioning work.

Do you offer your fitness or training services to others?
Yes, I am a personal trainer.

What sports do you play?
I don't play any organised team sports, I let my playfulness and competitiveness out on the mats during sparring.

STRENGTHS, WEAKNESSES & OUTSIDE INFLUENCES

What do you think is the biggest misconception about vegans and how do you address this?
That we are all militant, "alternative" types who either know nothing about health and fitness and live off boiled potatoes, or that we are crazed new-age health fanatics who live off expensive raw super foods.

What are your strengths as a vegan athlete?
Because of the high levels of vitamins, minerals and antioxidants present in a plant-based diet, I find my immune system is stronger than that of my non-vegan training partners. My blood sugar levels are more stable throughout the day and I am more focused and alert.

What is your biggest challenge?
Combating misconceptions and misinformation about healthy eating and a balanced lifestyle.

Are the non-vegans in your industry supportive or not?
Surprisingly so! So far everyone I have encountered has been very respectful of my diet, and often curious to find out more and to try my food.

Are your family and friends supportive of your vegan lifestyle?
Yes, and I feel incredibly lucky to be surrounded by a network of open-minded and respectful individuals. My family regularly try out new vegan recipes when I visit, and my friends are always happy to visit vegetarian and vegan places with me.

What is the most common question/comment that people ask/say when they find out that you are a vegan and how do you respond?
It's always about how and where I get my protein from. I normally explain that I do take protein supplements, but purely for the convenience, as do many athletes and gym-goers. If they seem curious, I go into more detail of my recommended protein requirements and my current protein intake, to reassure them that I do know what I'm doing.

Who or what motivates you?
The thought of other vegan athletes out there achieving great things is great motivation. Also, the feeling of being part of a worldwide team and community who all fight for a common purpose.

"Because of the high levels of vitamins, minerals and antioxidants present in a plant-based diet, I find my immune system is stronger than that of my non-vegan training partners. My blood sugar levels are more stable throughout the day and I am more focused and alert."

FOOD & SUPPLEMENTS

What do you eat for Breakfast?
Soy yoghurt with fruit, seeds, nuts, cinnamon and agave nectar, or porridge with banana, cinnamon, and nuts, nut butters or seeds, if I'm after something heartier.

What do you eat for Lunch?
If I'm at home and have a well-stocked kitchen, often a big salad loaded with colourful tasty ingredients like avocado, sundried tomatoes, and toasted seeds; or it could be an oven-baked sweet potato with scrambled tofu. Often I'll just graze throughout the day on whatever I feel like.

What do you eat for Dinner?
This is usually my first post-training meal and quite late in the evening, so I'm after something quick, full of nutrition, and easy to digest; usually a spicy collection of vegetables with tofu, tempeh or vegan mince (could be grilled, sautéed, braised, or stir-fried depending on my mood and hunger levels), often drizzled with tahini and hot sauce.

What do you eat for Snacks - healthy & not-so healthy?
Lots of fresh fruit, occasionally dried fruit, almonds, Brazil nuts, soy yoghurt, and dark chocolate.

What is your favourite source of Protein?
Tempeh, tofu, quinoa, vegan sausages.

What is your favourite source of Calcium?
Kale, broccoli, tahini, tofu.

What is your favourite source of Iron?
Spinach, tofu, blackstrap molasses, dried figs.

What foods give you the most energy?
Oats, dark chocolate, fresh and dried fruit.

Do you take any supplements?
Along with protein shakes, I take a daily multivitamin, Iron, and occasionally B12 or vegan D3 when I remember to buy them.

ADVICE

What is your top tip for gaining muscle?
Focus on developing strength in your big muscle groups by building your programme around compound exercises like squats and bench press, eat heartily and often, ensure you are getting protein and carbohydrates into your body within 30mins of training, limit steady-state cardiovascular workouts, and be sensible with your recovery and sleep.

What is your top tip for losing weight?
Mix up your programme with interval training, steady-state cardiovascular endurance work, try to go for a walk or a light jog before breakfast and after dinner, drink plenty of water and green or oolong teas, avoid high sugar foods before bed, get plenty of sleep. Identify your cravings and make sure you're not just eating out of boredom.

What is your top tip for maintaining weight?
Listen to your body. Stay active, enjoy your training, eat a varied diet full of colours and textures and flavours, take time to stretch and unwind and spend time with friends and family, enjoy life.

What is your top tip for improving metabolism?

Build muscle by lifting weights, mix up your training programme, work on increasing your power and explosivity, drink green tea and oolong tea, stand and walk whenever you can.

What is your top tip for toning up?

Focus on building up full-body strength with bodyweight exercises like pull-ups, chin-ups, pushups, planks, and progressively build in more explosive exercises like squat-jumps and burpees. Fill up on lean protein, stay active throughout the day, drink plenty of water, and pay attention to your sleeping pattern.

How do you promote veganism in your daily life?

Mainly I just try to stay healthy and happy. I train hard and stay fit and strong, enjoy a varied diet with its fair share of treats, engage in social activities with other vegans, cook for friends and family and take them out to vegetarian and vegan restaurants. I aim to be respectful, inspiring, and lead by example.

How would you suggest people get involved with what you do?

Find your nearest martial arts gym and just give it a go. Remember we are not born lean, strong, explosive, and technically skilled, and the most advanced people always remember what it was like to be a beginner. Leave your comfort zone at home - it will still be there when you finish training.

"The thought of other vegan athletes out there achieving great things is great motivation. Also, the feeling of being part of a worldwide team and community who all fight for a common purpose."

Eat for the Body you Want
Not the Body you Have

CRISTIANO PEREIRA
VEGAN ULTRA-ENDURANCE CYCLIST

Salt Lake City, Utah, USA
Vegan since: 2005

animalliberationracing.com
SM: *FaceBook, Twitter*

Cristiano Pereira is a vegan ultra-endurance cyclist and founder of Animal Liberation Racing. He spends most of the year training, racing ultra-endurance races, and supporting teammates. He is passionate about animal rights and promoting a vegan lifestyle by leading by example.

WHY VEGAN?

I feel a deep compassion and devotion to animals everywhere. The suffering that is inflicted upon them for the selfish reasons of man, are highly offensive to me. I choose to lead by example and hope that others will follow in my path.

How and why did you decide to become vegan?
I have always felt a connection to animals and that I didn't fit into society's view of animals being used for consumption. After high school, I volunteered at The Humane Society and things starting falling into place. I made the conscious decision to no longer support the exploitation of animals, and I started phasing them out of my diet. I was vegetarian for a period of time and then went fully vegan.

How long have you been vegan?
Since 2005.

What has benefited you the most from being vegan?
I have more energy and I feel like I am running more cleanly. I also recover more quickly from physically demanding training and competitions.

What does veganism mean to you?
Living in a conscientious way that is respectful of animals.

"I feel a deep compassion and devotion to animals everywhere. The suffering that is inflicted upon them for the selfish reasons of man, are highly offensive to me. I choose to lead by example and hope that others will follow in my path."

TRAINING

What sort of training do you do?
I ride my bike at least 6 days a week, year-round. Depending on what time of year it is, I am riding 20-30+ hours a week.

How often do you (need to) train?
6 days a week.

Do you offer your fitness or training services to others?
I am always willing to help others who are interested.

What sports do you play?
Mostly cycling, but I enjoy other endurance sports such as backpacking or hiking.

STRENGTHS, WEAKNESSES & OUTSIDE INFLUENCES.

My strengths are my ultra-endurance, I can ride 24 hours a day, and hill-climbs. Weaknesses are cake and Oreo cookies.

What do you think is the biggest misconception about vegans and how do you address this?
Biggest misconception is that all vegans are malnourished, weak, and protein deficient. I address this by telling those who doubt me, to come ride with me.

What are your strengths as a vegan athlete?
I recover fast, have more energy, and have a higher level of endurance.

What is your biggest challenge?
None.

Are the non-vegans in your industry supportive or not?
I honestly have not paid attention. I don't race for them and am not concerned with their viewpoints.

Are your family and friends supportive of your vegan lifestyle?
Yes.

What is the most common question/comment that people ask/say when they find out that you are a vegan and how do you respond?
"Where do you get your protein?" My response is, "What's protein?" Usually they can't adequately define protein and the conversation ends abruptly.

Who or what motivates you?
Animals. My motivation is to go out and perform my best, which ultimately causes pain during ultra-endurance races. I am able to push through the pain by focusing on the pain the animals suffer on a daily basis. I also get a great deal of satisfaction by doling out copious amounts of pain to my competitors.

FOOD & SUPPLEMENTS

What do you eat for Breakfast?
Fruit smoothie with chia seeds.

What do you eat for Lunch?
It varies. I eat a lot of rice and vegetables.

What do you eat for Dinner?
Same as lunch. I do eat a lot of bananas as well.

What do you eat for Snacks - healthy & not-so healthy?
I eat a lot of nuts. I also eat a lot of Oreos and cake.

What is your favourite source of Protein?
Beans or hummus.

What is your favourite source of Calcium?
Vegetables like broccoli and kale.

What is your favourite source of Iron?
Spinach and pepitas.

What foods give you the most energy?
Rice.

Do you take any supplements?
I use Plant Fusion products.

ADVICE

What is your top tip for gaining muscle?
Lifting weights.

What is your top tip for losing weight?
Long rides.

What is your top tip for maintaining weight?
Eat a balanced diet - not too much cake or Oreos.

What is your top tip for improving metabolism?
Eating a nutritionally dense, balanced diet.

What is your top tip for toning up?
Ride your freaking bike.

How do you promote veganism in your daily life?
I am always out doing stuff with the team, Animal Liberation Racing. By riding my bike 6 to 7 days a week, I lead by example while remaining in the public eye.

How would you suggest people get involved with what you do?
Check our website and our FaceBook page.

"My motivation is to go out and perform my best, which ultimately causes pain during ultra-endurance races. I am able to push through the pain by focusing on the pain the animals suffer on a daily basis. I also get a great deal of satisfaction by doling out copious amounts of pain to my competitors."

CYRUS KHAMBATTA
VEGAN EXERCISE ENTHUSIAST

San Francisco, California, USA
Vegan since: 2003

mangomannutrition.com
SM: *FaceBook, Twitter, Yelp*

Dr. Cyrus Khambatta received his PhD from the University of California at Berkeley in 2012, and started Mangoman Nutrition and Fitness in 2013 to teach people with diabetes the fundamentals of lifestyle management through informed nutrition and exercise. By providing nutrition and exercise coaching, he aspires to positively influence the lives of people with both type 1 and type 2 diabetes.

WHY VEGAN?

How and why did you decide to become vegan?
When I was 22, I was diagnosed with type 1 diabetes in my senior year of college. It flipped my world upside down. I had grown up as a very active kid, playing soccer, baseball, basketball, running and generally being a rambunctious child. At the time of diagnosis, I had no idea what diabetes was or what it meant for my life. At that time in my life, I was ignorant about everything related to diabetes, and therefore listened to everything the doctor and nutritionist told me because I was afraid that something bad could happen if I did not listen to them.

I was afraid that I would go blind. I was afraid that I would lose my vision. I was afraid that my kidneys would fail. I was afraid that I would develop heart disease. Worst of all, I was afraid that I would lose my ability to be active. Beyond everything else, compromising my ability to play sports scared me the most. I followed the advice of my doctor and nutritionist, and adopted a low carbohydrate diet, the one-size-fits-all prescription for people with diabetes. At that time I was unaware about any of the health effects of low carbohydrate diets, I simply followed the advice of my doctor and nutritionist out of fear.

I followed the low carbohydrate diet to a tee, and modified my cooking and eating habits significantly. I increased my consumption of eggs, turkey, chicken, salmon, peanut butter, milk and cheese. I did this because in the diabetes world, carbohydrates are the enemy and should be minimized or avoided at all costs. As a result, I ate foods high in protein and fat. In a short period of time, I lost all my energy. I was constantly lethargic, and severely dehydrated. Even though my blood sugar was supposed to be easy to control in the absence of carbohydrates, I experienced chronically high blood sugars all day long, and bringing my blood sugar into the normal range required large injections of insulin. I knew that something was terribly wrong, I just wasn't educated enough to make a change for the better.

Following about 1 year on a low carbohydrate diet, I hit "rock bottom." On that day, I lay on the couch, depressed, anxious, dehydrated, confused, and alone. I knew I needed to make a change, but I didn't know what to do. I listen to the voice in the back of my head that said, "You should learn how to eat." At that point, I started reading everything under the sun about nutrition. I attended scientific lectures, and I started talking to everyone I encountered, in search of more information. Before I knew it, I was introduced to the idea of being either a vegetarian or a vegan, and all the stories that I had heard from people made me believe that if I transition to a plant-based diet, I would experience significantly improved blood sugar control.

I was still nervous about becoming a vegan because I had not met any vegans who were athletes. Yes, I wanted better blood sugar control and improved insulin sensitivity, but I did not want to sacrifice my ability to be active - very active. Therefore, I hesitated in adopting a vegan lifestyle until I could be convinced that it was the right approach for maintaining an active lifestyle.

After a short period of time I met Dr. Douglas Graham, the creator of the 80/10/10 diet. He took me under his wing and taught me the principles of eating a high-carbohydrate, low fat and low protein vegan diet. He assured me that not only would I be able to remain active, but that transitioning to a vegan diet would actually increase my level of activity. I had nothing to lose at this point, so I followed his guidance and made the transition.

I told myself that I could commit to the 80/10/10 vegan approach for 1 month before evaluating it's effects. After two weeks on the 80/10/10 diet, my insulin usage had fallen by 30%, my blood sugar values had normalized, I was no longer dehydrated, my muscles felt limber, and I had significantly more energy. At the time, I remember feeling as though the 80/10/10 lifestyle charged me with energy in the same way that a computer battery gets charged when plugged into a wall power outlet. The increase in my energy level was noticeable, pronounced and incredibly empowering.

The results were so quick and dramatic that I was absolutely convinced that there was something fundamentally important happening within my body. At that point, I got so excited about nutrition that I decided to study towards a PhD in Nutritional Biochemistry, so that I could understand the scientific and molecular level details of nutrition to feed my "scientist" brain.

How long have you been vegan?
I was first diagnosed with diabetes at the age of 22, in 2002. I transitioned to being a vegan in 2003. It is now 2015, and this marks my 12th year as a 100% 80/10/10 raw food vegan.

What has benefited you the most from being vegan?
When I first transitioned to a vegan diet, I wanted improved blood sugar control. Controlling diabetes was my main objective. There is no doubt that adopting a low-fat, high-carbohydrate raw food diet has significantly improved my insulin sensitivity, reduced my insulin-dependency, and reduced my blood sugars significantly. I now maintain blood sugars that are technically classified as "non-diabetic."

Despite these obvious improvements in blood sugar control, being a vegan has fundamentally changed my body from the inside out. Having grown up as an avid soccer player, I am very familiar with muscle soreness, muscle tightness, and frequent injury. All throughout my childhood and high school career, I felt as though I was constantly battling injury, jumping from one sore muscle to the next. As a result, I would stretch daily, sometimes for an hour at a time.

Now, having been a vegan for a sufficient period of time, I can safely say that I experience a level of athleticism that is well beyond what I ever dreamed possible. My muscles are extremely limber. I am constantly well hydrated. I can perform exercise at an extremely high intensity whenever I want. I can push harder for longer periods of time, and my muscles recover from intense exercise extremely rapidly.

If I do get injured, maintaining a strict vegan diet has significantly shortened my injury recovery. I no longer have anxiety about how long it will take to fully recover, because I know that by maintaining a strict vegan diet, I can accelerate the recovery process and return to sport in a much shorter time than previously possible.

What does veganism mean to you?
To me, veganism means making a series of conscious decisions about what you put in your body. As a vegan, I think twice about every food that enters my body, and am now a 100% conscious eater. If I don't have the option of eating a plant, I will fast until I find the next opportunity.

True, veganism is a way of life. But more importantly, veganism is a philosophy of nutrition and environmental awareness.

TRAINING

What sort of training do you do?
On a weekly basis, I strength train four times per week. I play soccer twice per week for a total of about 150 minutes. I run once per week for about 3 to 5 miles (4.82-8km). When I strength train, I perform a series of multi-joint compound movements, such as squats, dead lifts, pull-ups, push-ups etc. I focus on getting full body workouts as often as possible, and deemphasize isolation movements that were popular back in the 1980s and 1990s.

How often do you (need to) train?
Exercise is my favorite part of being human. To me, movement is everything. If I had 24 hours left on this planet problem, I would spend 10-12 of them exercising. I choose to train for about one hour per day, seven days per week. By paying attention to my body, I can tell when it is time to rest, and therefore I take rest only as needed. My overall goal is to exercise seven days per week.

Do you offer fitness or trading services to others?
Yes, I am a personal trainer and small group fitness instructor. I train people individually, and I lead small group Boot Camp classes. I absolutely love inspiring other people to enjoy this as much as I do, and I trying keep all my sessions fun, high intensity, and difficult - extremely difficult. One of my favorite things to do is to push people beyond their mental limits, and watch when they get excited about how far they can push themselves.

What sports do you play?
I play soccer, weight train, run, and swim. In truth, I love playing all sports, but these are the sports that I train on a weekly basis.

"My understanding is that when people think of being a vegan, they think about all the foods they can't eat, and rarely focus on the foods that they can eat. Given that we have grown up in a meat- and dairy-heavy society, the concept of veganism seems like a radical approach to nutrition, when in reality it's simply about eating a large amount of whole fruits and vegetables."

STRENGTHS, WEAKNESSES AND OUTSIDE INFLUENCES

What do you think is the biggest misconception about vegans and how do you address this?

In my experience, many people view veganism as a "restrictive" lifestyle. Often, people make statements like, "I could never be a vegan because I can't give up cheese." My understanding is that when people think of being a vegan, they think about all the foods they can't eat, and rarely focus on the foods that they can eat. Given that we have grown up in a meat- and dairy-heavy society, the concept of veganism seems like a radical approach to nutrition, when in reality it's simply about eating a large amount of whole fruits and vegetables.

To me, veganism is also a mindset. If you open your mind to the idea that being a vegan can be delicious and fun, then that will be your experience. On the other hand, if you view veganism as a restrictive and socially isolating diet, you are likely to experience just that. In other words, your experience is often influenced by your preconceived notions.

What are your strengths as a vegan athlete?

The most noticeable strength as a vegan athlete is my ability to push at high intensity. Up until I was in my early 20s, I felt as though I was always operating at about 70% of my maximum. The top 30% was incredibly difficult to access, and I'm not convinced that I ever actually accessed the top echelon of my athleticism. I knew that my athleticism was being slowed down by something and that I was capable of more than I was consistently performing. The problem was that I simply didn't know how to access that top 30%.

Another noticeable strength of being a vegan athlete is significantly improved recovery time. Currently, when I exercise, I try to exercise at the highest intensity level possible. Following demanding workouts, I find that my muscles certainly get sore, but the soreness feels less debilitating than the soreness I experienced on an omnivorous diet. Even brutal workouts leave me with moderate tightness, and after a full day's rest, I am often fully recovered and ready to exercise within 24 hours. As an omnivore, sometimes it took me up to 72 hours to recover from high-intensity exercise, leaving me sidelined for longer than I wanted. Fortunately, this is no longer the case, and I count my blessings every single day.

What is your biggest challenge?

When I first became a vegan, I had a difficult time communicating to friends and family about why I choose to be this way. I would often get interrogated about my food choices, and conversations with friends often devolved into having to defend my position as a vegan. Overall, I found these types of conversations to be very uncomfortable and frustrating.

Over time, I have noticed that my friends and family understand that being a vegan is not a phase, but a long-term approach. It is a decision that I have made - and choose to stick to - because of the benefits that it provides for my diabetes and athletic health. Now, when I communicate my experience of being a 100% 80/10/10 raw food vegan for the past 12 years, people usually respond with "Wow, 12 years is a very long time."

Interrogation sessions do not happen nearly as frequently as before, and when they do, I simply tell people that I eat like a monkey. That usually makes the situation lighthearted and more enjoyable for everyone. When in doubt, I make fun of myself and others follow.

Are the non-vegans in your industry supportive or not?

Yes, even the non-vegans in my industry are very supportive of a vegan diet, because they understand the profound benefit that it has given to me, and they understand the benefits it has had on my clients as well. I believe the support has come with time, as people have seen that I have an unwavering commitment to being a vegan, as opposed to trying out a fad diet for six months and then transitioning to whatever else was popular at the time.

Are your friends and family supportive of your vegan lifestyle?

Yes, absolutely. All of my friends and family are now in full support of the vegan lifestyle. People often ask me questions about what they should be eating, and when I give them gentle recommendations, they incorporate them and usually report back to me about how great they feel.

What is the most common question/comment that people ask/say when they find out you are a vegan and how do you respond?

The most common question I get from people when I find out that I am vegan is "Where do you get your protein?" I know that is a common question that many vegans get, and I don't feel alone in answering this question. I respond by telling them that I get my protein from marijuana. I tell them that I eat about 1 pound of hemp protein per week, and that it keeps me feeling like a million bucks. I tell them that there are many protein choices on the market, and hemp protein is anti-inflammatory, easily digestible and tastes great.

Who or what motivates you?

I am motivated by the stories of people who I interact with who have transitioned to a plant-based diet and felt significantly more energy. Every time I hear about somebody who has made the transition to eating a more plant-focused diet, I add a tally mark in my head. I think it is only a matter of time before vegetarian and vegan diets are as common as meat-eating diets. Perhaps that will happen in my lifetime, perhaps it will take another 50 years. Regardless, slow progress makes me extremely happy.

FOOD & SUPPLEMENTS

What do you eat for Breakfast?

For breakfast, I usually eat the equivalent of 4-5 fruits, 4 tablespoons of hemp protein powder, 2 tablespoons of chia seeds hydrated in water, and cinnamon, cardamom or cocoa powder. I construct a fruit bowl in which the fruit is sitting at the bottom, hemp protein powder and chia seeds are poured on top, and the spices are then sprinkled on top of that.

If I have extra time, I will construct an açai bowl. I will blend in one packet of açai with a banana, and then I will construct a massive bowl including mangoes, papayas, dates, raisins and figs. I will then pour the açai mixture on top, sprinkle on some cinnamon and go to town.

What do you eat for Lunch?

For lunch, I generally eat about 1500 calories in 10 minutes. Lunch is my favorite meal of the day, because I am ravenously hungry following an intense exercise session. Generally, I eat 5 or 6 bananas, a handful of medjool dates, 1 or 2 mangoes, and 4 tbsp. hemp protein powder. I like to see how fast I can eat this giant bowl, because I eat like a caveman and love shoveling food into my mouth.

In the middle of mango season, I go crazy. It is not uncommon for me to eat 5 mangoes at lunchtime, on top of a heaping pile of bananas. In the height of mango season, I try to eat at least 10 mangoes per day, because I am addicted to them.

In 2007 I applied to the Guiness Book of World Records to set the record for the most mangoes eaten in 24 hours. I had practiced diligently in the preceding months, averaging 23 mangoes per day or a total of 1,750 mangoes in a 2.5-month period. My plan was to eat 50 mangoes in 24 hours, and exercise as much as possible during that time to burn off the excess energy. The Guiness Book of World Records promptly denied my request, claiming that they "do not sponsor food-eating records because it promotes unnecessary one-upsmanship." So for now I claim to hold the "unofficial mango eating world record" although I have absolutely no documentation to back up this invented claim.

What you eat for Dinner?
Dinner is also very fun meal for me. The reason is because dinner is my opportunity to be extremely creative. I enjoy making green papaya salads, kale salads, iceberg lettuce tacos. I have gained a reputation for making giant salads with a ton of hot spices, and people often ask me to make a "Cyrus salad" and bring it to their house for dinner. I think my friends are using me!

What do you eat for Snacks - healthy & not-so healthy?
For snacks, I usually eat 1 or 2 pieces of fruit, or a giant handful of medjool dates. I am addicted to dates, and will eat pounds of them unless you take them away for me.

What is your favorite source of Protein?
Manitoba Harvest Hemp protein powder.

What is your favorite source of Calcuim?
I like to pretend that mangoes have a ton of calcium.

What is your favorite source of Iron?
I also like to pretend that mangoes have a ton of iron.

What foods give you the most energy?
Bananas, dates and mangoes. Sometimes I eat up to 12 or 14 bananas a day, especially when I am very active. I have a serious addiction to medjool dates, and I can easily eat 1 pound (450g) at a sitting without even thinking about it. Mangoes are my weakness. Clearly, I have a sweet tooth.

Do you take any supplements?
Yes, I eat mangoes.

"Train like your life depended on it. Be diligent, be consistent, surround yourself with people who are superior athletes, push yourself beyond what you think is possible. Your body is a machine: treat it like one and you will be pleasantly surprised."

ADVICE
What is your top tip for gaining muscle?
In the bodybuilding world, protein is king. Bodybuilders constantly nitpick how much protein they are consuming with every meal. I have found that focusing on carbohydrates from whole foods (especially fruits) significantly increases glycogen storage.

I like to think of glycogen as rocket fuel for humans. The more glycogen you store in your muscles, the more responsive your muscle tissue will behave. Therefore, in order to build muscle tissue, I instruct my clients to consume a large quantity of readily available and easily digestible carbohydrates from fruits and starchy vegetables, and then to increase their protein intake from either beans or lentils or hemp protein powder. The combination of a significant quantity of carbohydrates and a high-quality protein from whole foods is a winning combination for increasing strength, power, quickness, recovery, and endurance. No questions asked.

What is your top tip for losing weight?
In graduate school, I studied the effects of calorie restriction and intermittent fasting. There is no question in my mind that intermittent fasting is the single most effective long-term strategy for weight control, and an incredibly fun mental and physical exercise. Performing a once-per-week 24-hour fast is a very easy way to control bodyweight, and promote weight loss at a reasonable weight rate of about 1 pound (450g) per week.

What is your top tip for improving metabolism?
In my experience, the term "metabolism" is thrown around loosely, even though most people do not know what the word actually means. The term "metabolism" technically means "the sum total of all biological reactions," therefore developing a strategy to improve all chemical reactions is theoretically not possible. That being said, when it comes to improving metabolism I have two general recommendations:
1) Significantly reduce the amount of dietary fat from all sources in your diet. Focus on eating a large proportion of carbohydrates, between 70% and 80% of total calories.
2) Eat multiple servings of high antioxidant content foods on a daily basis. These foods include raw onions, mangoes, squash, berries, açai berries, cinnamon, turmeric, and anything with a purple color.

We've all heard the term "eat the rainbow." I could not agree more, the rainbow is nutritious and quite delicious.

What is your top tip for toning up?
Train like your life depended on it. Be diligent, be consistent, surround yourself with people who are superior athletes, push yourself beyond what you think is possible. Your body is a machine: treat it like one and you will be pleasantly surprised.

How do you promote veganism in your daily life?
I promote veganism in my daily life by eating ridiculous quantities of fruits and vegetables. I love eating large piles of mangoes, papayas, dates, raisins, and bananas in public places. I enjoy acting like a monkey, because I often feel like one.

How would you suggest people get involved with what you do?
I would suggest that people open their mind to experiencing exceptional health by making small changes to the way that they eat. The first step in making a transition to a vegan lifestyle is believing that dietary change is possible, the second step is pure execution. Without believing that eating a plant-based diet can lead to exceptional health, reduced disease risk and abundant energy, nothing will happen. When you believe, anything and everything is possible.

"I believe the support (from my industry) has come with time, as people have seen that I have an unwavering commitment to being a vegan, as opposed to trying out a fad diet for six months and then transitioning to whatever else was popular at the time."

DAVID RAPHAEL HILDEBRAND
VEGAN MASTERS SWIMMER

New York City, New York, USA
Vegan since: 2003

drhildebrand.com
SM: *FaceBook, Twitter*

David Raphael Hildebrand is a vegan of over ten years and a nationally ranked Masters Swimmer in New York. He races middle-distance freestyle and individual medleys and he coaches the Fashion Institute of Technology swim team as well as fellow Masters Swimmers at Team New York Aquatics. Away from the pool, he is an author and a model. His first novel, "Walking Marina," is an exposé of the male modeling industry, and his current project is about swimming. He also contributes regularly to the vegan blog, The Discerning Brute.

WHY VEGAN?

How and why did you decide to become vegan?
I grew up vegetarian, though my family ate fish sporadically. Sometime during college, I began to sense that eating dairy, eggs, and anything else from animals was antithetical to my morals. From then on I gravitated more and more toward veganism, until the transition was complete.

How long have you been vegan?
Over ten years.

What has benefited you the most from being vegan?
Veganism heightens my inner consciousness as well as my global consciousness. It awakens me. It requires me to think, to stay engaged, to take responsibility. It encourages me, multiple times a day, to make active choices rather than passive ones.

What does veganism mean to you?
Respect.

"Veganism heightens my inner consciousness as well as my global consciousness. It awakens me. It requires me to think, to stay engaged, to take responsibility. It encourages me, multiple times a day, to make active choices rather than passive ones."

TRAINING

What sort of training do you do?
Mostly middle-distance, combining aerobic and anaerobic conditioning.

How often do you (need to) train?
In general, I swim about four or five days a week, usually about 4500 yards (4.11km) over 90 minutes. Anything more than that and I lose interest - anything less and I get antsy. I lift and run as well, depending on my schedule and the season.

Do you offer your fitness or training services to others?
I coach and give private instruction, though I don't actively seek clients.

What sports do you play?
Swimming.

STRENGTHS, WEAKNESSES & OUTSIDE INFLUENCES

What do you think is the biggest misconception about vegans and how do you address this?
Many omnivores view vegans as more committed to the wellbeing of non-humans than humans, and they find this attention misplaced. The majority of vegans, however, are not at all dismissive of human suffering, just as the majority of omnivores are not dismissive of non-human suffering. Everyone is different. So when I discuss veganism with non-vegans I try to focus on the things that they, as individuals, are most interested in. If that involves them - their diet, their health - rather than animals, pollution, water conservation and so on, then that's what I stick to: them.

What are your strengths as a vegan athlete?
Mentally, I'd say discipline, consistency and resolve. Physically, I probably recover quicker.

What is your biggest challenge?
Finding, as theologian Reinhold Niebuhr said, "the serenity to accept the things I cannot change, the courage to change the things I can, and the wisdom to know the difference."

Are the non-vegans in your industry supportive or not?
Some are and some aren't. I only discuss it with other athletes when they ask me what I eat. Either way, I didn't establish my diet to win others' support. I maintain a lifestyle that I believe is sound.

Are your family and friends supportive of your vegan lifestyle?
If they weren't I doubt I would think of them as family and friends.

What is the most common question/comment that people ask/say when they find out that you are a vegan and how do you respond?
"So, like, you can't eat bacon?" It's amazing how often I hear this word "can't" as if the choice I've made has somehow become an intrinsic part of me, as though it were physically impossible for me to consume flesh. I can. I simply don't. Veganism is a choice; no different than carnism is a choice. They appear different only because carnism is so culturally engrained that we take it as "natural." We do not stop, think, and realize that omnivores, just like vegans, make choices. All of us can eat just about anything. Some of us choose not to.

Who or what motivates you?
Honesty. I'm an addict for the truth.

"Everyone is different. So when I discuss veganism with non-vegans I try to focus on the things that they, as individuals, are most interested in. If that involves them – their diet, their health – rather than animals, pollution, water conservation and so on, then that's what I stick to: them".

FOOD & SUPPLEMENTS

What do you eat for Breakfast?
Generally cereal with almond milk and fruit. Sometimes oatmeal. Sometimes a toasted bagel with hummus. I've gotten back into juicing a few times a week, which I love. It clears my head.

What do you eat for Lunch?
For lunch I usually have leftovers from dinner. If not I'll have a sandwich of roasted veggie or seitan, avocado, tomato or a mushroom burger with arugula and caramelized onion. It varies.

What do you eat for Dinner?
The gamut: whole wheat pasta with miso pesto sauce, just about any sort of stir-fry, curry dishes, burritos, pizza, salad, roasted Brussels sprouts with onion and garlic no less than once a week, anything with kale, quinoa, chickpeas, tempeh, you name it. It's always changing.

What do you eat for Snacks - healthy & not-so healthy?
My number one snack is an apple with peanut butter. I sometimes make vegan shakes or cookies. If I'm at a good vegan restaurant, I might get chocolate cake. I really love dates, dried fruit, caramelized bananas, coconut rice pudding. Usually, though, it's an apple with peanut butter.

What is your favourite source of Protein?
I guess peanut butter. Beans, nuts, leafy green vegetables. I don't usually think about protein since it's in practically every imaginable whole food I eat, in more than sufficient servings.

What is your favourite source of Calcium?
Dark greens, nuts, flaxseeds, and sesame seeds.

What is your favourite source of Iron?
More dark greens, rice and bean dishes, pumpkin seeds, whole grain bread.

What foods give you the most energy?
Probably dates, raisins, and other dried fruits for quick energy. Fresh oranges and bananas too. Granola is another good one.

Do you take any supplements?
No. I don't understand supplements. A diet in need of supplements is a diet in need of change.

ADVICE

What is your top tip for gaining muscle?
Increasing lifting and increasing protein.

What is your top tip for losing weight?
Increasing cardio and decreasing calories, including those from alcohol and processed sugar.

What is your top tip for maintaining weight?
Determining your own personal intake to output balance.

What is your top tip for improving metabolism?
Increasing high-intensity aerobic training and decreasing processed sugars and similar junk.

What is your top tip for toning up?
A combination of cardio, consistent weights, and smart eating.

How do you promote veganism in your daily life?
By inviting others to ask questions, then encouraging them to explain and defend their choices just as soundly as they ask me to explain and defend mine. It is more effective to let someone figure out for himself that his diet is detrimental than it is to shout it at him.

How would you suggest people get involved with what you do?
Buy a bathing suit. Swimming is a full-body workout. It relaxes as well as stimulates the mind. It cleanses the soul. It opens the lungs. It stretches every muscle. Find a pool, a river, a lake. Go solo or in a group, and let the water move you.

"It's amazing how often I hear this word "can't" as if the choice I've made has somehow become an intrinsic part of me, as though it were physically impossible for me to consume flesh. I can. I simply don't. Veganism is a choice; no different than carnism is a choice. They appear different only because carnism is so culturally engrained that we take it as "natural." We do not stop, think, and realize that omnivores, just like vegans, make choices. All of us can eat just about anything. Some of us choose not to."

"In talking with people, don't begin by discussing the thing on which you differ. Begin by emphasizing—and keep on emphasizing—the things on which you agree. Keep emphasizing, if possible, that you are both striving for the same end and that your only difference is one of method and not of purpose."
- Dale Carnegie

What you do and how you do it reflects the WHOLE movement.
So, ACT like it!

DEEARNAH DE MARCO
VEGAN YOGA TEACHER

Brisbane, Queensland, Australia
Vegan since: 2012

SM: FaceBook, Instagram

Deearnah De Marco is a yoga teacher, Personal Trainer, and group fitness instructor who teaches a variety of group fitness classes from hard-core training to relaxation classes. Dee is a 48-year old mother of two, who is extremely passionate about helping people achieve their health and fitness goals to improve their quality of life - for life. She strongly believes it all starts with what we eat. Dee shares information, and encourages people to research for themselves how eating meat and dairy products is not only affecting their health in a negative way, but also the animals and our environment. Dee is a firm believer in the Albert Einstein quote "nothing will benefit health and increase the chances for survival of life on earth as the evolution to a vegetarian diet."

WHY VEGAN?

How and why did you decide to become vegan?
I have actually never tasted red meat. I was a vegetarian from birth. I ate some fish as a child, not much and then first tasted chicken and other seafoods (the only other meats I have tried) in my late twenties. I have been a vegetarian mainly for most of my life and now vegan. I am very passionate about health and fitness and decided to become a vegan for my own overall wellbeing. Initially my motivation was for my own health, but now even if I really loved meat and dairy products but had to stop eating them to stop the cruelty to animals I would immediately.

How long have you been vegan?
Over 2 years.

What has benefited you the most from being vegan?
My mind is clearer. I have more focus and motivation. I am a more positive person. My daily energy levels are high and overall health and vitality is much better. I virtually never get sick and if so it would be for one day, maximum. I have heaps of energy to get through my busy days. I look and feel healthier.

What does veganism mean to you?
It means I am doing the best I can to not support the meat and dairy industries and the cruel treatment of animals. It also means I am doing my best to not support the pharmaceutical industry. I do not have a doctor and have not had a doctor since leaving home at a very young age. I provide my body with the best nutrition I can and find it heals itself when needed. It also means I am giving myself the best possible chance at a great quality of life.

TRAINING

What sort of training do you do?
I do yoga almost every day. I train weights, kettlebell training, jog, body-weight training and dancing.

How often do you (need to) train?
I normally train 5 times a week for 1-2 hours a day, as I enjoy the feeling of training regularly. I can feel healthy, strong, vital, and remain lean with training as little as 2-3 times a week for an hour because of what I eat. When I was not vegan I trained 7 days a week for longer periods to feel this good.

Do you offer your fitness or training services to others?
Yes. I am a personal trainer, yoga teacher and group fitness instructor teaching a variety of classes from boxercise classes, kettlebell training, circuit classes, spin, aqua classes, ChiBall, pilates, yoga and a low impact women's-only workout I have developed over the years. I offer one-on-one or small group PT sessions, private or small group yoga sessions, and dietary advice.

What sports do you play?
At the moment, I don't play any sports. One of my greatest passions is sailing and I sail 1-2 times a week. I love being out on the water.

STRENGTHS, WEAKNESSES & OUTSIDE INFLUENCES

What do you think is the biggest misconception about vegans and how do you address this?
Where we get our nutrition from - and I address this by sharing the knowledge I have gained and directing people to where to find and research this information themselves.

What are your strengths as a vegan athlete?
My energy levels, stamina, recovery time, and my body's ability to heal itself quickly.

What is your biggest challenge?
Finding food to eat out that is as good as the food I make myself.

Are the non-vegans in your industry supportive or not?
Generally, they are, especially if they know me well before they find out I am vegan, as they know how fit and healthy I am and are surprised I have the energy levels I do on a vegan diet. I find generally people are just uneducated on the subject and if you are a living positive example, they are interested to know more.

Are your family and friends supportive of your vegan lifestyle?
Yes, very supportive. I find my close friends and family are not only supportive but inspired to change things in their diet as well to feel better. Both my daughters, now 22 and 19, have been brought up mainly on a vegetarian diet and have chosen to try everything over time, and have now - naturally of their own accord - come back to vegetarian or vegan diets as they feel so much better.

What is the most common question/comment that people ask/say when they find out that you are a vegan and how do you respond?
They ask me where I get my protein and calcium from, and I respond by informing them of how much protein and calcium is in the different organic foods I eat - compared to processed meat and dairy products - without the harmful things that are in these foods. I also like to discuss that the reason why most people think they know

where to get protein and calcium from, is because that's what mainstream media has always told us. The meat and dairy industries have a lot of products and want to sell them, but now as its costing governments more money as people are so overweight and so sick, the truth is starting to slowly come out in mainstream media as well. If these products had what we needed to be healthy, we would not have the current level of diseases we have today.

Who or what motivates you?
For most of my life the burning desire I have had from a very young age is to have the best quality of life. The longest life I can motivates me to eat well and move a lot. In addition to that, now not wanting to support the dairy and meat industries also motivates me to be vegan.

"Veganism means I am doing the best I can to not support the meat and dairy industries and the cruel treatment of animals. It also means I am doing my best to not support the pharmaceutical industry. I do not have a doctor and have not had a doctor since leaving home at a very young age. I provide my body with the best nutrition I can and find it heals itself when needed. It also means I am giving myself the best possible chance at a great quality of life."

FOOD & SUPPLEMENTS

What do you eat for Breakfast?
Generally a smoothie. My favourite smoothie is: 1-2 bananas, half an avocado, 2 tablespoons of my organic pea protein powder, 2 tablespoons of organic cacao powder, handful of frozen berries (whatever I have) blackberries and blueberries are my favourite. I mix just enough coconut water for the blender to mix the ingredients. So thick you eat with a spoon. Yummy.

What do you eat for Lunch?
I eat a lot of raw food, a lot of dark leafy greens. Sprouts are also a favourite. I make big salads, mixed with a choice of chickpeas, lentils, rice, nuts and seeds, seaweeds, tofu and tempeh.

What do you eat for Dinner?
Generally I would eat the same for dinner as lunch. Otherwise, I also love organic rice and curries. Chickpea and potato, or tofu and tempeh curries with a lot of greens and chilies.

What do you eat for Snacks - healthy & not-so healthy?
Generally I snack on seeds and nuts, seaweed, raw carrots, capsicums, apples or organic vegan cacao bars. My not so healthy snacks would be organic corn chips, sweet potato chips, wasabi peas and organic vegan chocolate.

What is your favourite source of Protein?
Lentils, tofu, tempeh, chickpeas and nuts.

What is your favourite source of Calcium?
All the dark leafy greens I eat - particularly love rocket, mint, coriander, spinach, and

kale - plus tempeh and tahini.

What is your favourite source of Iron?
Legumes, (tofu, tempeh, lentils), brown rice, nuts and seeds.

What foods give you the most energy?
Cacao powder – in my morning smoothies - legumes, dark, leafy greens, seeds, nuts and chilies.

Do you take any supplements?
Occasionally I will take some supplements, but feel great without them.

ADVICE

What is your top tip for gaining muscle?
Go vegan. Train hard, eat well, and get enough sleep.

What is your top tip for losing weight?
Go vegan. That's my tip for everything. Better for you, better for the animals, better for the planet, everyone's a WINNER.

What is your top tip for maintaining weight?
Go vegan, train regularly, and eat according to how much you move.

What is your top tip for improving metabolism?
Go vegan, eat spicy foods, especially chilies, train regularly, and do not overeat.

What is your top tip for toning up?
Go vegan. Train hard, eat well and eat according to how much you move around. Energy in equals energy out.

How do you promote veganism in your daily life?
Via social media channels and through conversations with people.

How would you suggest people get involved with what you do?
See my Facebook page. There and the Internet are great ways to find out about the benefits of veganism. Two great YouTube videos to watch if interested in veganism: Dr Michael Greger's "Uprooting the Leading Causes of Death" and Gary Yourofsky's "Best Speech you will ever Hear."

"The reason why most people think they know where to get protein and calcium from, is because that's what mainstream media has always told us. The meat and dairy industries have a lot of products and want to sell them, but now as its costing governments more money as people are so overweight and so sick, the truth is starting to slowly come out in mainstream media as well. If these products had what we needed to be healthy, we would not have the current level of diseases we have today."

DEREK TRESIZE
VEGAN COMPETITIVE BODY BUILDER

Richmond, Virginia, USA
Vegan since: 2007

veganmuscleandfitness.com
SM: *FaceBook, Twitter*

Derek Tresize is a competitive vegan bodybuilder residing in Richmond, Virginia, USA. He holds a Bachelor of Science in Biology, is a personal trainer through the American Council on Exercise, has a certificate in Plant-Based Nutrition through Cornell University, and is co-author of Vegan Muscle & Fitness. Derek has followed a plant-based diet since 2007 and promotes it to his clients and in the fitness and bodybuilding community as the best means to long-term health. Find Derek on Facebook, or follow @veganmuscle on Twitter.

WHY VEGAN?

How and why did you decide to become vegan?
In 2007, I was presented for the first time with the substantial evidence about the detrimental effects animal products have on our long term health, especially with regards to heart disease and cancer, when my wife Marcella gave me "The China Study" book as a gift. Cancer and heart disease both run in my family (as they do with all Americans), and that combined with my passion for healthy living compelled me to eliminate animal products from my diet.

How long have you been vegan?
Since 2007.

What has benefited you the most from being vegan?
Everything. I feel better, I perform better, I recover faster, I get leaner faster - you name it. And it has given me a tremendous appreciation for how we impact the world around us through our dietary choices there's really nothing you do that affects the world as much as what you choose to eat.

What does veganism mean to you?
Veganism means living a healthy and compassionate life. Choosing foods, occupations, and activities that nourish your body, helping others and doing as little harm to the world around you as possible is all part veganism to me.

TRAINING

What sort of training do you do?
I am a bodybuilder, so I do a lot of weightlifting, as well as various forms of cardiovascular exercise such as running and swimming.

How often do you (need to) train?
I lift weights 5 days per week and do some sort of cardio activity at least 2 days per week.

Do you offer your fitness or training services to others?

Yes! My wife and I created the website veganmuscleandfitness.com where we have an online subscription portal featuring videos of cooking, mini lectures and exercise demonstrations, and we offer group and individual personal training both online through our website and at our Richmond, VA training studio Root Force Personal Training. You can get in touch with us though our website, Facebook or Twitter if you'd like to learn more.

What sports do you play?

I don't play any sports recreationally, but I love the time I spend training in the gym - and I have fun competing in bodybuilding contests once or twice a year.

"I feel better, I perform better, I recover faster, I get leaner faster – you name it. And it has given me a tremendous appreciation for how we impact the world around us through our dietary choices there's really nothing you do that affects the world as much as what you choose to eat."

STRENGTHS, WEAKNESSES & OUTSIDE INFLUENCES

What do you think is the biggest misconception about vegans and how do you address this?

There is still a misconception out there that vegans are skinny, weak, and undernourished. This is changing rapidly as more and more mainstream celebrities and athletes go vegan, but it's still an idea that needs to be challenged regularly. I address this by being the most muscular, strongest and healthiest person I can possibly be, and by making myself visible through contests and online media so the world can see that vegans have no problem being fit, strong and healthy. I think in time it will even become apparent that vegans have the advantage over a more traditional omnivorous diet, rather than the other way around.

What are your strengths as a vegan athlete?

My performance and recovery are better than they ever were on an omnivorous diet, so I am able to train hard and bounce back better than a non-vegan athlete could. I also have a much easier time shedding body fat that most non-vegans, which is essential as a bodybuilder.

What is your biggest challenge?

If I had to pick one, I'd say gaining muscle mass is potentially more challenging as a vegan athlete. This is for the simple reason that since these foods are so clean and metabolically stimulating you have to eat much more volume than you would as a meat eater, and all that eating can get tough.

Are the non-vegans in your industry supportive or not?

I've come across both supportive and antagonistic non-vegans in my industry, but I'd have to say the larger part is supportive. Once they see my physique and what I've been able to accomplish, they are more likely to ask me questions about my methods than to tell me it can't be done.

Are your family and friends supportive of your vegan lifestyle?

Yes, for the most part. In a perfect world, they would all be vegan too, but they understand how passionate I am about it and have never tried to talk me out of it.

What is the most common question/comment that people ask/say when they find out that you are a vegan and how do you respond?
Definitely: "Where do you get your protein?"

Who or what motivates you?
Everyone and everything motivates me. My wife, my son, my friends, my clients - I want them all to be fit and healthy and free of chronic disease. Likewise, the animals and the environment motivate me to protect them. The vegan fitness community and my sponsor Vegan Bodybuilding and Fitness motivate me to lead by example and be a role model. That's the beautiful thing about a plant based-diet: it impacts everything. That's also why I could never go back to my old way of eating.

FOOD & SUPPLEMENTS

What do you eat for Breakfast?
Oatmeal with blueberries, and a protein shake with strawberries, banana, spinach, soymilk, and Plantfusion protein powder.

What do you eat for Lunch?
A big green salad, and red lentil dhal soup with a blackened tofu salad and a sweet potato.

What do you eat for Dinner?
A variety of dishes that center around beans, whole grains and vegetables. And always a big green salad.

What do you eat for Snacks - healthy & not-so healthy?
My patented bean shakes! Basically the same as my breakfast protein shake, but with added oats and white beans. There's a recipe on my website.

What is your favourite source of Protein?
Food ie beans, tofu, whole grains and green vegetables.

What is your favourite source of Calcium?
I've never worried about it and never will. I get tons from all my whole plant foods.

What is your favourite source of Iron?
Same as calcium.

What foods give you the most energy?
Probably fruit. I love fruit and feel great after eating it. A hearty helping of beans and greens is a close second.

Do you take any supplements?
I get the vast majority of my nutrition through whole foods like beans, whole grains, nuts, seeds, fruit and green vegetables, but I also like to supplement my diet with quality plant protein, especially after weight training to aid in recovery and promote growth. My favorite is Plantfusion, or Sunwarrior's raw brown rice protein; both taste great and are minimally processed so there are still intact nutrients. I also take creatine on and off, which I've found to help me make strength gains.

"Veganism means living a healthy and compassionate life. Choosing foods, occupations, and activities that nourish your body, helping others and doing as little harm to the world around you as possible is all part veganism to me."

ADVICE

What is your top tip for gaining muscle?
Stick to compound barbell exercises, and train as hard and heavy as you can without deviating from perfect form. Eat a lot, then eat some more and gains will come.

What is your top tip for losing weight?
Stick to whole, low-fat, unprocessed foods and reduce calories as slowly as you can. Train your whole body with weight lifting circuits to work your muscles and cardiovascular system at the same time, and get in regular intense cardio like timed 5ks, hill sprints, and fast biking or swimming to really stimulate your metabolism.

What is your top tip for maintaining weight?
Just eat healthy whole plant-foods and perform both strength and cardiovascular exercise of your choice more days than not during the week - it's that simple.

What is your top tip for improving metabolism?
Eat lots and lots of whole, unprocessed plant foods, perform intense compound barbell exercises, and get in regular intense cardio like sprinting and your metabolism will be flying.

What is your top tip for toning up?
The same a losing weight really, except you will want to eat more. Get in lots of healthy food and work up a hard sweat several days a week.

How do you promote veganism in your daily life?
I challenge my clients' dietary habits on a daily basis, I post information about plant-based nutrition on our blog and our Facebook and Twitter pages, and I wear vegan apparel wherever I go.

How would you suggest people get involved with what you do?
Get in touch! As I said above, please feel free to contact us through our website, through our FaceBook page or through our Twitter page. Thanks in advance.

"There is still a misconception out there that vegans are skinny, weak, and undernourished. This is changing rapidly as more and more mainstream celebrities and athletes go vegan, but it's still an idea that needs to be challenged regularly. I address this by being the most muscular, strongest and healthiest person I can possibly be, and by making myself visible through contests and online media so the world can see that vegans have no problem being fit, strong and healthy."

DREW McCALL BURKE
VEGAN FITNESS TRAINER

Murrells Inlet, South Carolina, USA
Vegan since: 2005

sexyrawfoodandfitness.com
SM: *FaceBook, Instagram, Pinterest, Twitter, YouTube*

Drew McCall Burke has been involved in the health and fitness industry in various ways. She is a fitness trainer, physical therapist assistant and raw food coach, speaker and the author and co-author of six raw food and juice cleansing books and eBooks.

WHY VEGAN?

How and why did you decide to become vegan?
I went vegan when I read a book called "Skinny Bitch" 7 years ago by Rory Freedman and Kim Barnoiun. By page 2, I was vegan.

How long have you been vegan?
Over 8 years.

What has benefited you the most from being vegan?
By going vegan, I improved my health, opened my compassionate heart, and focused on a mission and passion that has given me the most satisfaction in my life.

What does veganism mean to you?
Veganism is an end to the suffering of all creatures, human and animal, towards abolition, and not exploiting or harming any animal for the gain of human pleasure or appetite.

TRAINING

What sort of training do you do?
I run 10km just about every other day, practice yoga 4-6 days a week and train with my clients every day - a large variety of fun plyometric, acrobatic and strength training exercises.

How often do you (need to) train?
I like to play every day I can. The world is my gym.

Do you offer your fitness or training services to others?
I have been a professional fitness trainer for 20 years. From kickboxing to kettleballs, Pilates, yoga and athletic conditioning. I know how to train the complete person with nutrition, health and physical fitness.

What sports do you play?
I play whatever sport I can. I really enjoy all sports. I love to run, cycle and rollerblade.

STRENGTHS, WEAKNESSES & OUTSIDE INFLUENCES

What do you think is the biggest misconception about vegans and how do you address this?
Many people think that vegans are extreme, weak and hippies. A misconception would be assuming vegans are not healthy. Through my website and FaceBook page, we give every example of healthy living and transformations and testimonials of the wealth of health in a Sexy Raw Vegan (SRV) diet.

What are your strengths as a vegan athlete?
I can run fast longer and more than ever before. Recovery time is much quicker and I feel energy longer when I eat well.

What is your biggest challenge?
Running faster for longer and more than ever before. I am really enjoying the athleticism of running and cycling.

Are the non-vegans in your industry supportive or not?
We are in the midst of enormous change in the athletic diet, so many are open to a raw vegan lifestyle because the results have been very impressive.

Are your family and friends supportive of your vegan lifestyle?
Some in my family are supportive and some not so much but all are very interested and all have questions.

What is the most common question/comment that people ask/say when they find out that you are a vegan and how do you respond?
"What do you do to get enough protein?" I tell them I don't I eat amino acids every day.

Who or what motivates you?
People I train and coach motivate me, my SRV Crew and our future motivates me. My family and the potential to be part of the movement towards a Vegan Planet.

"By going vegan, I improved my health, opened my compassionate heart, and focused on a mission and passion that has given me the most satisfaction in my life."

FOOD & SUPPLEMENTS

What do you eat for Breakfast?
Juices, smoothies, banana, oatmeal, fruit, and coconut water.

What do you eat for Lunch?
Fruit, stackers, wraps, smoothies, and soups.

What do you eat for Dinner?
Raw pastas, stews, and SRV creations.

What do you eat for Snacks - healthy & not-so healthy?
SRV decadent desserts, which are healthy and low fat.

What is your favorite source of Protein?
Amino acids are in almost everything I eat.

What is your favorite source of Calcium?
Is in all the greens I eat.

What is your favorite source of Iron?
Greens and some seeds.

What foods give you the most energy?
What gives me the most energy are the carbs from what I ate the day before.

Do you take any supplements?
No.

ADVICE

What is your top tip for gaining muscle, losing weight, maintaining weight, improving metabolism and toning up?
Train hard and smart, eat a lot of raw food, hydrate well and sleep a lot.

How do you promote veganism in your daily life?
Through social networking, what I wear and what I promote.

How would you suggest people get involved with what you do?
Facebook and the Internet are fabulous places to meet people and get aligned with vegan and raw vegan meet ups near your town.

"Veganism is an end to the suffering of all creatures, human and animal, towards abolition, and not exploiting or harming any animal for the gain of human pleasure or appetite."

Is Veganism Enough?

How can we promote veganism in the most inclusive way?

What can we do to participate more in other social justice issues, and support their causes?

How can we encourage others to support our movement?

How can we become better examples of compassion in action?

ED BAUER
VEGAN CHAMPION BODY BUILDER

Oakland, California, USA
Vegan since: 1996

plantfitstrength.com
SM: *FaceBook, Instagram, Twitter*

Ed Bauer is a Champion Vegan Bodybuilder and owner of PlantFit Strength & Conditioning in Oakland, CA. He is a Certified Personal Trainer through The American Council on Exercise (ACE), and National Exercise and Sports Trainers Association (NESTA), with over 2000 sessions serviced. He is a Fitness Nutrition Coach through NESTA and also holds a Cross Fit Level 1 Certificate. He recently competed in the 2012 Reebok Cross Fit Games Open.

WHY VEGAN?

How and why did you decide to become vegan?
When I was 15, a few friends I knew through skateboarding were vegan. I could figure why people would be vegetarian, but I thought vegan sounded "extreme." After reading "Diet For a New America" by John Robbins and doing some soul searching, I decided that veganism was the only way to live a truly compassionate lifestyle. I haven't looked back ever since.

How long have you been vegan?
I went vegan in 1996 as a junior in high school.

What has benefited you the most from being vegan?
Veganism has given me a sense of purpose. Encouraging others to follow a plant-based diet seems to be the most profound impact I can have on people, animals, and the environment. In addition, I feel great!

What does veganism mean to you?
Veganism means living for the greater good in kindness and harmony with all living beings. It means being responsible and honest about how our actions affect others.

TRAINING

What sort of training do you do?
I currently train using CrossFit methodologies as well as traditional strength and Olympic lifting principles.

How often do you (need to) train?
I train 5 or 6 days a week, 2 Power Lifting days, 1 Olympic lifting day, and 2 or 3 CrossFit workouts

Do you offer your fitness or training services to others?
Yes, I own PlantFit Strength & Conditioning in Oakland, CA. I offer personal training, group classes, as well as nutritional consulting and program design, in person or online.

What sports do you play?
For the 2012 Reebok CrossFit Games Open, a worldwide event, I did one workout per week for six weeks. It was 7 minutes with as many reps as possible of burpees. I completed 111 reps. CrossFit summarizes all components of fitness so I find this to be ideal for cardiovascular endurance, stamina, strength, flexibility, power, speed, coordination, agility, balance, and accuracy.

STRENGTHS, WEAKNESSES & OUTSIDE INFLUENCES

What do you think is the biggest misconception about vegans and how do you address this?
The biggest misconception of vegans is that they are weak and unhealthy because of some missing essential nutrients. This has been proven many times over that all nutrients can be obtained on a 100% plant-based diet. As a champion bodybuilder turned CrossFit athlete, I break this stereotype every day.

What are your strengths as a vegan athlete?
Better recovery between workouts, better oxygen uptake and blood flow, better assimilation of nutrients and healthier digestion.

What is your biggest challenge?
My biggest challenge is challenging myself to always work harder. All essential nutrients including fatty acids and amino acids can be met with a varied whole foods plant-based diet. Once all nutritional requirements are met, the physical challenges out there are the same across the board, vegan or not. I am stronger and faster than a lot of meat eaters, just as there are meat eaters out there stronger and faster than me. What is important is that they see they have no advantage over me because of diet. They may see that I actually have an advantage over them because of diet, and that is what changes perceptions. A big challenge for me is spreading compassion to others. Once compassion for all living creatures is in a person's heart, they will work hard to stay vegan, even if they faced any health challenges. Proper nutrition does take some practice. Just going vegan isn't enough for health. People need to do their homework, live healthy and be a good representation of what a plant-based lifestyle can offer.

Are the non-vegans in your industry supportive or not?
They are once they see what I look like and what I can do.

Are your family and friends supportive of your vegan lifestyle?
Yes, my family and friends are very supportive. They see how veganism has helped shape me into the person I am today. My father eats vegan as well.

What is the most common question/comment that people ask/say when they find out that you are a vegan and how do you respond?
"Where do you get your protein?" still comes up. I usually say something like "Tempeh, tofu, seitan, lentils, rice protein, pea protein, hemp seeds, chia seeds, flaxseeds, pumpkin seeds, Tofurky, black beans, garbanzo beans, veggie burgers, pinto beans, peanut butter, almond butter, and walnuts. Where do you get your protein?"

Who or what motivates you?
This culture motivates me through it's continual belief that animals need to be confined, exploited, tortured, murdered, then consumed for our "well being." This ritual continues for no one's benefit except the meat and dairy industries financial gain while animals die, our health deteriorates, and our environmental resources are depleted.

In terms of individuals that motivate me, Robert Cheeke who got me to do my first bodybuilding competition, Brendan Brazier, Mike Mahler, T. Colin Campbell, Caldwell

B. Esselstyn, Neal Barnard, etc. All fitness and health professionals who promote the vegan lifestyle continue to motivate me and make me work harder.

FOOD & SUPPLEMENTS

What do you eat for Breakfast?
Protein shake with Vega powder, spinach, blueberries, rice and pea protein, and flax oil.

What do you eat for Lunch?
Veggie sausage with broccoli, kale and a handful of mixed raw nuts.

What do you eat for Dinner?
Huge salad with lots of veggies, beans, nuts, a little dried fruit, and goddess dressing. After Dinner Dessert: I eat homemade protein pudding with rice and pea protein, cocoa, unsweetened almond milk, stevia, and peanut butter.

What do you eat for Snacks - healthy & not-so healthy?
Vega Protein Bar, Organic Food Bar, hummus and veggies, nuts, dried fruit, vegan jerky, mixed bean salad, and protein shakes. I aim for some combination of protein, complex carbs and healthy fats.

What is your favourite source of Protein?
Tofu, black beans, and quinoa.

What is your favourite source of Calcium?
Leafy greens, raw nuts, and almond milk.

What is your favourite source of Iron?
Leafy greens and beans.

What foods give you the most energy?
My morning smoothie with Vega protein powder always gives me plenty of energy. I am also a big fan of coconut milk for medium-chain triglycerides (MCTs).

Do you take any supplements?
I take a multi-vitamin, flax oil as well as DHA algal oil, glutamine, zinc, and magnesium.

ADVICE

What is your top tip for gaining muscle?
It takes big weights to make big muscles.

What is your top tip for losing weight?
Do morning cardio and get to know intensity.

What is your top tip for maintaining weight?
It is all about balance.

What is your top tip for improving metabolism?
Work hard and rest just as hard. Stress kills your metabolism.

How do you promote veganism in your daily life?
I promote veganism in my daily life by working out with partners who are not vegan or vegetarian even. I also workout in four different gyms per week. When people know that I am vegan and I perform well, this sends a clear message that most likely changes their view on the issue.

How would you suggest people get involved with what you do?
Check out my website and let me know how I can help.

Elaine Brent
VEGAN LONG DISTANCE TRIATHLETE

Auckland, New Zealand
Vegan since: 1995

SM: *FaceBook, Twitter*

Elaine Brent is a long-distance triathlete from New Zealand. Originally born in England, she immigrated with her family to NZ at an early age. Before arriving in NZ, Elaine had already changed to a vegetarian diet and as her thought patterns progressed, she later became vegan. She became a triathlete in 2009 and after dabbling with different distances, is now aiming at Ironman 70.3 (half Ironman) World Championships 2016 over the next year of racing.

WHY VEGAN?

How and why did you decide to become vegan?
I became vegetarian when I was 9 after visiting a fish factory. Then became vegan permanently at around 19 after making the decision based on four grounds:
1) general industry cruelty standards that I believe should not be tolerated,
2) the fact that to use strictly only organic and/or free range dairy and/or eggs would be too hard for me to do at the moment,
3) the overriding principle that I don't believe I should take anything from anything without being able to ask (whenever possible),
4) I have read and listened to many different health arguments and my own conclusion is that I will be healthier without dairy.

How long have you been vegan?
Since 1995.

What has benefited you the most from being vegan?
Benefits include fat loss/muscle gain and elevated energy levels. Becoming vegan was the catalyst for the beginning of really looking after myself. It motivated me to delve in to other aspects of my health and even the smallest changes have led to large changes in my overall wellbeing. For example, having to check ingredients gave me an insight to just how much additives and un-needed ingredients are in food that I presumed only included what the title label suggested. Since being vegan, I have also become gluten-free once I found out I was intolerant. I have also cut back on raw cane sugar which has had endless positive impacts on my life. I have cut down alcohol and I am overall happier and appreciative of my life which I take as the best gift I was ever given.

What does veganism mean to you?
Veganism, I think represents strength of mind body and soul. Everything from the way I've learnt to react to criticism and standing by my decisions, to becoming the athlete that I am today is owed largely to being vegan.

TRAINING

What sort of training do you do?

As a triathlete my training is always working towards increasing my swimming, cycling and running abilities - even when stretching and popping out some squats in the gym.

How often do you (need to) train?

I was not from a swimming background so I am currently swimming 7–9 times per week averaging approximately 5km (3miles) per set (broken into repetitions) to play a "bit" of catch up. I spend the rest of my hours at the gym, running and cycling. I train just over 30 hours per week and have one day off per fortnight. This has been a very gradual increase and I can now balance this healthily whilst working part time.

STRENGTHS, WEAKNESSES & OUTSIDE INFLUENCES.

What do you think is the biggest misconception about vegans and how do you address this?

Being vegan definitely carries a huge stereotype and honestly, I can see why. Whenever anything surrounding veganism is brought up, there is usually a voiced opinion from a strongly outspoken vegan, which does not help the cause. Despite that kind of attitude being a minority among vegans, it is the one that is heard and remembered the most. That is why I always try to encourage a more peaceful approach. I believe the biggest influence comes from example rather than accusations and anger.

What are your strengths as a vegan athlete?

I can't really answer this one too well as I've only ever been a vegan athlete. I can say that I am just as strong as a non-vegan with no restrictions on what my body needs and I suppose I have less chance of food poisoning!

What is your biggest challenge?

Eating abroad and language barriers.

Are the non-vegans in your industry supportive or not?

I haven't had any experience of anyone being unsupportive emotionally from either vegans or non-vegans in regards to my racing, but I do think omnivores struggle to understand where I am getting my nutrients from to support my lifestyle.

Are your family and friends supportive of your vegan lifestyle?

My immediate family are all vegan or vegetarian and I have some other family members who are also vegetarian. The rest don't question how I choose to eat and maybe think it's strange at worst.

What is the most common question/comment that people ask/say when they find out that you are a vegan and how do you respond?

"How do you get enough protein/iron?" My response is "Protein and iron are in almost everything I eat, and I couldn't avoid it if I tried."

Who or what motivates you?

Understanding that pain and suffering is the same no matter who you are, and the fact that pain and suffering need to have no part of my diet is what motivates me to be vegan. The adrenaline of competition and the desire to win is what motivates me to train and race.

"Muscle helps burn fat but this does not mean if you do some hamstring curls you will dissolve your thigh fat. It will mean however, that you have more muscle working toward burning your overall fat and when you do strip fat, you will have shapely hamstrings waiting."

FOOD AND SUPPLEMENTS

What do you eat?
Here's my general daily diet.

Snack: Two rice cracker sandwiches with yeast free vege spread, 2 apples and 2 oranges.

Lunch: Gluten-free pasta, rice or potato meal including chickpeas, lentils or beans, tofu etc. and a variety of vegetables.

Snack: Gluten-free vegan bar or second serve of meal from lunch depending on third training session.

Dinner: Protein salad with plenty of vegetables, and including beans, lentils, chickpeas, falafel with large sprinkling of ground almond nuts, and chia, sunflower, and sesame seeds. Options of dressings include lemon, mustard, olive oil, tamari sauce, vinegar and sweet chilli. I might add a potato if I've had a very hard day.

Snack: Fruit, and of course the occasional dark chocolate or potato chip total cave in.

What is your favourite source of Iron?
Spinach or really anything dark green.

What is your favourite source of Protein?
Lentils, chickpeas, tofu and chia seeds.

What is your favourite source of Calcium?
Beans, nuts and broccoli.

What foods give you the most energy?
I have a naturally very high carbohydrate diet which fits well with my training. Apart from the occasional treats, it is all "good" carbs though and all contain vital nutrients. My energy is gained from having a mainly carbohydrate diet with the rest made up of fat and protein. The fact that I eat around double the amount of calories someone else my size would eat due to training, means my diet is still very high in protein and fat also ensuring my body functions well.

Do you take any supplements?
I take a women's multi-vitamin and chlorella powder mixed in water. Previous to this amount of training, I was on no supplements.

ADVICE

What is your top tip for gaining muscle?
Heavy weights and resistance training and, of course enough protein - plus everything else.

What is your top tip for losing weight?
14-hour fast from last meal at night. Cut out unnecessary sugars and processed food whilst watching portion size.

What is your top tip for maintaining weight?
Just eat more whilst still avoiding unnecessary sugars and processed food. If you want to gain weight, I presume you will want "good" weight, not excess fat. This goes without saying that muscle building is a must.

What is your top tip for improving metabolism?
All of the above.

What is your top tip for toning up?

I find this a funny one and I have often pondered it over the years but basically, I believe it's fat loss. We all have abs under fat but most of us will never show them because you have to be of a very low fat percentage to do so. Depending on your goals, I would be more focused on muscle development (and that doesn't have to be bulky muscle) whilst maintaining a healthy fat percentage. Muscle helps burn fat but this does not mean if you do some hamstring curls you will dissolve your thigh fat. It will mean however, that you have more muscle working toward burning your overall fat and when you do strip fat, you will have shapely hamstrings waiting.

I do remember the best advice I was ever given - in regards to fat loss: As I was sitting on a couch, probably devouring cake, I was doing my daily moan of "poor me, why am I so fat – how am I ever going to get rid of it?" I was confronted with an answer, which was slightly broad but never the less the eye-opener to my own self-indulgence and generally slack attitude. The advice was thus: Eat less, exercise more. As is obvious, my top tips weren't really vegan-specific and that's because I believe you can be fat, thin or a bit of both on any diet.

How do you promote veganism in your daily life?

I promote veganism in my daily life by just being vegan. I believe that the fight against animal cruelty needs to be a peaceful and factual one. More aggressive approaches may well have worked for other battles, but I have seen too many walls thrown up in defence to think that yelling and screaming my views will make any changes. I have known many people try veganism or vegetarianism and stick with it just because they see that it can work.

When questioned, I respond as factually and emotionally detached as possible. There has been a long build-up to make vegans appear as losers and emotionally weak individuals in society however slight the insinuations. It's the same technique used against feminists and environmentalists, and so I believe we do need to rise above the immediate impulse to anger when attacked about our beliefs and understand that to become vegan for some people means more than just changing their diet. I've noticed that some almost take the act of veganism as an attack on their own character, which I think is one of the many reasons that people are not always welcoming to the idea. It is a very different concept for most to understand and will not be understood overnight. I do believe that changes are happening, especially in the Western world.

Veganism is an act of moral standing but also a representation of a concept that can be implemented throughout many other aspects in our world. As a vegan, I am an individual taking my place in large-scale shift of mind-set and I hope this is just the beginning.

How would you suggest people get involved with what you do?

Have a search for your local triathlon club, cycling club, running club or check if your pool runs swim squads or lessons. Any one of those is bound to be packed with triathletes and you'll easily find people who are willing to help you to get started or have a go. The great thing about triathletes, for some strange reason, we want the whole world to do triathlons so you'll never be short on a helping hand.

"Veganism is an act of moral standing but also a representation of a concept that can be implemented throughout many other aspects in our world. As a vegan, I am an individual taking my place in large-scale shift of mind-set and I hope this is just the beginning."

ELLA MAGERS
VEGAN FITNESS TRAINER

Miami Beach, Florida, USA
Vegan since: 1995

sexyfitvegan.com
SM: *FaceBook, Instagram, Twitter*

An 18-year vegan veteran, Ella Magers, MSW (Masters in Social Work) has been helping people get fit and healthy with a plant-based diet and active lifestyle for over 11 years. She is a certified fitness trainer, wellness coach, and muay thai practitioner based out of Miami Beach, Florida, USA. Founder of SexyFitVegan.com, Ella is passionate about living life to its fullest while keeping true to her values of a healthy, fit body, and compassion for animals. Her mission is to educate, inspire, and empower people with tools to make conscientious choices and live a life they love.

WHY VEGAN?

How and why did you decide to become vegan?
My journey started with an "aha" moment in third grade when I connected my love of animals to the food on my plate. My Mom picked me up from school and asked, as she did every day, "How was school today?" I told her that we learned about American explorer Daniel Boone and I thought he was a horrible man because he killed animals. My mom said that Daniel Boone was actually being responsible for feeding and clothing himself, and that today we just go to the store. I was silent for a moment then told my mother that I was not going to do that anymore. Despite my mother's initial protest, I never ate meat again and she soon became proud and supportive of my decision. My path to a vegan lifestyle started with a deep sense of compassion for all living creatures. My continuing exploration of animal rights issues led me to adopt a totally vegan diet in middle school, when I discovered the connection between the meat, dairy, and egg industries. I learned that the life of a dairy cow for example, is just as horrific than that of a cow raised for beef, and upon this discovery, I became 100% vegan for life.

How long have you been vegan?
Over 18 years.

What has benefited you the most from being vegan?
Living a vegan lifestyle has benefitted me in every way possible. Not only am I extremely healthy physically, but also, refraining from ingesting animals and by-products from animals who have suffered and died keeps me emotionally and spiritually healthy as well.

What does veganism mean to you?
Veganism means to live a lifestyle that considers all life to be equally valuable. It means moving through the world in a way that is compassionate and full of love for yourself and other animals (human and non-human). It means dedication toward making the

world a better place. It means educating others about how the meat, dairy, egg, leather, and fur industries affect animals, the environment, and our health, and living by example so as to inspire others.

TRAINING

What sort of training do you do?
I do a wide variety of types of training. My favorite exercise "hobby" is muay thai, which I have been practicing for 10 years. I have done Mixed Martial Arts (MMA) and jiu-jitsu training, a lot of functional and bodyweight training, running, cycling, spinning, park workouts, track workouts, interval training, cross-training, swimming etc. I am always mixing it up to be challenged and prevent getting bored or hitting a plateau.

How often do you (need to) train?
I train 6 days per week, sometimes doing yoga on day 7.

Do you offer your fitness or training services to others?
I am National Academy of Sports Medicine (NASM) certified and have been training clients for 11 years.

What sports do you play?
I do muay thai - sparring but not competing - and I enjoy playing volleyball recreationally. As a child and teen, I competed in swimming, gymnastics, and volleyball.

STRENGTHS, WEAKNESSES & OUTSIDE INFLUENCES

What do you think is the biggest misconception about vegans and how do you address this?
The stereotype of vegans as being either "hippie-dippy," "radicals" and/or unhealthy, scrawny people is definitely changing. I created "Sexy Fit Vegan™" to bring attention to the fact that vegan can mean strong, beautiful, sexy, healthy, with a fighter spirit.

What are your strengths as a vegan athlete?
My strength is simply living by example, sharing what I know, inspiring, and motivating others to make the transition to a plant-based diet and vegan lifestyle while staying on a path of constantly improving their fitness level.

What is your biggest challenge?
My biggest challenge is taking the time to do therapeutic bodywork that will help prevent injury and help with injuries I have already. I am go-go-go all the time and it really takes conscious effort to schedule in down time and time for long stretching sessions, massage, physical therapy, etc.

Are the non-vegans in your industry supportive or not?
Yes, for the most part they are supportive. I take a gentle approach (different than my approach when I was younger), of educating, sharing, and inspiring, so it does not threaten non-vegans and instead, generally makes them curious and willing to learn more.

Are your family and friends supportive of your vegan lifestyle?
Absolutely! I am extremely fortunate to have an amazing family who has always been supportive of decisions I make based on my beliefs and who I am. In fact, my father and sister followed my lead and are also vegan, and my mother eats very little animal products. One of my best friends also went vegan within a year of us meeting each

other. My other friends see my passion and support me in whatever ways they can.

What is the most common question/comment that people ask/say when they find out that you are a vegan and how do you respond?
"How do you get your protein?" is probably the most common question I get since I am fit and strong. My response is, "It's easier than you think!" I refer them to my website where I give tips through my blog and newsletter. I also let them know I offer individual nutrition coaching and consulting, and do workshops periodically to help people with vegan nutrition basics and meal planning.

Who or what motivates you?
My number one motivating factor is the pain I feel deep within me for the horrendous suffering of innocent sentient beings that is taking place every second of every day. The environmental destruction that is a direct result of the meat & dairy industries also motivates me a great deal. The fact that eating a well-balanced whole foods-based vegan diet is the healthiest way to live, preventing diseases and disorders that ruin the quality of life of so many people including loved ones, is icing on the cake.

FOOD & SUPPLEMENTS

What do you eat for Breakfast?
My favorite breakfast is a shake I make in my Vitamix with flax or almond milk, hemp seeds, chia seeds, flax meal, alma powder, banana, and either berries or a splash of coffee and raw cacao. Occasionally I enjoy scrambled tofu or cultured coconut (coconut milk yogurt) with nuts, seeds, and berries. On very special occasions, I love vegan blueberry pancakes and waffles.

What do you eat for Lunch and Dinner?
I love eating huge, hearty salads of all different types! Different types of greens, legumes (especially garbanzo beans), nuts and seeds, grilled mushrooms, quinoa, etc. I also love mung bean pasta (over 20g protein per serving!) and when the craving hits I add Daiya cheese for a delicious, high protein vegan mac and cheese.

I like a wide variety of cuisines including Tex-Mex, Indian, and Thai, as long as it's cooked clean with healthy oil in moderation and with whole food ingredients. I stay on the low side when it comes to carbs, sticking with quinoa and legumes as my main source of carbohydrates.

What do you eat for Snacks - healthy & not-so healthy?
Healthy snacks include raw veggies with hummus, celery and apples with almond butter, kale chips, raw cashews, fresh green juices, fresh fruit - especially pineapple, mango, all berries, cherries, nectarines, and peaches. Not-so-healthy snacks are lentil chips, okra chips, coconut milk ice cream and vegan brownies.

What is your favourite source of Protein?
I love edamame (organic, non-GMO of course.) The seeds I add to my shakes are also a source I rely on daily, like hemp, chia, and flax. When I travel, I bring organic protein powders (mostly made from pea, hemp, and brown rice) and a shaker bottle so I never have to worry about finding quality plant-based protein when I'm somewhere without many healthy options.

What is your favourite source of Calcium?
The vegan milk substitutes I use with my shakes daily are all fortified with a ton of calcium so I know I'm getting enough.

What is your favourite source of Iron?
I love lightly sautéed spinach with olive oil and garlic (but I don't recommend it if you are on a date!)

What foods give you the most energy?
Fresh fruit as well as the shakes I make seem to give me the most energy - they don't weigh me down and they seems to give me a quick boost.

Do you take any supplements?
I take B12 daily, magnesium (as an oil you spray on your skin) regularly, and zinc if I feel run-down or like I'm catching a cold.

ADVICE

What is your top tip for gaining muscle?
Adding shakes to your daily healthy, whole foods-based routine is the easiest way to dramatically increase your protein intake to help you gain muscle. There are several clean, organic, protein powders on the market made with pea protein, brown rice protein, hemp protein, etc, that make it simple to get in a ton of complete protein in one easy step.

What is your top tip for losing weight?
TRAIN YOUR ASS OFF and be aware of the amount of grains you consume (carbs you may not be able to burn off), nuts and seeds (high calorie and fat intake even though they are a good fat), and beans - yes they contain protein, but also a lot of carbs and can be rough on some people's digestive systems.

What is your top tip for maintaining weight?
Consistency is key. Train hard, and always challenge yourself. Eat a wide variety of whole foods daily. Become body-aware. Everyone is different and it's important you find the exercises and vegan food habits that make you feel the best, while taking in all the essential nutrients we all need to be healthy for years to come.

What is your top tip for improving metabolism?
Consistency. Create positive eating and exercise habits and stay consistent with those habits. Overeating and then starving yourself or over-exercising is not helpful to keeping your machine (your body) running as it is meant to.

What is your top tip for toning up?
First, you must build lean muscle if you are lacking it through strength training-type of exercises, sports, or activities. From there, the key is eliminating the body fat that covers that lean muscle, leaving you feeling your hard work is not paying off. Cardio can help, but a balanced, healthy vegan diet is the primary way you can get the fat off, leaving the lean muscle visible and your body looking toned.

How do you promote veganism in your daily life?
Almost every step I take I find ways to promote veganism through sharing my life with those around me. I love being asked, "How do you get those legs?" by a random person at the grocery store so I can share that I have been vegan for 18 years! I wear my Sexy Fit Vegan™ promotional shirts, and am constantly finding ways to bring the topic into conversation with anyone and everyone. People are so interested in improving their bodies and health it's not hard to do.

How would you suggest people get involved with what you do?
Visit my website, check out the forum, connect with me on FaceBook, Twitter, and Instagram. I do my very best to stay connected to people all over the world through social media, my blog and newsletter.

ELLEN JAFFE JONES
VEGAN SPRINTER

Holmes Beach, Florida, USA
Vegan since: 2004

vegcoach.com

SM: *FaceBook, Twitter, YouTube*

Ellen Jaffe Jones is an Aerobics and Fitness Association of America nationally certified personal trainer, a Road Runners Club of America nationally certified running coach, and the author of her publisher's #1 bestseller, "Eat Vegan on $4 a Day". As an Emmy-winning TV investigative reporter and anchor for 18 years, Ellen got tired of seeing stories on the news with obese food stamp recipients saying, "You can't eat well on a budget." Vegan for most of the past 30 years trying to dodge a family history of breast cancer that got her Mom, Aunt and both sisters, Ellen continues to place in 72 5km races for her age group (60-64) in the Tampa, Sarasota, Bradenton area since 2006. She didn't get all the good genes and has blood tests that show a vegan diet saved her from pending heart disease and a life of doctor-prescribed medicines for colon disease.

WHY VEGAN?

How and why did you decide to become vegan?
Initially, for health and animal rights. I began going to meetings in the 1980s and saw some of the first undercover videos about circus elephants being abused during training. When I was 28, I almost died of a colon blockage. The same year my sister got breast cancer for the second time. I began eating a macrobiotic diet that included fish. I found the rules too restrictive for my busy schedule, so I morphed to a vegetarian diet.

How long have you been vegan?
For most of the past 30 years, with several regressions. When I worked at Smith Barney as a financial consultant, we had many catered meals and working lunches where there was only one choice of what topping we had on our pizza. I gained weight and when we moved to Florida, I had hemorrhaging fibroids that caused the ER doctors to say I needed an immediate hysterectomy. My regular obstetritian got on the phone and said, "Go back to that plant-based diet and call me in the morning." 3 weeks later, all signs of menopause were gone, including the hot flashes. Even my skeptical hubby was blown away.

What has benefited you the most from being vegan?
Avoiding being on medications for colon issues, the doctors said I would need to, and avoiding a hysterectomy. Peace of mind, knowing no animals were harmed. As technology has improved, with the amazing documentaries shot inside factory farms, it is hard to stick our heads in the sand and pretend that we don't see.

What does veganism mean to you?
Life-saving, healthy, enhances athletic performance and gives me enjoyment of life.

TRAINING

What sort of training do you do?
Certified Personal Trainer (AFAA - Aerobics and Fitness Association of America), Running Coaching (RRCA - Road Runners Coach of America Certification). For myself, I try to run at least 3 miles (3.8km) every day or every other day, with a long run 5-6 miles (8-9.6km) on weekends. Due to a metatarsal arch stress fracture several years ago from running on the beach (did too much too soon, even though I didn't think so), I try to run on soft surfaces like trails and the beach when it is flat and ideal, as much as possible.

How often do you (need to) train?
I've been running and/or walking since 28. I try to take a rest day in my old age, once a week. I try to do a 5km race once or twice a month during the running season, which is about 8-9 months long. The biggest question I had when I moved to Florida was, "How do you workout or run during the summer here?" Answer: At sunrise.

Do you offer your fitness or training services to others?
I used to work at the local gym, but I don't have time now. Since my second book came out, I've been on the road most weekends at the request of my publisher doing trade shows and the largest vegetarian festivals in the US and Canada. My publisher tells me I'm unusual as an author because I really do engage with the public and enjoy public speaking. With 18 years in TV news, and subsequent media consulting for some of the most well-known vegan doctors and their organizations, the public speaking was second nature.

What sports do you play?
Running, swimming, biking - mostly running. I did my first marathon in 2010 and was the 5th oldest female to finish - Palm Beaches Marathon). I did my first marathon (Palm Beaches Marathon) in 2010 and was the 5th oldest female to finish. I enjoy racing because it really helps you improve performance and maintain your health and level of fitness.

STRENGTHS, WEAKNESSES & OUTSIDE INFLUENCES

What do you think is the biggest misconception about vegans and how do you address this?
They don't get enough (fill in the blank). Protein, calcium, variety, fun in life. All so not true!

What are your strengths as a vegan athlete?
I usually "smoke" my age group in 5km. Though there are some faster than me, but when I look at them, their legs are usually up to my neck or they are just built differently. At 5'3", I've been very pleased with my performance. When I started running again after a long break and did races, I would often answer the post-race question, "How did you do?" with, "Finished without injury." Because I have been injured, I understand how difficult that can be, especially as we age.

What is your biggest challenge?
Avoiding the family genetic and environmental history that gave my Mom, Aunt and both sisters breast cancer. We were part of the original breast cancer gene studies. My sister, both parents and all grandparents had diabetes and major heart disease.

Are the non-vegans in your industry supportive or not?
They all see what it has done for me. My clients know about me before they sign up.

Even if they have no interest in going vegan or vegetarian, they know I'll require them to keep a food diary. Part of what I do with clients is discussing how motivated they are to change and what they are willing to do to make that happen.

Are your family and friends supportive of your vegan lifestyle?
I'm the youngest in my family of origin. I've had a lifetime to figure out what works and what doesn't in our family. Do the terms "black sheep" or "cult member" ring a familiar bell? I've been called it all. My husband is not vegan but has seen how it has improved my health and helped me lose 25 pounds (11.3kg) over 6 months.

What is the most common question/comment that people ask/say when they find out that you are a vegan and how do you respond?
"What do you eat?" In addition, "How do you get enough to eat or to do all that racing?"

Who or what motivates you?
My best friend Lori died of breast cancer about 12 years ago. We took Lamaze classes together. She tried to change her diet the last year of her life, but it was too little too late. She said to me on her deathbed, "Take care of my kids." She had a great husband, so I didn't need to really take care of her kids. However, I honor her request by trying to spread the word that a vegan diet can do incredible things. Health is just one of them. I'm convinced it has helped me to avoid our family history of breast cancer. I've yet to meet anyone as I travel, who has my identical history with a Mom, Aunt and both sisters having breast cancer. I'm still waiting for someone to study me. However, as I say in my book, when you understand there's no money in broccoli, you understand why you have to be your own investigative reporter and figure out what works for you.

"When you understand there's no money in broccoli, you understand why you have to be your own investigative reporter and figure out what works for you."

FOOD & SUPPLEMENTS

What do you eat for Breakfast?
Oats, berries and green tea.

What do you eat for Lunch?
Huge salad, beans and fruit.

What do you eat for Dinner?
Huge salad, beans, grains and fruit.

What do you eat for Snacks - healthy & not-so healthy?
Love Larabars. Many smoothies, some with protein powder after a race or hard training. Don't laugh, one plain vegan chocolate chip, by itself.

What is your favourite source of Protein?
Black beans or any beans.

What is your favourite source of Calcium?
Kale and collards.

What is your favourite source of Iron?
Beans.

What foods give you the most energy?
Fruit smoothies with greens, bananas, berries, and mangoes.

Do you take any supplements?

Occasionally a multi-vitamin, if I feel like I need one after heavy training or a race. B12, of course.

ADVICE

What is your top tip for gaining muscle?

Weight training or dynamic, plyometric exercises.

What is your top tip for losing weight?

Juicing, lots of salads, ramping up exercise. For me, running is the only thing that works now. Walking will help me maintain, but I've found that women my age really need to ramp up the exercise routine to maintain or lose weight.

What is your top tip for maintaining weight?

Exercising at least every other day, preferably aerobic workouts during that time. However, aerobic cross-training works on alternate days too. I'm a big fan of the Jeff Galloway books for starting a walking or run/walk program. As I certified personal trainer and running coach, I custom design programs for individuals based on their injuries, history and goals. Many clients don't care about losing weight, they just want their clothes to fit better, improve energy or fitness.

What is your top tip for improving metabolism?

Walk or run bursts. Getting up out of the chair.

What is your top tip for toning up?

Spot weight training. Generally, not a fan, but it is amazing how much the arm flab comes running back when you let the upper body workouts slide.

How do you promote veganism in your daily life?

Every waking minute it seems. One of the reasons my publisher believes my book has been so successful is because of my social media presence. He's asked me to coach other authors on doing the same. I also do big cooking classes twice a month at a large independent health food store in St. Petersburg and Tampa, both in Florida.

How would you suggest people get involved with what you do?

My website, Facebook, Twitter or YouTube. I also have additional Facebook pages: Vegan Athletes, Ellen Jaffe Jones-Author and Personal Trainer.

"The benefits for me are avoiding being on medications for colon issues, when the doctors said I would need to, and avoiding a hysterectomy. Peace of mind, knowing no animals were harmed. As technology has improved, with the amazing documentaries shot inside factory farms, it is hard to stick our heads in the sand and pretend that we don't see.

EMILIE TAN
VEGAN EXERCISE ENTHUSIAST

Melbourne, Victoria, Australia
Vegan since: 2011

evolvedgeneration.com
SM: *FaceBook, Instagram*

Emilie Tan was born in Montreal, Canada and has been living in Melbourne, Australia for more than 7 years. With her husband Luke, she is the co-founder of Evolve'd Generation, a website that aims to spread positive change to the world through connection and inspiration. For 12 years, Emilie competed in short track speed skating for both Canada and Australia at an international level. She considers her 5th place at the 2003 World Junior Championships, along with her five medals at the 2003 Canada Winter Games, highlights of her career. She also participated in national level track competitions and recently competed in her first bodybuilding/bikini show at the International Federation of Bodybuilding and Fitness (IFBB) Victoria titles.

WHY VEGAN?

How and why did you decide to become vegan?
Since a young age, I had been interested in vegetarianism as I never really liked the taste of meat. I was always cooking tofu or lentil-based dishes for my family and knew I would one day forgo meat completely. I tried a "pescatarian" diet around the age of 22-23 but failed as I was also following a very unhealthy lifestyle (binge drinking, social smoking, etc) and replaced meat with lots of eggs and cheese.

I had been suffering from pre-menstrual syndrome and digestive problems since my teen years and just could not get to the bottom of it. Even after taking gluten out of my diet, things had not really improved and got even worse when following a low carbohydrate "paleo" style diet. I had enough and started looking for answers.

My eye caught the frequent FaceBook posts of an acquaintance about veganism. I had a gut feeling that it might be the answer. I started watching videos from Freelee and Durianrider from 30 Bananas a Day, bought John Robbins' "The Food Revolution" and was convinced pretty quickly. I started by eliminating dairy, red meat and poultry, then fish and seafood and finally, I gave up eggs, honey and other animal by-products for good. I also pledged to never buy leather, wool, fur or silk garments again.

How long have you been vegan?
Over 3 years.

What has benefited you the most from being vegan?
My digestion has improved greatly and I do not suffer from pre-menstrual syndrome anymore. I have also connected with so many new amazing people who share veganism as an interest.

What does veganism mean to you?
Making an informed decision to do my best to not participate in industries that cause the suffering of any of my fellow earthlings.

TRAINING

What sort of training do you do?
I am training under the guidance of an amazing running coach and mentor, Sally McRae, an American professional ultra runner. I run probably around 100km (62miles) a week, 6 days a week. I typically do one long run of 20-40km (12-24miles) a week and my other runs are 10-15 km each. Some of my runs are at an easy, conversational pace and others, more challenging and hard. I swim and bike a few times a week as well and do about 3 strength sessions in the gym.

How often do you (need to) train?
I train 6 days a week.

Do you offer your fitness or training services to others?
I like to answer any fitness and training related questions to the best of my knowledge. I would love one day to become a running coach and communicate my passion.

STRENGTHS, WEAKNESSES & OUTSIDE INFLUENCES

What do you think is the biggest misconception about vegans and how do you address this?
That vegans are malnourished and scrawny due to a lack of nutrients people believe are only available through consumption of animal products. I believe in preaching by example and use my body, positive attitude and unlimited energy as a proof that it is not true at all!

What are your strengths as a vegan athlete?
My stamina. I have a very good cardiovascular endurance and coupled with a high carbohydrate fruit diet I get through the most gruesome workout.

What is your biggest challenge?
I do not have the best coordination and my flexibility is quite challenged to say the least! I find yoga, when practiced regularly, really helps with that.

Are the non-vegans in your industry supportive or not?
People are always very curious at work and love to see what I eat for lunch. It is always funny to see people's expression when you tell them you can eat more than 15 bananas a day! It is always nice when a colleague tell me I have inspired them to eat less meat and more fruits and vegetables. I really feel like I'm reaching my goal, which is preaching by example.

Are your family and friends supportive of your vegan lifestyle?
Yes. They know it is the right thing to do and they love sharing a vegan meal with me, however to them it's "extreme" and I believe they have no intention to follow my footsteps in the near future.

What is the most common question/comment that people ask/say when they find out that you are a vegan and how do you respond?
Them: "Wow, that's extreme!" Me: "And factory farming is not?"

Them: "What do you eat?" Me: "Plants".

Them: "Where do you get your protein from?" Me: "From everything I eat... Do I look protein deficient to you?"

Who or what motivates you?
Feeling like I am making a difference. Knowing that I am a part of a movement, which is saving our planet from a grim future. I also look up to other vegan endurance athletes like Scott Jurek, Hillary Biscay and Rich Roll.

FOOD & SUPPLEMENTS

What do you eat for Breakfast?
I have a banana before my morning run. After my run, I have a massive green smoothie made with lots of green leaves and veggies, a couple bananas, one pear, chia seeds and some Fresh Greens from Prana ON.

What do you eat for Lunch?
Fruits! My favorite is a mono-meal of mangoes, dragon fruit or watermelon, but most of the time it ends up being bananas as they are the easiest to get.

What do you eat for Dinner?
A massive salad made with a lot of lettuce, a few tomatoes, mixed raw veggies, olives and some avocado and lemon juice.

What do you eat for Snacks - healthy & not-so healthy?
Healthy: "ice cream" made with either frozen bananas, berries or mangoes; my special trail mix made of dehydrated coconut, goji berries, raisins and pepitas; any fruit in its most simple form.

Not so healthy: I am not a fan of junk food, however I love anything Mexican including tequila and margaritas. A restaurant in Melbourne called La Tortilleria has the best vegan cheese I have ever tasted! I swear it tastes better than what I remember of cheese. I also love Vegie Bar's vegan nachos and enjoy a raw desert once in a while.

What is your favourite source of Protein?
In general, I get my protein from the high volume of fruits and vegetables I eat which is enough. However, I do enjoy some legumes once in a while like lentils, chickpeas or black beans. I rarely eat soy, but I do enjoy a bit of tempeh in a dragon bowl and vegan miso soup.

What is your favourite source of Calcium?
Kale.

What is your favourite source of Iron?
Spinach, beetroot and tahini.

What foods give you the most energy?
Bananas.

Do you take any supplements?
B12, Fresh Greens from Prana ON, and once in a while, I will add a scoop of Prana ON protein powder to my post long run smoothie.

"Doing what you love is most important. Forget the trends, experts and magazine articles. Consistency is most important and it is easy to achieve when you are passionate about something."

ADVICE

What is your top tip for gaining muscle?

Eat enough calories from whole food only sources. At the beginning, it is a great idea to keep track of the calories you eat as it is easy to not eat enough while on a vegan diet as plant food is not as calorie dense as animal products.

Training wise, make sure to mix things up a little to keep your body guessing. Weight training is king to make muscle gain. You should definitely work with a strength coach to point you in the right direction if you are serious about getting results. It makes a world of difference.

What is your top tip for losing weight and toning up?

Carbs, Carbs, Carbs, preferably from fresh fruits whenever you can and whole starches like brown rice, sweet potatoes and gluten-free pasta when fruits are hard to find or not in season. I also find that a big salad at night helps with elimination and detoxification.

Keep fats fairly low and chose them carefully: avocado, seeds, olives, coconut meat and small amounts of nuts are best. Avoid oils and other refined fats. For a lot of people, keeping soy to a minimum will make a difference. Only have it once in a while and stick to organic and whole tofu, tempeh, edamame or miso.

For training, doing what you love is the most important. Forget the trends, experts and magazine articles. Consistency is most important and it is easy to achieve when you are passionate about something.

What is your top tip for maintaining weight?

Make moving and eating well a part of your life. When you eat enough carbohydrates coming from fruits and/or starches and vegetables, your cells are satiated and happy. You then do not crave junk food. Do not restrict the calories coming from low-fat sources of carbohydrates. If you are craving bad stuff, it means you are not eating enough fruits or starches.

Do activities you like, as training should be fun, not a chore. Take a few classes at the gym like Body Pump, spinning, Body attack, etc. Go for a run and listen to you favorite music, take a dance class, organize a trekking holiday with a few friends, etc.

What is your top tip for improving metabolism?

Eat enough carbohydrates. It is proven that low-carbohydrate diets will cause metabolic damage. Do read this great book on the subject from Canadian coach Scott Abel, "Metabolic Damage and the Danger of Dieting."

How do you promote veganism in your daily life?

As mentioned before, I preach by example. People are always impressed with how much energy I have and how I am rarely sick. I like to talk about the way I eat and try and keep it positive. I also try to inform people with facts about factory farming and the dairy and egg industries. I do believe that a lot of people ignore completely what is really happening and would probably start considering the lifestyle if they only knew. To get a conversation started, I also love to wear t-shirts with vegan messages. At my first ultra-marathon, I had "Em Plant Power" written on my race bib. It got a lot of attention, which was amazing!

How would you suggest people get involved with what you do?

First have a look at our website where you can find information about training and veganism and a lot more. We have a list of different resource related to veganism: documentaries, books, website, etc. Get informed!

Erin Fergus

VEGAN PERSONAL TRAINER

Greer, South Carolina, USA
Vegan since: 2013

definitionfitnessmagazine.com
SM: *FaceBook, Instagram*

Erin Fergus is the Academic Program Director of the Personal Training Department at Greenville Technical College in Greenville, South Carolina, and a member of Team PlantBuilt competing in physique. She is a regular contributor to the online magazine, Definition Fitness, which circulates positive information for plant-powered fitness enthusiasts. You can follow her journey as a self-proclaimed "girly bodybuilder" on Facebook or Instagram.

WHY VEGAN?

How and why did you decide to become vegan?

I grew up in the country surrounded by animals and raised by parents who taught me to love animals and appreciate nature. My diet was not meat-heavy to begin with, but I decided to stop eating beef, chicken, pork and turkey after seeing People for the Ethical Treatment of Animals (PETA) posters and demonstrations on a vacation to Washington, DC, right after high school graduation. I took another step by eliminating milk, cottage cheese, fish and eggs in October 2007, and I always said I couldn't go 100% because it was expensive and I didn't have the resources. I realized that those were just excuses, and I made a full commitment in March 1, 2013. I have always loved all animals, and my choice is rooted in animal rights, but the undeniable health benefits are an added perk.

What has benefited you the most from being vegan?

I am easily able to complete my heavy training load and recover more quickly from it. I can maintain a lower body fat percentage year round and do not have to go to the extreme levels that most non-vegan bodybuilders have to do to prepare for a show, and I never, ever get sick!

What does veganism mean to you?

It means caring for all animals and the environment and trying to do as little as possible to harm or exploit either. I am becoming more ethically driven. I eliminated palm oil this year, and I try to stay informed on those types of issues so I can educate myself and others. I view myself as a walking billboard for the lifestyle, so I do my best to let the fact that I'm incredibly healthy and happy speak for itself. I focus on spreading the message in a caring and educational manner instead of a condescending one. In the end, it's all about compassion for all life.

TRAINING

What sort of training do you do?
I train for the women's physique division of bodybuilding competitions, although I have also dabbled in powerlifting and strongman-style training. I have a background in endurance running and triathlon, but I doubt I'll ever go back to it. If I could train for anything at all it would either be for pole fitness competitions or America Ninja Warrior - opposite ends of the spectrum, I know.

How often do you (need to) train?
I lift weights six to seven days a week, and I do some form of cardio at least five days a week, but it's usually low intensity such as elliptical, riding my hot pink cruiser bike, or walking my dog. I choose not to take a true rest day because I enjoy the mental challenge so much, and I meticulously plan my training splits to make sure no muscles get over-trained. When I am in contest prep I also add high-intensity interval training (HIIT) cardio such as stepmill, battle ropes, tire flipping or sled pushes to help torch fat. I also use stretching, foam rolling and massage for injury prevention.

Do you offer your fitness or training services to others?
I do offer in-person and online services, and I can be found in the Vegan Health & Fitness Magazine directory or connected with via my Social Media outlets.

What sports do you play?
I grew up playing basketball and softball, and taking dance and gymnastics. I don't play any organized sports now, but I have recently completed adventure races including the Tough Mudder and Spartan Beast, and taken trapeze and silks classes at a circus school. I'm serious enough about hiking and geocaching that they may as well be sports!

STRENGTHS, WEAKNESSES & OUTSIDE INFLUENCES

What do you think is the biggest misconception about vegans and how do you address this?
A lot of people think vegans are deathly pale, anemic, sickly and weak. I have clear, smooth, olive toned skin, thick shiny hair, and have been told several times, "You look so healthy...for a vegan" or "You are the healthiest looking vegan I've seen." I hope one day that people will say, "You look so healthy" and leave it at that.

What are your strengths as a vegan athlete?
I add strength and muscle very easily. I went vegan and began my bodybuilding journey at the same time. My body looks drastically different from two years ago, and all my gains can be attributed to plant power. This makes an even more effective argument for vegan bodybuilding because naysayers often ask how much of the muscle was gained before the athlete went vegan.

What is your biggest challenge?
One of my biggest mental and emotional challenges is that I live in the South (of USA) and don't have a vegan fitness community here. Thank goodness it is thriving online. My biggest physical challenge is that I have a naturally thick waist and compete in a sport that favors narrow waists and bodies that create an "X" shape. I have to work that much harder to create a wider upper back and thicker legs to create the illusion of a smaller waist. I also have several old injuries to my right leg that I am constantly rehabbing while I train.

Are the non-vegans in your industry supportive or not?

Meat is "the way" in South Carolina, but I have had mixed reactions here. Females tend to be more supportive than do males, and all the women who I went to posing clinics with last year before my figure competition thought it was fascinating. I have even connected with some vegetarians who compete, and I encourage them to make the transition. One of the biggest knowledge gaps is that when people say "that must be so hard" or "that takes so much dedication," it proves that most people still view veganism as a diet and not a lifestyle. I just tell them it's not hard at all to do something you believe in.

Are your family and friends supportive of your vegan lifestyle?

My parents have always been my number one fans. Although they do not follow the same lifestyle, their support of my choices grows every year. I have taken over more of the holiday cooking so I can expose extended family to my delicious food. I teach personal training at a community college, and my students are some of my biggest supporters. Most of them had no idea what a vegan was, but I have inspired them to incorporate more plant-based eating and have debunked all the myths that plants can't build muscle. They also love the vegan cupcakes and other treats that I bring them.

What is the most common question or comment that people ask/say when they find out that you are a vegan and how do you respond?

It used to be "Where do you get your protein?" but that one has died down. Recently it's more, "But cows make milk anyway or bees make honey anyway," and I use that as an opportunity to educate them on factory farming and other forms of animal exploitation. Sometimes I'm shocked at some of the basic knowledge people lack. For example, almost every time I talk about eggs I find out that some people don't know that chickens lay unfertilized eggs every day and that not every egg turns into a chicken. I'm also saddened that people think that claims such as "free range" and "grass fed" eliminates the cruelty. I believe that unless every animal who is petted, hugged, or loved, we have a problem.

Who or what motivates you?

Right now I am obsessed with adding strength and muscle for the animals. I know that the more size I can gain and the more weight I can lift, the more seriously vegan bodybuilding (and other sports) will be taken. I wait for that moment when I am on stage and the announcer reveals that I'm vegan. I love wearing vegan gear and striking up conversations with it. When I'm in the most intense stages of contest prep, I am fueled by animal cruelty. I think about how much is taken away from so many animals, and I think about how they never have a choice. I have a choice, and I choose to put my 100% into my training and diet. It's so much more motivating and meaningful to know that I am training to save the animals and to change people's perspectives instead of just to look "perfect" one night on a stage.

FOOD & SUPPLEMENTS

What do you eat for Breakfast?

Usually oats with banana and peanut or almond butter, and then my "second breakfast" is a protein shake and grapefruit.

What do you eat for Lunch?

Sweet potato, tofu and green veggies such as kale, broccoli, lima beans or Brussels sprouts sprinkled with nutritional yeast and spritzed with Braggs liquid aminos.

What do you eat for Dinner?

"First dinner" is quinoa and homemade seitan (Vital Wheat gluten) with green veggies. "Second dinner" is brown rice, tofu, avocado and more green stuff, usually a blend of spinach, mushrooms and onion with black pepper.

What do you eat for Snacks - healthy & not-so healthy?

Berries blended with nuts and protein powder to make a protein pudding is my favorite last meal of the night, but I also love experimenting with making my own variations of hummus and pesto as well as layering all sorts of combinations of foods on top of rice cakes.

What is your favourite source of Protein?

My favorite shakes are made with Raw Fusion or Plant Fusion protein powders because I like the fun flavors of banana nut, chocolate peanut fudge, cookies 'n cream and chocolate raspberry, but I also love tofu, tempeh, seitan and quinoa.

What is your favourite source of Calcium?

Almond milk, tofu and green veggies.

What is your favourite source of Iron?

I love pepitas and usually add them to my aforementioned spinach, mushroom and onion blend.

What foods give you the most energy?

I have felt better after adding at least two cups of kale per day into my diet and also love the natural energy from bananas.

Do you take any supplements?

For daily vitamins, I take a multivitamin, Iron, B12, calcium, magnesium, and CoQ10 for headache prevention, and turmeric and glucosamine with MSM for joint health. I take CLA and L-carnitine to help me lean out for my show, and I also take creatine at pre-workout, and BCAAs when I am training intensely.

"I am becoming more ethically driven. I eliminated palm oil this year, and I try to stay informed on those types of issues so I can educate myself and others. I view myself as a walking billboard for the lifestyle, so I do my best to let the fact that I'm incredibly healthy and happy speak for itself."

ADVICE

What is your top tip for gaining muscle?

Lift HEAVY! Go for weights that you can only lift six to twelve times, and make sure to increase to the next weight up when those become easy. I also really like to use drop sets, which is stripping off weight when I have reached failure and making myself continue with more reps at a lighter weight. Increasing pyramids, which is lifting with a moderate weight to failure and then increasing the weight for fewer reps, is another favorite. Make sure to take in complex carbohydrates and protein after a workout to begin recovery and repair the tissues.

What is your top tip for losing weight?

For me, it is making sure I'm not eating too much right before bedtime and reducing the amount of fats I'm eating - I like nut butters and coconut oil too much. But, also spacing food out throughout the day so I'm never too hungry or too full and making sure I eat when I'm hungry instead of letting my appetite take over.

What is your top tip for maintaining weight?
One of the easiest ways to maintain weight is to not obsess about it! Enjoy exercise and enjoy eating, making sure to only eat treats in moderation. Trying to restrict too much leads to overeating and all sorts of added stress that won't do your efforts any good.

What is your top tip for improving metabolism?
As I said before, don't get too full or too hungry, also drink plenty of water and add high-intensity interval training (HIIT) into your program.

How do you promote veganism in your daily life?
I wear slogan shirts when I can (I practically lived in my PlantBuilt vegan muscle team hoodie this winter) because I know they are good conversation starters. I try to keep a lot of positive things on my social media channels, such as showing how delicious my food is (I have a "food porn" album on my FaceBook page) and commenting about how wonderful my health and performance are as a vegan.

How would you suggest people get involved with what you do?
If someone wants to compete in any form of bodybuilding, then he or she needs to figure out which division best matches his or her physique. Connect with other vegan competitors and possibly find a vegan trainer or coach, even if the training has to be online. Watch bodybuilding shows in person or through videos to see what it really looks like. Set a goal competition date in your mind and start training for it. You can wait farther along in the journey to pay the registration fee, buy a suit and do all the other required things, so you can always change your mind without losing money. Lastly, if you want to do figure, physique or bodybuilding, get off the cardio machines, lift heavy weights, and eat whole foods!

"When I'm in the most intense stages of contest prep, I am fueled by animal cruelty. I think about how much is taken away from so many animals, and I think about how they never have a choice. I have a choice, and I choose to put my 100% into my training and diet. It's so much more motivating and meaningful to know that I am training to save the animals and to change people's perspectives instead of just to look "perfect" one night on a stage."

Always Encourage, instead of Judge (yourself and others)

ESTHER OAKLEY
VEGAN FITNESS FANATIC

Germantown, Maryland, USA
Vegan 2009

abcvegan.com
SM: *FaceBook, Pinterest, Twitter*

Esther Oakley is a Vegan Lifestyle Coach and plant-based nutritionist, offering personalized coaching for individuals looking to go vegan or merely to incorporate some meatless meals and learn about eating healthier. She also offers menu consultation services, helping restaurants add meatless items to their menus to make more restaurants accessible for everyone.

Esther works and blogs at A,B,C,Vegan, where she helps new vegans, experienced vegans, and the merely curious explore this wonderful new world, giving inspiration, motivation, and community for a vegan lifestyle. She teaches the hows (recipes), the whys (health and compassion for animals), the whats (ingredients), and anything else readers want to see.

WHY VEGAN?

I'm vegan because now that I know all of the information about the health benefits, disease prevention, and animal compassion, it's impossible to ignore.

How and why did you decide to become vegan?
I did it as an experiment over 4 years ago after reading about the health benefits, and I never stopped. The more I learned and the more I saw how my body felt on this diet, the more I wanted to keep going.

How long have you been vegan?
Over 5 years.

What has benefited you the most from being vegan?
Now I feel like I'm truly living for the first time ever. My body has more energy and I want to do more. I've become an athlete in at least 6 different activities. I was never an athlete before in my life. On the mental side of things, the compassion towards animals extends to compassion to people, and I feel like my mind is much more at peace than ever before.

What does veganism mean to you?
I think it comes down to health - both physical and mental. My body feels wonderful now, and I also know that I am living in a way that will keep my healthy for a long time to come. Mentally I feel that I am doing the best I can to live in harmony with every other being on the planet, and that allows for a much more calm, even, steady approach to life.

"Any time I have a moment of craving based on some nostalgic memory or good smell wafting by, I'm motivated to stick with it by everything I've learned about compassion for animals and meat, dairy, and egg industries."

TRAINING

What sort of training do you do?
Depends what new activity I've gotten involved in. I do strength and cardio through rock climbing, pole dancing, triathlons (swimming, biking, running), and yoga. I also did a program recently that focused on high intensity training, through bodyweight exercises and cardio.

How often do you (need to) train?
After the program I did recently I try to do some form of training 6 out of 7 days a week.

Do you offer your fitness or training services to others?
Not yet, though I hope to offer pole dance lessons soon, and to teach at a pole studio.

I do however offer Vegan Lifestyle Coaching, and exercise is absolutely a component of the coaching program. I work on helping others eat healthier, whether that means going fully vegan or just exploring the Meatless Monday idea. I work with where people are and where they want to go.

What sports do you play?
See above.

STRENGTHS, WEAKNESSES & OUTSIDE INFLUENCES

What do you think is the biggest misconception about vegans and how do you address this?
I think it's two-fold:
1. That we're not healthy, that we're weak, etc. I address this by living through example. I'm stronger and healthier than ever, and people see that. They see that I can climb walls and flip upside-down on the pole and that my diet is only helping me build strength - certainly not hindering me.
2. That the food is terrible. Again, addressed by living through example. I bring wonderful dishes to any gathering I attend, and have people who know that anything I bring is just going to be good. I even have one friend who has told me she would go vegan if I would be her personal chef.

Are your family and friends supportive of your vegan lifestyle?
I am extraordinarily lucky to be blessed with incredibly supportive family and friends. They may not have been convinced (yet), but everyone in my life goes out of their way to make sure there's always vegan food available, to bring vegan food when they come to my house, etc. They love what I make and food is never an issue. That being said, I have people who question the idea, who challenge me on it, but it's never in a critical way, just in a learning-from-each-other way, and I value their input highly. Keeps me learning, keeps me thinking.

Who or what motivates you?
Any time I have a moment of craving based on some nostalgic memory or good smell wafting by, I'm motivated to stick with it by everything I've learned about compassion for animals and meat, dairy, and egg industries.

FOOD & SUPPLEMENTS

What foods give you the most energy?
Greens. Leafy greens, and my green smoothie. It's amazing how much I start craving greens when I'm eating them on a regular basis.

Do you take any supplements?
B12.

ADVICE

What is your top tip for gaining muscle?
Work at it, and track your progress. We live in a culture where we want immediate results, and that doesn't happen here. It takes time to build up muscle, and you might not notice the small incremental changes - but when you suddenly can do 10 pushups no sweat when 4 weeks prior you couldn't do a single one - that resonates, that means something. And then it builds on itself, to keep you going for the next milestone.

How do you promote veganism in your daily life?
Leading by example. Being passionate about what I believe in, while not being pushy. If people get me started talking about veganism or my different exercise activities, they can't get me to shut up! I try to be conscious of where are other people are at, and respect that we all started out as not vegan, so everyone's on their own journey.

How would you suggest people get involved with what you do?
Find me at A,B,C,Vegan, on FaceBook and Twitter. Check out my blog, comment, share, and contact me if you're interested in coaching. I would love to help anyone out there begin to explore, get more committed, learn how to cook better - whatever your personal need is, I'm here to help.

Now I feel like I'm truly living for the first time ever. My body has more energy and I want to do more. I've become an athlete in at least 6 different activities. I was never an athlete before in my life. On the mental side of things, the compassion towards animals extends to compassion to people, and I feel like my mind is much more at peace than ever before.

To Supplement, or Not?

- Vitamin B12 is the only vitamin that you cannot get from a 100% plant-based diet. Supplement with tablets or spray. A lot of vegan products also have fortified B12 added.
- Unless you live in a place where it's sunny (and you are outside) most of the year, you may need to supplement Vitamin D - just like non-vegans do - or eat fortified products.
- Also be aware of Iodine, Calcium and Iron levels.
- Please don't share misleading or incorrect vegan health information that may jeopardise another person's health. It's important that vegans are aware of real FACTS about the diet. People with health and nutrition credentials are the people to listen to.
- For factual, evidence-based nutrition information, please see theveganrd.com and veganhealth.org

FIONA OAKES
VEGAN MARATHON RUNNER

Asheldham, Essex, England, UK
Vegan since: 1972

towerhillstables.com
SM: *FaceBook*

Fiona Oakes is a Vegan Marathon Runner and fire fighter from the UK, who also cares for over 400 rescued animals at Tower Hill Stables Animal Sanctuary in Asheldham, UK. Fiona has come top 10 in several international marathons (Florence, Moscow, Amsterdam and Nottingham) and top 20 in London and Berlin. In 2013, Fiona broke three marathon world records – all certified by Guinness and is the fastest female to run a marathon on each continent – something she achieved in less than 24 hours (23h 27m.) She also won the North Pole marathon and the Antarctic Ice marathon in 2013 – both in new course records.

WHY VEGAN?

When and why did you decide to become vegan?
I became vegan at around 6 years old. It was just a natural progression from vegetarianism. I decided to become vegetarian at the age of 3 or 4, as soon as I was able to make a conscious decision. I have been vegan all of my adult life.

What has benefited you the most from being vegan?
Obviously, the health benefits of being vegan are written in stone but I honestly believe the most benefit to me being vegan is that I do not carry the burden of guilt that I would have to endure knowing that I abused others for my own 'benefit'.

What does veganism mean to you?
Veganism is everything to me. It touches every part of my life. It is my life. I could not begin to imagine living my life any other way. It's not just the diet, but also the lifestyle and the life choices I have made through my veganism, such as starting the Tower Hill Stables Animal Sanctuary and my marathon running.

TRAINING

What sort of training do you do?
I run a maximum of 90 to 100 miles (144-160 kilometers) a week when seriously training for a Marathon.

How often do you (need to) train?
I split my training into 10 sessions divided between speed and endurance.

Do you offer your fitness or training services to others?
I always respond to anyone who is seeking advice regarding their running and combining it with a vegan diet, but I always say that everyone is different and I can only tell them what has worked for me.

What sports do you play?

I used to cycle competitively, row and now I run marathons. Recently I took up the ultimate challenge of the Marathon des Sables that I completed - the first ethical vegan woman to do so.

STRENGTHS, WEAKNESSES & OUTSIDE INFLUENCES

What do you think is the biggest misconception about vegans and how do you address this?

I think the biggest misconception of vegans is that we are weak - often people think we are weak in body and mind. They mistake our compassion for weakness. This is why I took up the ultimate challenge of the Marathon des Sables, the toughest foot race on the planet, which is renowned for making grown men cry!

What are your strengths as a vegan athlete?

My strengths as an athlete are that I am not an athlete for myself. I am doing it for the benefit of others, which makes me work much harder to achieve. I am not selfish enough to want something this badly for myself. It makes me push myself that bit harder knowing that by doing well I can possibly convince others to consider a vegan lifestyle. It does work too. Once, when I won a Marathon in a massive course record, the Mayoress who was presenting the prizes told me her daughter had wanted to go vegetarian but she was against it as she was not convinced it would be ideal for a young girl who was still growing. Seeing what I had just done on a vegan diet had convinced her that it was okay for her daughter, which was the biggest prize I could ever want!

What is your biggest challenge?

My biggest challenge is fitting everything I have to do into a day. I have the Tower Hill Stables Animal Sanctuary to look after with its 400 residents, my training and my work as a retained Fire Fighter.

Are the non-vegans in your industry supportive or not?

The non-vegans in my sporting and fire fighting life can be very skeptical of my veganism but when they see what I can do that usually shuts them up.

Are your family and friends supportive of your vegan lifestyle?

My family and especially my Mother have always been supportive of me.

What is the most common question/comment that people ask/say when they find out that you are a vegan and how do you respond?

The most common question I get asked is "Where do you get those enormous muscles from?" I answer "From my wonderful, healthy diet of course!"

Who or what motivates you?

The only motivation I need is to know that I am helping others. I don't care where or what, just as long as I can use my life to benefit someone else less fortunate than myself. That is all that matters to me.

FOOD & SUPPLEMENTS

What do you eat?

I don't actually have a set pattern of regular eating such as breakfast, lunch and dinner. Due to my lifestyle, it is impossible, as I never know what I am going to be doing or where I am going to be from one minute to the next. I only actually eat when I am hungry and when I do it tends to be nuts, fresh fruit, rice, pulses and bread. I do not spend too long analysing my diet. I know what works for me but that might not suit everyone.

I think people need to be less hung up about food, follow their own eating patterns and work out what their body needs rather than always being told what to eat by others. My biggest piece of advice is to know yourself and listen to your body. Ultimately, it will tell you all you need to know if you have the wisdom to listen.

What is your favourite source of Protein?
Mainly lentils and nuts. I swear by almonds and pine nuts.

What is your favourite source of Calcium?
Broccoli, kale, cabbage, almonds and figs.

What is your favourite source of Iron?
Sesame seeds, leafy vegetables and, of course, spinach.

"I think the biggest misconception of vegans is that we are weak – often people think we are weak in body and mind. They mistake our compassion for weakness."

ADVICE

What is your top tip for losing weight and toning up?
I don't actually really think about gaining or losing weight or weight training to tone up etc. I live a very, very active lifestyle getting up at around 3:30am and basically doing manual work all day, either at the Sanctuary, at the Fire Brigade or actually doing my running training. I guess my energetic lifestyle is my cross training. I only really train either with rowing on my Concept 2 rower or running.

My weight is pretty much static whatever I do but, if you do want a top tip to losing weight I would have to say enter the Marathon des Sables. I lost 6 kilos (13 pounds) in one week running it but this is rather extreme as it is 155 miles (249km) in the harshest Desert conditions you can imagine, crossing the toughest terrain carrying a backpack with all your supplies, weighing around 12 kilograms (26 pounds).

How do you promote veganism in your daily life?
I promote veganism through my daily life as a fire fighter, as a marathon runner and by rescuing animals at my Tower Hill Stables Animal Sanctuary.

How would you suggest people get involved with what you do?
I encourage people to get involved the best they can to help my sanctuary, and other animal sanctuaries continue to provide a safe and happy life for the animal inhabitants.

"The only motivation I need is to know that I am helping others. I don't care where or what, just as long as I can use my life to benefit someone else less fortunate than myself. That is all that matters to me."

FRANZ PREIHS
VEGAN ULTRA-ENDURANCE CYCLIST

Graz, Austria, EU
Vegan since: 2008

franzpreihs.at
SM: *FaceBook*

Franz Preihs is a professional vegan ultra-endurance cyclist who spends most of the year training and participating in different ultra-endurance events worldwide. He has completed most of the world's longest and toughest endurance cycling races like RAAM (Race Across America 3000 mile nonstop), Le Tour Ultime (the tour of France nonstop), XX-ALPS (crossing the alps nonstop with over 50000 meters of vertical climbing), Crocodile Trophy in Australia, Race Around Slovenia, Alpentour and many more.

WHY VEGAN?

I grew up in the hardcore music scene, with lots of vegan straight-edge bands. When I was about 20, I started to become straight edge and simultaneously became vegetarian then vegan after a couple of months.

How and why did you decide to become vegan?
It went hand in hand with becoming straight edge.

How long have you been vegan?
I have been on a vegan diet from 2000 until 2006 and again from 2008 until now.

What has benefited you the most from being vegan?
I simply feel more comfortable with myself and I can look into every animal's eye with respect.

What does veganism mean to you?
For me, being vegan and living straight-edge is a personal way of life. I don't actually care too much about humans, but I am very active with animal liberation work.

TRAINING

What sort of training do you do?
I am a professional cyclist, so most of my training is cycling. I also do a lot of climbing and mountaineering.

How often do you (need to) train?
I train about 20-30 hours per week endurance, plus around 10 hours a week climbing or pumping iron.

Do you offer your fitness or training services to others?
I do a lot of motivational speeches for public audiences and I am also involved in a campaign for "sober" living.

STRENGTHS, WEAKNESSES & OUTSIDE INFLUENCES

What do you think is the biggest misconception about vegans and how do you address this?
Most people are curious that I am able to ride my bike 3000 miles (4828km) nonstop on a vegan diet – they wonder if I can get enough calories and protein from a plant-based diet. But basically I don't explain too much. It's my life, my way, my rules.

What are your strengths as a vegan athlete?
I feel "cleaner" somehow and I burn thing easier.

What is your biggest challenge?
Being vegan is no challenge at all.

Are the non-vegans in your industry supportive or not?
I really don't care about the support of non-vegans. They can do whatever they like to do – as long as they don't want to argue with me.

Are your family and friends supportive of your vegan lifestyle?
Basically, it's the same as above. Since I was a kid, I've lived it my way. I really don't care too much about this kind of support.

What is the most common question/comment that people ask/say when they find out that you are a vegan and how do you respond?
I don't discuss - I do my own thing. If they ask, I tell them that I am vegan. If they ask, I tell them that I am vegan. If they are not vegan, they will not understand it anyway.

Who or what motivates you?
My performance in endurance sports motivates me.

FOOD & SUPPLEMENTS

What do you eat for Breakfast?
Soy milk and banana shake, two slices of wholegrain bread and some cashews.

What do you eat for Lunch and Dinner?
All sorts of pasta, rice and potatoes, with vegetables and bread.

What do you eat for Snacks - healthy & not-so healthy?
Cashews, macadamia nuts, bananas, apples and smoothies.

What foods give you the most energy?
I think I can go really well on wholegrain pasta.

Do you take any supplements?
I don't add any supplements to my diet except a vegan multi-mineral supplement.

ADVICE

What is your top tip for gaining muscle?
Maximum strength training 3 times, maximum 8 repeats with maximum weight.

What is your top tip for losing weight?
Endurance training.

What is your top tip for maintaining weight?
Eat a lot of carbohydrates eg rice and pasta.

What is your top tip for improving metabolism and toning up?
Endurance training mixed with a low-fat and low-carbohydrate diet.

How do you promote veganism in your daily life?
I work close together with Austrian vegan platform vegan.at and I support Animal Liberation Racing. Their jerseys are available to athletes worldwide supporting the same cause. My goal is to raise awareness of the unethical treatment of animals helping the guys with my promotion work.

How would you suggest people get involved with what you do?
Check me out on FaceBook or on my website and watch me perform in the world's toughest endurance races!

Keep Going!

It takes 4 weeks
For You to see your Body Changing.

It takes 8 weeks
For your Friends and Family.

It takes 12 weeks
For the rest of the world.

GEORGES LARAQUE
VEGAN RETIRED ICE HOCKEY PLAYER

St-Hubert, Quebec, Canada
Vegan since: 2009

georgeslaraque.com
SM: *FaceBook, Twitter*

Georges Laraque is a former 13-years National Hockey League (NHL) player, best selling author, motivational speaker and Deputy Leader of the Green Party Canada. His best-selling biography, "The Story of The NHL's Unlikeliest Tough Guy", goes well beyond the stereotype of the tough guy. It is the story of a true humanitarian, an engaged citizen not only in his immediate community, but on the global stage as well. Since his retirement, Georges has been very active as a speaker. He has been invited to hundreds of events and has spoken on various topics such as sports, motivation, racism, bullying, veganism, business, charities and politics.

WHY VEGAN?

How and why did you decide to become vegan?
After watching the documentary "Earthlings".

How long have you been vegan?
Since 2009.

What has benefited you the most from being vegan?
I recovered from asthma and high blood pressure where I no longer need medication. I'm also stronger, healthier and have more energy.

What does veganism mean to you?
Consuming or wearing no animal products, being compassionate towards animals, beneficial to our own health and the best way to help our planet.

TRAINING

What sort of training do you do?
Running, biking, skating, weight lifting and cross training.

How often do you (need to) train?
5 days a week.

Do you offer your fitness or training services to others?
Yes, see my website.

What sports do you play?
Hockey, soccer, also I run half and full marathons.

STRENGTHS, WEAKNESSES & OUTSIDE INFLUENCES

What do you think is the biggest misconception about vegans and how do you address this?

People think we don't eat anything. A typical question is "what do you guys eat?" then I give a whole list of various foods I do eat. They're surprised when they realize it's even more then what they're eating.

What are your strengths as a vegan athlete?

Definitely my physical abilities.

What is your biggest challenge?

Doing a full Ironman, which I intend to do someday.

Are the non-vegans in your industry supportive or not?

The majority are, yes.

Are your family and friends supportive of your vegan lifestyle?

Yes, but they like making jokes about it. For example, if they bring me dinner, they cut their grass and put it in a bag for me. I always respond, "I'd rather eat your grass then eat dead animal corpses." They then change the subject!

What is the most common question/comment that people ask/say when they find out that you are a vegan and how do you respond?

"How you get your protein?" or "How you keep your muscle?" Then I go on and on about how I eat quinoa almost everyday, lots of grains, all kind of beans, green vegetables, a lot of Vega products especially the 100% protein powder after every work out etc.

Who or what motivates you?

The fact that everyday more and more people are becoming more conscious about the real issues in our world. They are becoming more open to veganism, understanding animal cruelty, understanding what meat and dairy product does to their body, understanding the impact on our environment. Every day, the number of vegans grows as well as restaurants adjusting their menus to cater to vegans. I think we're on the right path.

FOOD & SUPPLEMENTS

What do you eat for Breakfast?

Vega shake with fruit.

What do you eat for Lunch?

Quinoa salad.

What do you eat for Dinner?

Chilli.

What do you eat for Snacks - healthy & not-so healthy?

Vega bars.

What is your favourite source of Protein?

100% Vega protein powder.

What is your favourite source of Calcium?

Green vegetables, mostly kale.

What is your favourite source of Iron?
Green vegetables.

What foods give you the most energy?
Fruits. Everything with sugar gets me hyper.

Do you take any supplements?
No.

ADVICE

What is your top tip for gaining muscle?
Vega protein shake.

What is your top tip for losing weight?
Adopting a raw vegan diet.

What is your top tip for maintaining weight?
Eating healthy.

What is your top tip for improving metabolism?
Eating healthy.

What is your top tip for toning up?
Adopting a raw vegan diet and working out.

How do you promote veganism in your daily life?
I speak at conferences all over the place but also I have discussions with people every day about veganism.

How would you suggest people get involved with what you do?
Email me through my website, I do so many different things - pick your fight and join forces with me.

"My motivation is the fact that everyday more and more people are becoming more conscious about the real issues in our world. They are becoming more open to veganism, understanding animal cruelty, understanding what meat and dairy products does to their body, understanding the impact on our environment. Every day, the number of vegans grows as well as restaurants adjusting their menus to cater to vegans. I think we're on the right path."

GLENN MARTIN
VEGAN EXERCISE ENTHUSIAST

Brisbane, Queensland, Australia
Vegan since: 2008

glennmartin.blogspot.com.au
SM: *Instagram*

Glenn Martin is a 28-year-old Brisbane man who loves fitness, nature, yoga, cooking and travelling. He is always looking for a new challenge, enjoys illustrating and volunteering in social justice issues, and lives by the motto: "This, too, shall pass," encouraging one to appreciate each moment.

WHY VEGAN?

How and why did you decide to become vegan?
My brother was constantly telling me about the ethical dilemma of eating meat but I didn't want to hear about it. I knew it was wrong but I wanted to eat it. This was at the same time I started having some blood pressure problems. I tried reducing the amount of salt and fat in my diet (reduced a lot of meat and dairy) and as a result my blood pressure improved and I started feeling better. Once I realised that I didn't need to eat meat and dairy to be healthy, it became ethical, as I couldn't justify eating it.

How long have you been vegan?
I became vegan in May 2008 (vegetarian for a year before that). So this year will be 8 years. Almost ready for my 10 year badge!

What has benefited you the most from being vegan?
I feel more positive. I feel like I am making a worthwhile effort to tread lightly on this world and the creatures that we share it with.

What does veganism mean to you?
Veganism is a way of life. It influences what I eat, what I wear, what companies I support, and has made me a much more passionate and caring person.

TRAINING

What sort of training do you do? How often do you (need to) train?
I usually do resistance training 4 times a week, yoga 3 times a week, rock climbing once a week and do as many walks, cycles and stair climbs (at work) whenever I get a chance.

Do you offer your fitness or training services to others?
Not currently but I have studied a Certificate III & IV in fitness and a Bachelor of Nursing prior.

What sports do you play?
At the moment I am really into rock climbing and yoga. Both are a great physical and mental workout.

STRENGTHS, WEAKNESSES & OUTSIDE INFLUENCES

What do you think is the biggest misconception about vegans and how do you address this?

I have destroyed most of my friend's misconceptions that being vegan is boring or tasteless by cooking them awesome meals. I have destroyed the misconception that you can't be healthy and excel on a vegan diet by being a positive healthy role model. The one I am tackling at the moment is that even though people know it can be done and that it's healthier and you can be happier, they still think it's all too hard. They say they could probably go vegan, but couldn't give up cheese or other foods. They could easily do it; they just have to believe it is a worthy enough cause.

What are your strengths as a vegan athlete?

I am more positive and have more energy. I seem to recover fast.

What is your biggest challenge?

I've done a half marathon and that pushed me to my limit.

Are the non-vegans in your industry supportive or not?

Most people are very supportive and curious.

Are your family and friends supportive of your vegan lifestyle?

They are now. There were a lot of misconceptions and jokes to start with, but a lot of that has faded and there is a much more positive attitude towards not eating meat. It also seems more common now than in 2008.

What is the most common question/comment that people ask/say when they find out that you are a vegan and how do you respond?

I think a lot of people ask how long I have been vegan for to see if it's just a phase. When I tell them almost nine years they can see that it isn't a phase and that it is achievable and has great results.

Who or what motivates you?

I want to be happy, and eating great healthy food and exercising helps me achieve that. Thinking of the footage I saw in the documentary "Earthlings" is enough motivation to never eat meat again.

FOOD & SUPPLEMENTS

What do you eat for Breakfast?

Homemade bean patties with herbs, lemon juice, avocado, tomato, cucumber and kale.

What do you eat for Lunch?

Usually a salad or vegetables with rice or pasta.

What do you eat for Dinner?

Usually gluten-free toast with peanut butter, and a smoothie.

What do you eat for Snacks - healthy & not-so healthy?

Nuts, fruit and raw bars mainly. Sometimes I bake an orange and almond cake or fruit cake and polish that off pretty quickly - my weakness!

What is your favourite source of Protein?

At the moment I would say beans. Just can't get enough of them – and no I am not always farting!

What is your favourite source of Calcium?
Fortified soy milk. Mainly because a large portion of your Recommended Daily Intake (RDI) is in one easy hit.

What is your favourite source of Iron?
Beans! They are so so high in Iron. One tin of beans has 44% of your RDI. I always eat them with foods high in Vitamin C to aid absorption and avoid tea, coffee and calcium rich foods at the same meal as they inhibit the absorption.

What foods give you the most energy?
Salads, smoothies and fresh juices make me feel light and full of energy.

Do you take any supplements?
I take a multivitamin that's high in Iron and B12.

ADVICE

What is your top tip for gaining muscle?
Increase your weights slowly. A good baseline would be 3 sets of an exercise, 8-12 repetitions each set, 70% of your one rep maximum. Eat a good meal of protein afterwards to aid in rebuilding muscle.

What is your top tip for losing weight?
70% of weight loss is from the food you eat. Reduce highly processed foods. Go back to the basics of fresh produce. Where you can, cut back on adding sugar and oils or fats to cooking. Exercise is great too but you will never outrun a bad diet.

What is your top tip for maintaining weight?
Find the balance right for you between what you are eating and what you are expending. Eat in tune with your exercise - not out of habit or routine. If you exercise more, you eat more. If you get into a routine of eating more but stop exercising, the weight will pile on.

What is your top tip for improving metabolism?
Resistance training will increase your lean muscle mass. Lean muscle burns more energy than fat does, hence, you will be burning more energy throughout the day. Smaller, more regular meals also helps to speed up the metabolism.

What is your top tip for toning up?
Best way to tone up is a combination of resistance training to increase that muscle, and then cardio and eating healthy to reduce the layer of fat that is covering those beautiful muscles.

Don't look for quick fixes and diet fads. They will fail just as fast – they always do, that's why we always have new diet fads. The best diet and exercise tip is to live healthy.

How do you promote veganism in your daily life?
At work I always turn up with delicious looking meals that everyone comments on and asks questions about. I try to lead by example. If I am happy, looking fit and healthy, then people notice that.

How would you suggest people get involved with what you do?
I think everyone should really take a moment to evaluate what is important in life. People try to make their lives so busy. They want an expensive house, car or material items so they have to work harder and longer to get it. They aren't happy along the way and often compromise their fitness, health and social life. I believe people should go back to the basics. Simple food, simple exercise, work less, stress less and you will find people are happier and healthier. Live simply. Live in the now.

GLYNN OWENS
VEGAN EXERCISE ENTHUSIAST

Glendowie, Auckland, New Zealand
Vegan since: 1976

auckland.academia.edu/RGlynnOwens

Glynn Owens grew up in the post-war slums of the UK. As a small child he avoided exercise but took up judo when 16, going on to hold several titles, represent, Britain, fight in Japan at the age of 40 and finally retire aged 46 after taking second place in the 1997 New Zealand championships. He has also competed (with little success but lots of fun) in many other sports and spent several years as a contemporary dancer.

Since turning 60 his activities have been dominated by circus aerials, particularly flying trapeze and aerial silks, and more recently pole dance. Glynn helps other sportspeople, (he is a clinical psychologist, and a Professor at Auckland University) working with professional teams and Olympians. He lives in Glendowie with his partner, a distance runner (she has represented both Wales and New Zealand) and a cat who simply regards him as another staff member.

WHY VEGAN?

How and why did you decide to become vegan?
Easy one this - I'm generally soppy about animals, and when a former girlfriend explained to me what was involved in the dairy industry it made sense to go vegan completely.

How long have you been vegan?
Since 1976.

What has benefited you the most from being vegan?
Having a clear conscience. Perhaps also notable is when I turned vegan I was 58Kg (128lb). Yesterday I was 58Kg (128lb) - certainly an easy way to maintain a healthy weight.

What does veganism mean to you?
Perhaps surprisingly, these days, it's no big deal - it's so easy, with so many alternatives to meat, milk etc. Even the supermarket shelves are crammed with soy milk - though must admit that lately I've started making my own.

"Keep a 'benchmark' of things you think you should do. For example, if I could no longer bench press my own body weight, I'd start working on the weights until I could do so again; if I couldn't run 5km (3miles) in less than 25mins I'd do more running – so set your own goals, and ensure you keep within your own limits."

TRAINING

What sort of training do you do?

My sports have varied over the years - these days I'm mostly concentrating on rock climbing and various circus activities (especially flying trapeze), though as part of keeping in shape for that I also do some running, weights, stretches etc.

How often do you (need to) train?

When I was a serious competitor I'd train once or twice a day, e.g. run in the morning and perhaps a weights and gym session later in the day. But I'm not competing seriously now, and have reverted to doing things for fun! Which means I can take my training at a rather more leisurely pace.

Do you offer your fitness or training services to others?

My circus skills certainly aren't good enough to enable me to offer guidance to anyone else - but climbing is always a cooperative activity, so yes, basically those of us in our group all help and encourage each other.

What sports do you play?

These days mostly rock climbing and circus stuff. In the past I've competed in a whole heap of sports, most of which I was very bad at, a few at which I was okay and one or two I did quite well. My main success in sport was as a judo player - I was a national student champion and a Great Britain international competitor when I'd been vegan for at least three years. I made various comebacks at different times - I was North Wales champion at 39, toured Japan for a series of matches when 40, and had my last appearance in the New Zealand national championships (I took second place) when 46. At that point I really probably had to admit that it's more a sport for young people.

I was a sort of ordinary club-level distance runner for a while, with a marathon time somewhat under 2 hours 50 minutes and a 10mile (16km) time (sorry about the archaic units) of 57 minutes. Most sports, though I was pretty bad at, and some I enjoyed even though I was totally unsuited. As a decathlete, for example, a 1.65m (5'4") 58Kg (127lb) competitor isn't really going to have much impact on the 1.9m (6'2") 95Kg (209lb) bundles of muscle who usually do it - though at least I could beat some of them in the final event, the 1500 metres. I was also a modern pentathlete for a while in the UK, and a triathlete, but I'm a pretty terrible swimmer - I've done the Rangitoto to St Heliers (Auckland) swim 6 or 7 times, but always very slowly. These days I'm mostly having fun climbing and swinging through the air.

STRENGTHS, WEAKNESSES & OUTSIDE INFLUENCES

What do you think is the biggest misconception about vegans and how do you address this?

Hmmm, not sure I can say - most people I know are aware I'm vegan, and they don't seem to have any distorted view of me. Perhaps the biggest misconception is that it's difficult to be vegan!

What are your strengths as a vegan athlete?

Well, it does seem easy to maintain a constant body weight.

What is your biggest challenge?

Probably ensuring that I keep an adequate Iron and B12 intake.

Are the non-vegans in your industry supportive or not?
I work at the University of Auckland and seem to meet more and more vegans there every year.

Are your family and friends supportive of your vegan lifestyle?
Oh yes, I think quite a few would probably like to give it a try - but of course for some it's quite a big step.

What is the most common question/comment that people ask/say when they find out that you are a vegan and how do you respond?
At least these days, people know what it means. Usually it's just a question about protein, iron or something similar.

Who or what motivates you?
To be vegan? I can't imagine not being after all this time. To train? I love the things I do.

FOOD & SUPPLEMENTS

What do you eat for Breakfast?
Muesli and cereals usually with fruit (dried and/or fresh) added, and (now home-made) soy milk.

What do you eat for Lunch?
Sandwiches of some kind - Auckland's vegan shop has a wealth of possible fillings, and my home-made wholemeal walnut bread is very tasty - a testament to the automatic bread maker, not to any skill of mine.

What do you eat for Dinner?
Usually something involving tofu - very often with avocado - a splendid combination.

What do you eat for Snacks - healthy & not-so healthy?
Not sure I have many - occasionally a treat of vegan chocolate or the like, if I've visited the shop in town. Otherwise things like fruit - grapes, oranges etc.

What is your favourite source of Protein?
Definitely tofu - fresh, fried, marinated, firm, silky - I love them all.

What is your favourite source of Calcium?
Probably the almonds I put into my soy milk recipe.

What is your favourite source of Iron?
Hard to say, have always ensured I keep some iron supplements in the diet anyway.

What foods give you the most energy?
By definition those with the most calories!

Do you take any supplements?
Yes, iron, folic acid, B12, calcium - and multivitamins.

"I promote veganism by being me. I enjoy life - more so than most people I know. It's an example, I don't nag people to follow it but it's there if they think they'd like to try it - and if they do I'm more than happy to help."

ADVICE

What is your top tip for gaining muscle?
Heavy weights of which you can only do a few (3-4) repetitions.

What is your top tip for losing weight?
Not really an expert, but basically you can't beat distance running for cutting down fat.

What is your top tip for maintaining weight?
Match your intake to your activity - if you've slowed down the training, keep an eye on the calories.

What is your top tip for improving metabolism?
Lots of activity - don't miss an opportunity - walk instead of riding, take the stairs instead of the lift and so on.

What is your top tip for toning up?
Keep a 'benchmark' of things you think you should do. For example, if I could no longer bench press my own body weight, I'd start working on the weights until I could do so again; if I couldn't run 5km (3miles) in less than 25mins I'd do more running - so set your own goals, and ensure you keep within your own limits.

How do you promote veganism in your daily life?
By being me. I enjoy life - more so than most people I know. It's an example, I don't nag people to follow it but it's there if they think they'd like to try it - and if they do I'm more than happy to help.

How would you suggest people get involved with what you do?
With being vegan? Join the Vegan Society, talk to vegans, go to the vegan shop, do a bit of reading and so on. With climbing? Come along to the climbing gym (mine is Extreme Edge in Panmure, Auckland) and join in. With circus? Same sort of thing - come to Auckland's Dust Palace and have fun with the rest of us. Basically, just decide what you'd like to try and give it a go!

"Food is the most abused Anxiety Drug.
Exercise is the most Under-utilised Antidepressant."
- Bill Phillips

Don't start a diet that has an expiration date.

Focus on a lifestyle that will last forever.

Heather Nicholds
VEGAN EXERCISE ENTHUSIAST

Ottawa, Canada
Vegan since: 2008

heathernicholds.com
SM: *FaceBook, Google+, Instagram, Pinterest, Twitter, YouTube*

Heather Nicholds is a Registered Holistic Nutritionist, showing you how to have fun while making simple, fast, healthy and incredibly delicious meals that leave you and your family satisfied and full of energy. She shares vegan recipes and health tips in her free weekly videos, and offers more comprehensive information resources - like nutritionally-balanced online meal plans and health-oriented video cooking classes.

WHY VEGAN?

How and why did you decide to become vegan?
I decided to become vegan when I learned about the massive environmental impact of animal agriculture. I quickly learned more about the health benefits and ethical issues, which only made me even more committed.

How long have you been vegan?
I've been vegetarian since 2007, and vegan since 2008.

What has benefited you the most from being vegan?
I really enjoy cooking and eating a lot more than I did before. I think I've found I'm more creative in putting together plant-based meals, and I've started using a lot more interesting flavors, so I enjoy my food more.

What does veganism mean to you?
To me, veganism is a choice to live more consciously and have respect for life – the life of animals, the health of our ecosystem and respect for my own body.

TRAINING

What sort of training do you do?
Right now I'm not training for anything specific, just maintaining my strength and cardiovascular fitness. I've been a competitive synchronized skater off and on since I was 10 years old. I'm not currently competing, but have been since becoming vegan.

I've gotten into running more in the last couple of years. I've done a 12km (7.5miles) trail run, a 15km (9.3miles) race and a half-marathon. I'm not sure if I'll continue racing, but I really enjoy training towards a goal with running. I hope to get more into trail running in future if I live somewhere with good trails. I've also started training with a roller derby team - it's my new alternative to ice skating. I really like the physical and endurance challenge, and also the team building aspect.

How often do you (need to) train?

Training for skating was 2 days a week on ice. For my own personal fitness, I run 5-6 days a week (ranging from 5-10km/3-6miles), I do body weight strength training 4-5 days a week, and I cycle and practice yoga a few days a week.

What sports do you play?

I still figure skate whenever I can, play tennis occasionally and am a big fan of frisbee. I also do a lot of hiking, and last year did a big hike up a volcano in Peru called El Misti (of course eating vegan the whole way up) and had no fitness or altitude issues. We hiked from 11,200' to 19,000' in about 12 hours of hiking time, overnighting at 15,000'. It was an amazing, unforgettable experience.

STRENGTHS, WEAKNESSES & OUTSIDE INFLUENCES

What do you think is the biggest misconception about vegans and how do you address this?

That vegans can't be strong and fit. I address it by keeping myself in good shape without letting myself get too skinny, and by sharing the stories of amazing vegan athletes and bodybuilders.

What are your strengths as a vegan athlete?

I seem to have a lot of endurance – more so than before. I'm also able to recover fairly quickly, so I can keep doing some kind of training on a daily basis. I find that when I have meals, I don't feel heavy – I feel energized.

What is your biggest challenge?

My biggest challenge is maintaining my training when I travel and visit with people. I sometimes have trouble keeping up to my regular schedule when I'm on planes and trains and buses, and when I'm on someone else's time. The great thing about running is that I don't have to travel with any equipment, I can do it anywhere, and it doesn't take any extra time. That's the reason I stick with body weight workouts, although I would love to work out with some weights at some point. I have an audio podcast that I download to keep doing yoga on the road. It's helpful after a long flight, and is a good exercise if the weather's not good for running and I have to be quiet (i.e. no jump squats).

Are your family and friends supportive of your vegan lifestyle?

Totally – my family and friends are always curious about what I'm doing and what I'm eating, and have made major changes in their lifestyle and diet along with me. It's really fantastic to see, and I'm grateful to have such wonderfully supportive people in my life.

What is the most common question/comment that people ask/say when they find out that you are a vegan and how do you respond?

'Don't you get bored with the food?' My response – never! I have so much more fun making meals now – more than I did when I ate meat. I find the flavors are fresher, more vibrant. I taste my food more, and I enjoy every bite.

Who or what motivates you?

The way I feel – healthy, happy and energized – and the wonderful people around me (friends, family and clients/viewers) motivate me to keep being the best I can be.

FOOD & SUPPLEMENTS

What do you eat for Breakfast?
a) smoothie with a banana, berries, flaxseeds, sprouts (or another green) and protein powder or
b) porridge with flaxseeds and some fruit (apple, pear, plum, berries, etc).

What do you eat for Lunch?
A big salad with lots of veggies, some kind of bean or legume (chickpeas and edamames are my favorites) and tahini dressing.

What do you eat for Dinner?
A smaller salad or lightly steamed/sauteed vegetables with a cooked grain or sweet potato/squash and tahini or avocado dressing.

What do you eat for Snacks - healthy & not-so healthy?
I love making my own chocolate-protein spread with some mashed banana, protein powder, cocoa and/or carob powder and just enough almond milk or water to make a spread. Then I put that on a rice cracker – sometimes I mix in some crystallized ginger or dried cranberries. If I feel like salty, I spread some nut butter on a rice cake, sprinkle with sea salt and serve with lettuce, cherry tomatoes, cucumber or sprouts. This is also really nice with avocado in place of the nut butter.

I also love having fruit with some nuts, like an apple with almonds or a pear with Brazil nuts. I sometimes have dark chocolate, or make myself dark hot chocolate sweetened with maple syrup. Chai tea lattes with almond milk and a dash of maple syrup are also a regular treat. I do also like making healthy cookies and squares and muffins, but I don't make them too often because I wind up eating more than I should.

What is your favourite source of Protein?
Beans, legumes, grains, greens, nuts, seeds, spices and every single plant food. I do use protein powders for an easy source of calories and to increase the proportion of protein relative to carbohydrates and fats. I like brown rice, quinoa, hemp and pea proteins.

What is your favourite source of Calcium?
Sesame seeds, almonds, dried figs, broccoli, chickpeas, lentils, kale... again, beans, legumes, grains, greens, nuts, seeds, spices and every single plant food give a lot or a little.

What is your favourite source of Iron?
Beans (chickpeas, lentils), legumes, greens (spinach, parsley, chard, beet greens), molasses, quinoa, cocoa, seeds (sunflower, sesame), cashews. The key with iron is to make sure it gets absorbed properly, so I also make sure to have lots of vitamin C, and not have black tea or coffee at the same time.

What foods give you the most energy?
Fruits are my go-to for energy. They taste amazing, so they wake up my tastebuds, and they have easily-absorbed sugars to get me going. They also digest really well, so I don't have to wait long until I can get moving.

Do you take any supplements?
Yes – I take a low dose of a multivitamin (which includes vitamins B12 and D2 and calcium), a vegan DHA and occasionally a probiotic and/or digestive enzyme.

ADVICE

What is your top tip for gaining muscle?
Training (with weights or bodyweight) is the way to gain muscle, and your diet can only be a support. You can't eat your way to muscles.

What is your top tip for losing weight?
Keeping your diet in check with healthy whole foods in appropriate portion sizes is the key to losing weight. Training can support and speed up your metabolism and weight loss, but the key on this side is diet.

What is your top tip for maintaining weight?
Make sure you get enough calories and nutrients to fuel and nourish your body.

What is your top tip for improving metabolism?
Do cardio and strength training on a regular basis, and eat clean whole plant foods.

What is your top tip for toning up?
Start where you can, in a way that you'll stick with it. You don't have to be crazy about it at the start, and it's far more important to keep training long term than it is to follow a specific program.

How do you promote veganism in your daily life?
I post videos on my site every week to show how easy and fun it is to make simple, healthy meals. In my personal life, I try to be as healthy and positive as possible to show those around me the impact that a healthy vegan lifestyle can have.

How would you suggest people get involved with what you do?
They can sign up on my website for a free meal plan and transition guide and weekly updates from me.

"I decided to become vegan when I learned about the massive environmental impact of animal agriculture. I quickly learned more about the health benefits and ethical issues, which only made me even more committed."

"If it doesn't challenge you,
it doesn't change you."
- Fred Devito

If you wait for things to be perfect, you'll never get anything done.

HOLLY NOLL
VEGAN GO-KARTER AND FITNESS FANATIC

Bay Area, California, USA
Vegan since: 2005

fitquickmix.com
SM: *FaceBook, Google+, Instagram, Twitter*

Holly Noll loves Go Karts, Fitness and Food. Her journey began by growing up in the food industry, heavily inspired by her father, grandmother and their traditional styles, then learning to twist them into healthier, plant-based, versions. Along the way she's worked with some amazing restaurants and people including: Cafe Gratitude as the pastry chef, which changed her vision of what could be done with healthy, raw, food. In Seattle, she met and joined an awesome team and created Vegan Shortcake, an ongoing cooking and lifestyle show, then moved back to California, became certified in Plant-Based Nutrition from eCornell and started her most recent project Liberation Food and Lifestyle. Holly also became serious about racing shifter karts and much more dedicated to training both for her own fitness addiction as well as faster times and more laps.

WHY VEGAN?

How and why did you decide to become vegan?
I realized the insanity in killing for meat early in my teen years, which had been a huge step coming from the meat and butter loving chef family that I do, but in my late teens I got into anarchism and found myself in a house in the mission district of San Francisco, CA. I picked up a small feminist 'zine that had only a page or so article on the connection between women's struggle for sexual equality, reproductive rights and against violent sexual oppression and the female struggle of other species in the dairy industry. I realized I could not fight for the equality of my species/culture's women while actively oppressing another. That day I went vegan, against hypocrisy and oppression, and in solidarity.

How long have you been vegan?
Over 8 years.

What has benefited you the most from being vegan?
It has given me so much - it is beginning to sound borderline religious. At first I'd say that it gave me awareness, a sense of being awake to even more, though this was painful as it is still today. Consciousness is not an easy burden to carry. Then, I think, it gave me a connection to where in my career I wanted to go as a chef. Purpose. The next step was health and education, and now I know that it also gives me protection against so many chronic diseases that are so prolific in our world. Veganism has also given me the ability to recover my physical self faster as well as a much better awareness of what I'm putting in myself and how it effects me. Of course, it has certainly isolated me and made things more difficult in some regards but the benefits have far outweighed the challenges and in many ways the challenges are what I'm fighting to break down.

What does veganism mean to you?
Veganism, to me, means maintaining a lifestyle that better reflects the world I want to live in.

TRAINING

What sort of training do you do?
I do Crossfit-style workouts, weights, as well as trail running.

How often do you (need to) train?
6 days a week.

Do you offer your fitness or training services to others?
Nope, I'm a chef, but I am also deeply into fitness.

What sports do you play?
I race shifter karts. I would like to start competing in CrossFit soon as well.

STRENGTHS, WEAKNESSES & OUTSIDE INFLUENCES

What do you think is the biggest misconception about vegans and how do you address this?
Ya know, I think it's interesting just how many misconceptions there really are. As a chef the biggest is definitely that the food is boring and can't be made to be tasty, or at very least, even come close to as tasty as flesh food. In the rest of society the biggest one that I've come across is that it's very difficult. I think all movements have encountered this because people are afraid of sticking out. Being vegan is more difficult in that there is more thought that goes into it, but really, when you think about it in this context, do you wish to live your life with less thought going into your actions?

What are your strengths as a vegan athlete?
In the short term: definitely recovery time and drive.
In the long term: not consuming supplements and foods that will cause diseases in the future, shortening my ability to train.

What is your biggest challenge?
Not over-eating because healthy vegan food is delicious and I want to try everything.

Are the non-vegans in your industry supportive or not?
Nope, not really, but they are curious.

Are your family and friends supportive of your vegan lifestyle?
Yes, now they are. It took a good bit of time for them to come around that my career as a chef and my part of our family wasn't seriously diminished by my lifestyle but now they respect what I believe and how I want to live as well as the ground I'm part of breaking in cutting edge healthy, vegan, foods.

What is the most common question/comment that people ask/say when they find out that you are a vegan and how do you respond?
"But what do you eat?" This is usually connected with the obnoxiously over-asked protein question. My response varies from person to person. I try to tailor my responses to inquiries to the person so that I can be more effective with each individual, staying warm, understanding and helpful. I usually respond with describing a few delicious sounding meals quickly then briefly hit the protein centerpieces to ease their mind then go into quickly talking about protein sources and flavor profiles. My other favorite comment is "But... You don't LOOK like a chef" and that's when I

get to talk about how being a vegan chef makes me not have bad skin, awful body composition and a short, diseased, life.

Who or what motivates you?
My motivation comes from fighting for a better world, as well as those who fight beside me.

FOOD & SUPPLEMENTS

What do you eat for Breakfast?
Smoothie of cold-pressed coffee, almond milk, banana, cacao powder, a few berries, protein and ice with a touch of vanilla and cinnamon. Along with unsweetened oatmeal with fresh fruit or a homemade protein bar usually including nuts, seeds, protein, cacao, and dates.

What do you eat for Lunch?
Lunch is usually my post-workout and changes constantly but is always my big meal of the day. Some examples are chickpea fritters filled with caramelized peppers and onions, spinach, and herbs. Crimini mushrooms topped with eggplant hummus. Curry with quinoa fritters over fresh greens. Raw onion wrap full of greens, avocado and grilled asparagus. I like to have fun with food.

What do you eat for Dinner?
I don't really eat dinner. My bigger meals are stacked at the beginning and middle of the day and at night I usually just snack on something like Beyond Meat, greens, cucumber and oil-free hummus and some sweet chia protein soft serve.

What do you eat for Snacks - healthy & not-so healthy?
Greens or cucumber with oil-free hummus, apples with cinnamon, nuts or seeds bars, chia jam on bananas or chickpea bread, berries, kombucha. On race days my "snacks" are really important because they're what give me fuel at the track as eating big meals doesn't work well in this context. My track snacks usually consist of super nutrient-dense bars, lots of fruit, and chia kombucha.

What is your favourite source of Protein?
Cruciferous veggies, seeds or hemp, protein powder and Beyond Meat.

What is your favourite source of Calcium?
Dark leafy greens, figs and tofu.

What is your favourite source of Iron?
Spirulina, quinoa and lentils.

What foods give you the most energy?
Fruit, for sure. I love foods that have probiotics such as kombucha, but fast-digesting carbohydrates and a little fat do the trick perfectly. Lemon water and smoothie with chia seeds, fruit, a bit of fresh raw coconut milk, cold-pressed coffee and dates is the perfect whole food pre-workout.

Do you take any supplements?
I love PlantFusion protein powder, chocolate. It kills my chocolate craving and I make "frappuccinos" with it that make my heart beat faster. I also take zinc and magnesium before bed but in general I try to stay away from supplements, especially since reading Dr Campbell's book "Whole" and giving a lot of thought to how my body responds to the nutrients given to it and in what form that takes.

ADVICE

What is your top tip for gaining muscle?
Sleep, drink water, eat enough and high intensity workouts with heavy weight.

What is your top tip for losing weight?
Drop grains and sugar, add water, sleep, eat clean carbohydrates and do intense, heavy, workouts.

What is your top tip for maintaining weight?
Eat clean, drink water, sleep, and meditate.

What is your top tip for improving metabolism?
Green tea, lemon water, probiotics and time control of food.

What is your top tip for toning up?
Cut sodium, add green juice, sweat and sleep.

How do you promote veganism in your daily life?
My primary goal in promoting veganism is to show people that it's not a sacrifice. That you can eat delicious food, that is also clean, healthy and vegan that beats flesh foods out on all levels. I also believe in leading by example. Many of the people I know who have gone vegan were inspired by the amount of energy I have, how I look and how delicious the food I eat is. I find that this is more effective for me than telling them what they're doing wrong or being critical. Positive reinforcement is my favorite way of going about showing people the vegan lifestyle rules. By showing that vegan food can be more amazing than flesh foods and that vegans can be strong, active and awesome, I think, is a great way to promote the lifestyle. Many people are unhappy in their lives and if they see a better way - a way to look, feel and be better - and it just happens to help the world suck less, than they're likely to get into it

How would you suggest people get involved with what you do?
I keep everything updated on my Instagram account, so that would be the best way to keep up to date. Check out Definition for Ladies, an online magazine I'm part of. Also FitQuick my protein waffle business, or just go vegan and represent!

"In my late teens I got into anarchism and found myself in a house in the mission district of San Francisco, CA. I picked up a small feminist 'zine that had only a page or so article on the connection between women's struggle for sexual equality, reproductive rights and against violent sexual oppression and the female struggle of other species in the dairy industry. I realized I could not fight for the equality of my species/culture's women while actively oppressing another. That day I went vegan, against hypocrisy and oppression, and in solidarity."

Jaclyn Gough
VEGAN NPC FIGURE ATHLETE

Lauderdale-by-the-Sea, Florida, USA
Vegan since: 2013

theskinnyvase.com
SM: *FaceBook*

Jaclyn Gough is a triplet, floral designer and a National Physique Committee (NPC) figure athlete. She is extremely passionate about health and fitness and was actually going to become a personal trainer before becoming a floral designer in 2007. Some of her floral work can be seen on her blog The Skinny Vase. Jaclyn got into competing at the age of 19, completed three shows living in Maryland and one show in Florida where she currently lives. There she placed 1st at a National Qualifier. Currently, Jaclyn's boyfriend Nick Tumminello is her trainer and her nutrition coach is Claudia Lailhacar.

WHY VEGAN?

How and why did you decide to become vegan?
I made the final cut to stop eating animal products forever after crying over a slice of pizza, because I knew deep down by eating the cheese I was contributing to animal cruelty. I no longer wanted to associate myself and my lifestyle with cruel behaviors.

How long have you been vegan?
I've been vegan since May 2013.

What has benefited you the most from being vegan?
My mind is clearer, my heart is happy and my health continues to soar by feeding my body with plant-based foods.

What does veganism mean to you?
Veganism is a way of life. For me, it means not contributing to the pain and suffering of animals or other beings. Veganism means living compassionately.

TRAINING

What sort of training do you do?
Hybrid Training.

How often do you (need to) train?
4-5 times a week.

Do you offer your fitness or training services to others?
No. I am not a personal trainer.

What sports do you play?
I am an NPC (National Physique Committee) Figure Athlete.

STRENGTHS, WEAKNESSES & OUTSIDE INFLUENCES

What do you think is the biggest misconception about vegans and how do you address this?
That we need animal protein to gain muscle and animals were put here for us to eat so we can survive.

What are your strengths as a vegan athlete?
My strengths continue to go up in the gym through weight training almost every time I train. I also believe I can run better than before when I was a meat eater, because I am feeding my body with the nutrient-dense foods and no animal flesh to slow me down.

What is your biggest challenge?
Being better than I was the day before.

Are the non-vegans in your industry supportive or not?
Once someone in this industry finds out I am vegan they are surprised. Those who are not supportive I tend to weed them out of my life because I have no room for negativity.

Are your family and friends supportive of your vegan lifestyle?
Let's just say they are slowly coming around. At first, it was a big struggle and no one understood why I refused to eat animal products no matter how many times I would give them my reasons. My friends are used to it and become amazed when I tell them I too can eat pizza and nachos - mine just have different ingredients!

What is the most common question/comment that people ask/say when they find out that you are a vegan and how do you respond?
I've had people ask, "So does that mean no cheese or fish?" My response is anything that came from an animal I do not eat. When I show others photos of my physique, they are shocked but it is true a body can be built and run on plants.

Who or what motivates you?
I admire all athletes, people who are determined, set goals and chase after them. I am motivated by all the vegan athletes from Vegan Bodybuilding & Fitness - their posts, photos and support motivates me to be better. I am also motivated when I hear that I am an inspiration to others to become healthier.

FOOD & SUPPLEMENTS

What do you eat for Breakfast?
Oats, protein powder, berries & coconut oil.

What do you eat for Lunch?
Tofu, veggies, any type of carbohydrate eg sweet potato or rice.

What do you eat for Dinner?
Lentils with nutritional yeast and veggies.

What do you eat for Snacks - healthy & not-so healthy?
Healthy: Chia seed pudding. Not-So Healthy: Raw vegan chocolate mousse pie. Note: My diet varies every couple weeks, on and off-season of competition preparation.

What is your favourite source of Protein?
Lentils.

What is your favourite source of Calcium?
Soybeans.

What is your favourite source of Iron?
Pumpkin seeds.

What foods give you the most energy?
Bananas mixed with protein powder, berries and peanut butter before training.

Do you take any supplements?
I consume a plant-based protein powder and try to consume vitamins and minerals through whole foods. I don't like to think of myself as a "pill popper!"

ADVICE

What is your top tip for gaining muscle?
Lift heavy weights.

What is your top tip for losing weight?
Lift heavy weights, stop being a cardio bunny or like a hamster on a wheel.

What is your top tip for maintaining weight?
Eat wholesome foods, have a splurge meal if you want and stop depriving yourself.

What is your top tip for improving metabolism?
Interval training, gain muscle, add a cup of green tea with a meal or two and eat breakfast.

What is your top tip for toning up?
Lift heavy weights.

How do you promote veganism in your daily life?
Inform others of the benefits of a vegan diet, the downside of where their food actually comes from and I share what works for ME. I'm proud to be vegan but I also try not to preach my beliefs and put them on others as if my way of life is better than someone else. Lastly, share the love! If I choose to make a yummy treat, I'll bring to work and share or give a copy of Vegan Health & Fitness to a friend so they can learn about my lifestyle.

How would you suggest people get involved with what you do?
Check out Vegan Health and Fitness online and purchase the magazine. Connect and look up other vegans, athletes, activists or health enthusiasts. Don't be scared to approach a vegan and ask questions.

"I admire all athletes, people who are determined, set goals and chase after them. I am motivated by all the vegan athletes from Vegan Bodybuilding & Fitness – their posts, photos and support motivates me to be better. I am also motivated when I hear that I am an inspiration to others to become healthier."

Jaie Nelson
VEGAN PARKOUR PRACTITIONER

Adelaide, South Australia, Australia
Vegan since: 2013

facebook.com/groups/144536568987921

Jaie Nelson is a 25-year old male, who consider himself to be extremely active if not hyperactive. He has been vegan for over two years and feels amazing for it. Jaie works as a Health Consultant, is a practitioner of the discipline Parkour, the founder of the volunteer group Vertical Freedom Parkour, a martial artist and also recently become addicted to calisthenics.

WHY VEGAN?

How and why did you decide to become vegan?
My wife and I first became vegetarian to save money after our wedding, and two months after that I just woke up one morning turned to her and said, "I'm vegan from now on." My mind and body just told me to do so.

How long have you been vegan?
I have been vegan now for over two years.

What has benefited you the most from being vegan?
I feel the most functional and clean I have ever been, functional being in my training and mental state. Clean being internally. I also found that after 3 months of being vegan I grew in my already immense love of animals and really started noticing the debauched state we treat animals in society.

What does veganism mean to you?
Veganism for me was the next step in my physical and mental purification of my body. It was not just a change in diet, but a way of life and a new way to view the world.

TRAINING

What sort of training do you do?
I am a Traceur (Parkour Practitioner) and am also heavily involved in calisthenics.

How often do you (need to) train?
I feel I need to train every day. Personally, I don't believe in rest days.

Do you offer your fitness or training services to others?
I started a volunteer group, Vertical Freedom - we hold regular Parkour training sessions and all our work we do for free.

What sports do you play?
None.

"I feel the most functional and clean I have ever been, functional being in my training and mental state. Clean being internally. I also found that after 3 months of being vegan I grew in my already immense love of animals and really started noticing the debauched state we treat animals in society."

STRENGTHS, WEAKNESSES & OUTSIDE INFLUENCES

What do you think is the biggest misconception about vegans and how do you address this?
I feel the biggest misconception about vegans is that we all are unhealthily thin and non-functional. When I hear this said I can't help but jump up and show off a Parkour or Calisthenics technique that leaves the instigator speechless.

What are your strengths as a vegan athlete?
I have become more flexible, which helps a lot, and as I mentioned above I feel more functional and energized constantly.

What is your biggest challenge?
I don't believe I have any.

Are the non-vegans in your industry supportive or not?
Not particularly. I work at a gym so at times I get bombarded by the rubbish 'ideals' of other Personal Trainers.

Are your family and friends supportive of your vegan lifestyle?
They are. My wife is vegetarian however we always eat vegan, both my family and in-laws are hugely supportive, when we come around for tea they both make and eat vegan meals too.

What is the most common question/comment that people ask/say when they find out that you are a vegan and how do you respond?
We all know it's, "Where do you get your protein and iron?" I respond to this by explaining that there are plenty of other natural sources of both and that these are more easily absorbed by our bodies.

Who or what motivates you?
Three things: My constant striving to be the most functional I can be, my wife Shayli, and a colleague at work who is also vegan and has been a lot longer than myself.

FOOD & SUPPLEMENTS

What do you eat for Breakfast?
Hot cacao, and a fruit smoothie (only using fresh water system, reverse osmosis water.)

2nd meal: Something light and quickly digested eg. tabbouleh or quinoa salad.

What do you eat for Lunch?
A rice or rice noodle dish eg. Laksas, or vegan sushi.

4th meal – Again something light and also fruit.

What do you eat for Dinner?
Varies, but I do enjoy vegan Indian meals.

What do you eat for Snacks - healthy & not-so healthy?
Homemade hummus, and vege chips.

What is your favourite source of Protein?
Chickpeas.

What is your favourite source of Calcium?
Rice milk.

What is your favourite source of Iron?
Raw spinach or kale.

What foods give you the most energy?
If I have to pick one I'd say my smoothies.

Do you take any supplements?
Sometimes I experiment with trying to make my own non-caffeinated protein pre-workout shakes and drinks - always be cautious as a lot contain hidden animal products.

ADVICE

What is your top tip for gaining muscle?
Eat a lot, frequently, and train muscle groups till exhaustion.

What is your top tip for losing weight?
Eat frequently but in smaller portions and don't snack. Also end all your training sessions with a hard hitting cardio workout.

What is your top tip for maintaining weight?
The saying "eat like a king for breakfast, a prince for lunch and a pauper for tea" comes to mind. Try to get at least 3 -5 workouts in a week.

What is your top tip for improving metabolism?
Through my own experience I can say step up the amount of times you eat. Eat frequently but in smaller portions and don't snack.

What is your top tip for toning up?
See above for improving metabolism. Also I have found training 6-7 times a week works well - I don't believe in rest days.

How do you promote veganism in your daily life?
I talk to a lot of people due to working at a gym and when we discuss diets, I make myself available to answer any and all questions asked.

How would you suggest people get involved with what you do?
I have a lot of mottos to live by. One of my favourites being "shut up and deal with it" - so get yourself out there, and train to be strong and useful.

"Veganism for me was the next step in my physical and mental purification of my body. It was not just a change in diet, but a way of life and a new way to view the world."

James Aspey
VEGAN EXERCISE ENTHUSIAST

Sydney, New South Wales, Australia
Vegan since: 2013

voiceless365.com
SM: *FaceBook, Instagram, Twitter*

James Aspey is a 27-year old vegan health and fitness coach from Sydney, Australia who embarked on a 365-day vow of silence throughout 2014. He educates his clients on exercise, nutrition and positive thinking through various books, movies, meditations and his own personal experiences. It is a privilege for James to be a guide and service to others, and he is grateful every day to have such an amazing job.

WHY VEGAN?

How and why did you decide to become vegan?
I went vegetarian to experience the personal benefits, then during my research became aware of the harsh reality that is happening to animals today and knew I could never, nor would I ever want to go back to eating meat. A few months later after understanding more about the dairy industry, which I previously thought was in no way cruel to animals, I stopped purchasing dairy and only ate it if it was going to be thrown out anyway. A few months later I decided I didn't want to ingest the product of pain and suffering of another living being and have been a happy, thriving vegan ever since.

How long have you been vegan?
Over 2 years.

What has benefited you the most from being vegan?
The joy I get from eating food that isn't causing cruelty and violence towards other living beings.

What does veganism mean to you?
To me, being vegan means to be living in constancy with the belief that violence and unnecessarily inflicting pain, suffering and killing other beings is wrong. It means respecting life and seeing non-human animals as more than just a product to be taken advantage of. It's living the healthiest, most compassionate, most environmentally-friendly way to benefit the whole of nature and Earth's inhabitants.

TRAINING

What sort of training do you do?
Resistance and sprint.

How often do you (need to) train?
Since I've been vegan, far less to maintain a fit, strong and healthy body. I usually train at least three times a week.

Do you offer your fitness or training services to others?
Yes, I've been a Personal Trainer for the last 8 years.

What sports do you play?
Surfing, break dancing, tennis.

STRENGTHS, WEAKNESSES & OUTSIDE INFLUENCES

What do you think is the biggest misconception about vegans and how do you address this?
That what we are doing is extreme and unachievable for most people. I address it by often explaining that if any lifestyle is extreme, it is definitely not the vegans, it is the ones exploiting and murdering innocent animals. Also, by showing how easy and enjoyable it is to be vegan through delicious food and recipes.

What are your strengths as a vegan athlete?
It's so much easier for me to maintain a healthy physical appearance. I've done far less exercise than usual as of late though my body has maintained muscle mass and aerobic endurance far better than I would have in my previous meat and dairy eating lifestyle. Also, the food I eat energises me and makes me want to be active rather than making me feel bloated and wanting to lie down and do nothing.

What is your biggest challenge?
The constant disagreement from people who think they know what they are talking about when it comes to vegan nutrition or the "health benefits" of eating animal products.

Are the non-vegans in your industry supportive or not?
Some are, some are not. That's why it is important to be a shining example of the lifestyle.

Are your family and friends supportive of your vegan lifestyle?
Absolutely, my Mum and Dad are now both vegan and have both lost near 20kg (44lb) and are feeling and looking better than they did 30 years ago. Many friends have also gone vegan and the ones that haven't understand why I am and respect it.

What is the most common question/comment that people ask/say when they find out that you are a vegan and how do you respond?
People ask me, "What do you eat?" I say, "More variety and amazing food than ever before in my life. Veganised versions of everything you eat and then all the rest. Pizza, pasta, smoothies, curries, sandwiches, cakes, ice cream, muffins, stir-fries, burgers, noodles, fruit."

Who or what motivates you?
I'm motivated by the suffering of animals and inspired by every single vegan activist who speaks up on their behalf.

FOOD & SUPPLEMENTS

What do you eat for Breakfast?
Fruit feast, smoothies, oats with berries and nuts.

What do you eat for Lunch?
Zucchini pasta with avocado, chia seeds, sprouts, nutritional yeast. Lentil burgers and salad.

What do you eat for Dinner?
Satay tofu stir-fry. Curry and rice. Roast veg and soy sausages.

What do you eat for Snacks - healthy & not-so healthy?
Banana ice cream.

What is your favourite source of Protein?
Lentils, tofu and tempeh.

What is your favourite source of Calcium?
Tahini.

What is your favourite source of Iron?
Kale.

What foods give you the most energy?
Fruit, especially bananas.

Do you take any supplements?
No.

ADVICE

What is your top tip for gaining muscle?
Do weights slowly and in a controlled manner until you reach failure in each set. Eat a variety of high protein, whole-foods.

What is your top tip for losing weight?
Read "End Emotional Eating" by Dr. Jennifer Taitz.

What is your top tip for maintaining weight?
Figure out how many calories you burn in a day, consume around the same.

What is your top tip for improving metabolism?
Resistance training at least 3 times a week.

What is your top tip for toning up?
Full body and weight training program.

How do you promote veganism in your daily life?
For all of 2014, I was involved in a campaign called Voiceless365, where I took a 365-day vow of silence while travelling around Australia. My blog is about the experience, and about all aspects of animal exploitation, veganism, food, health and all things related. I promote it by being a shining example of a healthy, positive, thriving vegan. I bring up veganism at any given opportunity and strive to educate others on how to take on the lifestyle.

How would you suggest people get involved with what you do?
Visit my website, follow Voiceless365 on Facebook, Instagram and Twitter. Read as many books on veganism and animal ethics as possible. Join all the vegan groups on Facebook. Share all the enlightening quotes and videos. Educate, educate, educate and be the change you wish to see in the world.

I'm motivated by the suffering of animals and inspired by every single vegan activist who speaks up on their behalf.

JARED PALERMO
VEGAN EXERCISE ENTHUSIAST

Charlton, New York USA
Vegan since: 2007

motivecompany.com

Jared Palermo has been working out on and off his entire life through playing sports. In the last few years, he was into recreational weight lifting and now core strength lifting and cardio. Jared helps out with Motive Company, a vegan straight-edge clothing company based out of Upstate New York.

WHY VEGAN?

Why not vegan is the real question?!

How and why did you decide to become vegan?
I became vegan after being vegetarian for 2 years and seeing that while I was vegetarian, I was sort of living hypocrisy. I would not eat meat, but yet I would still purchase shoes that were made of leather or suede, or eat candy that had gelatin in it. After consuming more than my fair share of dairy in the form of cheese I realized I was even more unhealthy, as well as contributing to an industry that I do not see as right.

How long have you been vegan?
It's been over 8 years now since I went vegan and I would not change my decision.

What has benefited you the most from being vegan?
I feel so much healthier and connected to the environment around me.

What does veganism mean to you?
Veganism to me means a few things:
1) Not contributing to the murder, rape, and exploitation of living beings who feel the pain of these injustices and tortures.
2) It is a healthier lifestyle that has less impact on our environment.
3) Does not allow one to be fooled by big industry into believing that an animal's sole purpose is to be abused and consumed.

TRAINING

What sort of training do you do?
Used to be weight lifting and cardio. Now it's changed to more core strength lifting and cardio due to have some injuries from lifting heavier.

How often do you (need to) train?
I tend to try and train at least twice a week. My body tends to require a fair amount of recovery time. I am fortunate that when I am at the gym I am there for over 2 hours and that I have the body type that gains muscle fairly easily.

Do you offer your fitness or training services to others?
I do not currently offer my services to anyone - I am not a licensed fitness trainer. However, I will never turn down helping someone who asks for help or someone I see who may need some friendly advice.

What sports do you play?
I currently snowboard, skateboard, ride my bike, train, do karate, and weight lift. I used to play soccer, track and field, and baseball.

STRENGTHS, WEAKNESSES & OUTSIDE INFLUENCES

What do you think is the biggest misconception about vegans and how do you address this?
The biggest misconception is that vegans are malnourished, weak, and cannot gain muscle size. I try to be a living example to prove these people wrong.

What are your strengths as a vegan athlete?
I feel that because I am vegan I have a better energy level and my strength is 100% natural.

What is your biggest challenge?
My biggest challenge is my recovery time after lifting heavy weights. My body has had its fair share of injuries that I have acquired over the years from playing sports so young and so much.

Are the non-vegans in your industry supportive or not?
Many of my friends are supportive of my lifestyle - they know how passionate I am about what I believe in and live. So I think they are impressed at times to see the gains I've made from working out.

Are your family and friends supportive of your vegan lifestyle?
Yes, my family and friends are supportive of being vegan. Often times my immediate and extended family members are searching for new vegan recipes to try to get my approval of whether they taste good or not. Some of them have also become more aware of animal right issues and have altered their diets in response to it.

What is the most common question/comment that people ask/say when they find out that you are a vegan and how do you respond?
I think the most common question that is asked is "What do you eat?" or "Where do you get your protein from?" I simply just tell them I eat vegan food and get what I need from that. I then continue to inform them where they can buy vegan food and that I gain most of my protein from soy-based products or from beans etc.

Who or what motivates you?
I motivate myself, along with staying vegan for the animals. As well as helping out with Doug DeFriest and Linwood Bingham at Motive Company. A friend of mine, Ed Bauer is an absolute machine when it comes to vegan bodybuilding and fitness. Robert Cheeke has done wonders in bringing vegan bodybuilding and fitness to the mainstream. Those two guys, as well as anyone else involved in the fight for animal rights and veganism are my motivators.

"Do your research. There are countless books, people, and organizations out there to help you. There is even a little thing called the Internet that can be a great start to get your feet wet into an amazing lifestyle. As I like to say. GO VEGAN and STAY VEGAN."

FOOD & SUPPLEMENTS

Disclaimer: I do not have the healthiest eating habits.

What do you eat for Breakfast?

I was never much of a breakfast eater. When I do I will have tofu scramble, toast, or skip breakfast foods and have an early lunch which will either be a vegan burger, vegan chicken wings, vegan pizza, French fries, vegan chicken tenders, vegan nachos, vegan mac and cheese, vegan BLT or sandwich etc.

What do you eat for Lunch?

See breakfast foods above.

What do you eat for Dinner?

Tofu, stir-fry, vegan chili, vegan tacos, vegan chicken breast, vegan chicken or eggplant parm salad, burritos, soup etc.

What do you eat for Snacks - healthy & not-so healthy?

Potato chips, candy, wheat thins and salsa, vegan ice cream, iced tea, soda.

What is your favourite source of Protein?

Soy or beans.

What is your favourite source of Calcium?

Soy milk and multivitamin.

What is your favourite source of Iron?

Broccoli and multivitamin.

What foods give you the most energy?

Vegetables do, even though (as weird as this may sound) I am not the biggest vegetable fan when they are just by themselves. Vegetables provide a higher amount of energy and nutrients. Fruit is also a good energy source as well.

Do you take any supplements?

I take a multivitamin. I have been debating taking vegan protein powder, but have not done so yet.

ADVICE

What is your top tip for gaining muscle?

Take in a lot of calories and lift heavy weights, with low reps.

What is your top tip for losing weight?

Watch your calorie intake, and do cardio and light weights at high reps.

What is your top tip for maintaining weight?

Finding a calorie range that is suitable for you. Do weights and cardio that you are comfortable with and just stay level when doing them. If you don't want to gain more muscle, then don't lift heavier weights that will cause your muscles to grow. If you don't want to lose where you are now, then don't go below the weights and cardio time that you are maintaining now.

What is your top tip for improving metabolism?

I am no professional with diets and fitness training like I mentioned previously, but to improve metabolism eating 5-6 smaller meals a day will help keep your metabolism working, as well as doing cardio and exercise.

What is your top tip for toning up?

I am not very toned, because I go for more of the lift heavy to gain mass type of working out. For toning up, it's all about the foods you eat and the cardio and exercises you do. You want to burn the fat and unwanted calories to get the definition.

How do you promote veganism in your daily life?

I am always willing to talk to someone and have an intelligent conversation of why I live the lifestyle that I do. I do not talk down to people or force my views onto them - even though I'd love the world to be vegan. You have to be realistic and not so confrontational - at least for me I have found the most success that way. The more that I talk to someone on an equal level and explain the truths and benefits of veganism the more accepting those people are. I used to have co-workers who would come into work the next day and be more aware of what they were consuming and were cutting down on certain things after we had conversations the day before or earlier in the week. I know personally I don't want someone forcing upon me that I shouldn't be vegan, so the approach of civil communication has really proven beneficial for me. The more that people see how I conduct myself living this way and am easy to get along with, the more people have made efforts in the right direction.

How would you suggest people get involved with what you do?

Do your research. There are countless books, people, and organizations out there to help you. There is even a little thing called the Internet that can be a great start to get your feet wet into an amazing lifestyle. As I like to say. GO VEGAN and STAY VEGAN.

What is Straight-Edge?

The term means poison-free and comes from the punk and hardcore music scene (in America.) This includes drugs, alcohol, cigarettes, and also can include not engaging in promiscuous sex. A lot of people also agree that the term poison-free includes veganism.

Turn Your Anger into Action.

Lose Excuses to Get Results.

Jeff Golfman
VEGAN EXERCISE ENTHUSIAST

Toronto, Canada
Vegan since: 1998

thecoolvegetarian.com
stepforwardpaper.com
SM: *FaceBook, Google+, Twitter, YouTube*

Jeff Golfman has been an eco-entrepreneur for the last 24 years, is an Honours Graduate of the Ivey School of Business and the Co-Founder and President of Prairie Pulp & Paper Inc. His blog The Cool Vegetarian is a lifestyle site providing inspiration and tools on how to live a healthier, more sustainable lifestyle.

WHY VEGAN?

How and why did you decide to become vegan?
Health reasons. I was overweight and had chronic fatigue.

How long have you been vegan?
Vegetarian for over 24 years, Vegan 15, and raw vegan 9 years.

What has benefited you the most from being vegan?
Improved health, fitness, energy, skin, hair, and eyes.

What does veganism mean to you?
Healthy body, healthy mind, and healthy planet.

TRAINING

What sort of training do you do?
Run, walk, bike, weights and yoga.

How often do you (need to) train?
Run 5-6 times per week, upper body weights 1-2 times per week, daily yoga, walk 2-3 per week.

Do you offer your fitness or training services to others?
Not officially, but on my website, I feature many athletes for inspiration and advice for others at no cost.

What sports do you play?
I run in races for fun.

I am motivated by making the world a better place through a plant-based diet, exercise and environmental stewardship.

STRENGTHS, WEAKNESSES & OUTSIDE INFLUENCES

What do you think is the biggest misconception about vegans and how do you address this?
The protein myth is the biggest misconception. It is easy to get enough protein by eating enough fruits, vegetables, seeds, nuts, ancient grains, beans and seaweeds.

What are your strengths as a vegan athlete?
As an amateur, non-elite athlete I try to do my best to achieve my athletic goals by performing well in my age category. My raw and vegan diet gives me lots of energy, great cardio capacity and quick recovery times.

What is your biggest challenge?
Juggling full time career/work, 100 airplane rides per year and training.

Are the non-vegans in your industry supportive or not?
They are very curious, inquisitive and playful. Not negative but often poke fun.

Are your family and friends supportive of your vegan lifestyle?
Same as above, and they often come to me for health advice.

What is the most common question/comment that people ask/say when they find out that you are a vegan and how do you respond?
The protein question is # 1 by a landslide. I give the facts and do not judge or cause any discomfort for the person asking.

Who or what motivates you?
I am motivated by making the world a better place through a plant-based diet, exercise and environmental stewardship.

FOOD & SUPPLEMENTS

What do you eat for Breakfast?
Fruit and smoothies, or chia pudding and fruit.

What do you eat for Lunch?
Fruits, salads and juices.

What do you eat for Dinner?
Salads and juices or quinoa and veggies.

What do you eat for Snacks - healthy & not-so healthy?
Fruits and nuts.

What is your favourite source of Protein?
Greens, seeds and quinoa.

What is your favourite source of Calcium?
Seeds.

What is your favourite source of Iron?
Seeds and greens.

What foods give you the most energy?
Fruit smoothies and chia seeds.

Do you take any supplements?
Vitamin B and D, digestive enzymes, and probiotics.

ADVICE

What is your top tip for gaining muscle?
Increase calories and do weights.

What is your top tip for losing weight?
Increase calories, decrease fats, increase cardio, increase water.

What is your top tip for maintaining weight?
Eat good fat sources, exercise, get enough calories.

What is your top tip for improving metabolism?
Eat low fat, eat often, and consume raw vegan, local, organic, non-GMO foods.

What is your top tip for toning up?
All of the above and do lighter weights with more repetitions.

How do you promote veganism in your daily life?
Through my actions, attitude and website.

How would you suggest people get involved with what you do?
Go to the "Give Help" of my website.

Always Be Prepared:

- Pack snacks when travelling
- Ring restaurants beforehand
- Bring your own food to events

"Nobody makes a greater mistake than he who does nothing because he could only do a little."

- Edmund Burke

More Muscle = More Calories Burned.

Jennifer Moore
VEGAN EXERCISE ENTHUSIAST

Memphis, Tennessee, USA
Vegan since: 2005

vegwell.com
SM: *FaceBook*

Jennifer Moore is a plant-based Registered Dietitian and Certified Personal Trainer. She achieved undergraduate training in nutrition from Mississippi State University. She then went on to intern at Vanderbilt University Medical Center in Nashville, Tennessee. This is where plant-based nutrition was first introduced to her. Her Master's degree is also in nutrition from Central Michigan University where her research into plant-based nutrition pushed into full veganism. Professionally, Jennifer works as a clinic dietitian and personal trainer in the specialty of nephrology and wellness/prevention in the Memphis, Tennessee area. Personally, she eats a plant-based diet in the non-conducive environment of the deep South. Jennifer is the mother of four precious babies and the proud wife of a 20-year Air Force veteran.

WHY VEGAN?

How and why did you decide to become vegan?
Coming from the southern state of Mississippi, I never had a thought of eating only plants. As an intern in nutrition at Vanderbilt University Medical Center, I first learned of plant-based nutrition. My preceptor told me to read "Diet for a New America" by John Robbins. I did and the journey began. First, I was in and out of vegetarianism, then a strict vegetarian. After the birth of my third child and after reading "The China Study" by T. Colin Campbell and researching on my own for my Masters degree, I moved on to veganism.

How long have you been vegan?
Since 2005.

What has benefited you the most from being vegan?
My health. My cholesterol as a healthy omnivore was still 220. It is now 145. I dropped from a size 4-6 to a 0-2. I have more energy. My skin is clear. I feel alive!

What does veganism mean to you?
Conscious responsibility and stewardship. Being responsible for my health. Being a good steward of the body God gave me. I have one, no replacements. Being a steward of God's world. It is not mine to destroy. Not supporting factory farming represents a large step in that direction. Seeing humanity as everyone's responsibility including mine. If we would all avoid meat and eat only plants, we could feed the world.

TRAINING

What sort of training do you do?
I run, lift, and do a number of the Beachbody programs.

How often do you (need to) train?
I train 6 days a week. Everyone is different, some more fit than others. It is important to tailor your program to your own personal needs.

Do you offer your fitness or training services to others?
Yes, I am a Registered Dietitian. I work with end stage renal disease patients as well as those whose kidneys are damaged but not yet in need of renal replacement therapy. Additionally, I teach wellness classes and I am a healthy coach - both locally to the Memphis area and online.

What sports do you play?
I play soccer with my children in the yard.

STRENGTHS, WEAKNESSES & OUTSIDE INFLUENCES

What do you think is the biggest misconception about vegans and how do you address this?
With the public, of course, "Where do you get your protein?" which includes that we are weak. In the scientific community, a lack of knowledge of the large research base for plant-based nutrition. I have competed in figure competitions as a plant-based athlete. I am also on the Plantbuilt Team, which totally obliterates the "weak" idea. As for my colleagues, I direct them to plant-based research.

What are your strengths as a vegan athlete?
That I am lean after delivering four children into the world. People ask me what I do. I get to tell them I am vegan.

What is your biggest challenge?
Getting discouraged when people believe the arguments for plant-based nutrition and still don't adopt the diet and lifestyle.

Are the non-vegans in your industry supportive or not?
In the bodybuilding scene, not so much. They cannot fathom building muscle without chicken. As a registered dietitian, if I am given the opportunity to present the research, I gain respect fairly quickly.

Are your family and friends supportive of your vegan lifestyle?
Well, I live in the deep South, so I would say sometimes. I have had family invite me over for dinner and make chicken soup, knowing I won't eat it. I find that terribly rude. My current husband is vegetarian so he is extremely supportive. We have a blended family though and my former husband is not supportive, so that in itself is a huge challenge and a whole other conversation.

What is the most common question/comment that people ask/say when they find out that you are a vegan and how do you respond?
As I said, when people meet me and realize I have four children they are curious about "what I do". When I tell them, a barrage of questioning begins. A common one is, "What do you eat?" I tell them that they have fewer options than me: chicken, fish, beef, pork. I have broccoli, beans, peaches, bananas, Brussels sprouts, cucumbers, tomatoes - and the list goes on and on.

Who or what motivates you?
My children motivate me. I want to be a role model for them. My patients motivate me. I see the power of an unhealthy lifestyle every time I enter a dialysis clinic. My Savior Jesus Christ motivates me. I want to live a life worthy of his calling.

FOOD & SUPPLEMENTS

What do you eat for Breakfast?
Smoothie, with either Shakeology or Sun Warrior protein, and spinach, beet, strawberries, raspberries and peanut butter.

What do you eat for Lunch?
Various cooked veggies with beans or tofu or tempeh.

What do you eat for Dinner?
A large salad (I eat one every day) with soup or beans or tofu or tempeh, and dark chocolate for dessert.

What do you eat for Snacks - healthy & not-so healthy?
Usually fruit, flaxseed crackers, and sweet potato.

What is your favourite source of Protein?
Shakeology or Sun Warrior protein powder.

What is your favourite source of Calcium?
Almond milk.

What is your favourite source of Iron?
Beans, dark leafy greens - in my smoothies and salad.

What foods give you the most energy?
Raw veggies.

Do you take any supplements?
Tumeric, Vitamin D, and Vitamin B12.

ADVICE

What is your top tip for gaining muscle?
Lift heavy.

What is your top tip for losing weight?
More cardio, portion control and DO NOT OVEREAT.

What is your top tip for maintaining weight?
Consistent healthy lifestyle - consistency is key. Stop fad dieting.

What is your top tip for improving metabolism?
Never starve yourself. Never overeat. Avoid fad diets.

What is your top tip for toning up?
Mixture of lifting and cardio. Circuit type workouts are effective.

How do you promote veganism in your daily life?
My actions. People see what I eat at lunch. People learn what I eat when they are around me. I don't have to say a lot. They usually are curious. I also have a website and do a lot of promoting on my FaceBook page as well.

How would you suggest people get involved with what you do?
If they are not vegan, open their mind and read the facts. Just because they were raised one way does not mean it is right. I was raised in the Mississippi Delta - likely one of the unhealthiest places on earth. I am an unlikely vegan. For the vegans, educate. Send people to my website, friend me on FaceBook and let's educate together!

JEREMY MOORE
VEGAN SPEED SKATER

Milwaukee, Wisconsin, USA
Vegan since: 2001

E: *veganpotter@mail.com*
SM: *FaceBook*

Jeremy Moore is a long-time vegan – since October 2001 – who is always willing to speak with anyone about it. In the past, he was a 320lb (145kg) track and field athlete (shot put, discus, hammer) as a vegan and eventually an elite Time Trial specialist on the bike at 190lbs (86kg). For two years Jeremy was on the Philippine National Cycling Team but is now pursuing Long Track Speed Skating with plans to go back to cycling once he gets to the Winter Olympics for skating. He recently won CAT ½ State Time Trial Championships in Wisconson in August 2014. He also has a Bachelor in Fine Arts from Virginia Commonwealth University and plans to eventually go back to being a Studio Potter and hopefully run a vegan restaurant once he's through with his career in sports.

WHY VEGAN?

How and why did you decide to become vegan?
I became vegan after volunteering at an animal shelter in Philadelphia. Being Filipino I had eaten dog meat when I was a kid. I wouldn't have done it in my teens but when I worked at the shelter I saw piles of euthanized cats and dogs and that made me think of what I was eating. Cows, pigs, chickens die for the same reasons; humans create them for our "enjoyment". I didn't want to be a part of that anymore.

How long have you been vegan?
I went vegan in October of 2001 so over 14 years now. I was vegetarian for only 2 weeks before that.

What has benefited you the most from being vegan?
As an athlete, I gained a lot of strength upon becoming vegan but more than anything, I can now live with the choices I make at the dinner table.

What does veganism mean to you?
Killing an animal for selfish reasons is the worst thing anyone can do. To me veganism is a biggest step to living without any guilt - if that's possible. I couldn't imagine an animal being tortured for years of its life, only to be part of my life for a few minutes.

TRAINING

What sort of training do you do?
As an elite cyclist converted to speed skating, I'm an endurance skater which means I can still get away with riding my bike a lot in the off season along with lots of drills and weight training. In season I stick to shorter bike training sessions, along with weights and a lot of ice time.

How often do you (need to) train?

In the off-season I train around 25-30hrs a week - sometimes a bit more. In season the volume drops to around 22-25hrs a week but the intensity is much higher than when I was racing bikes. I could easily handle 35 hours of cycling a week but skating is much more taxing on the body.

Do you offer your fitness or training services to others?

I have advised many athletes on diet and general power and endurance. As a former 320lbs (145kg) national level shot putter I know what it takes to perform on vegan fuel for power sports. However due to injuries I decided to give bike racing a try. After a year, I got most of my weight off and a couple years after that I was winning bike races at 190lbs (86kg). I have experience on both spectrums of sport so I'm always willing to give training advice to athletes, especially young athletes or late vegan converts that my have questions with their diet.

STRENGTHS, WEAKNESSES & OUTSIDE INFLUENCES

What do you think is the biggest misconception about vegans and how do you address this?

Obviously I get a lot of crap about losing muscle or not being able to gain any as a vegan. Well being a 320lbs (145kg) shot putter made it easy to prove that wasn't true. As a cyclist I spend years and years trying to loose as much muscle as possible. I was still around 190lbs (86kg) when winning races, which is actually enormous for a cyclist at my level. Really losing muscle on a vegan diet is pretty difficult.

What are your strengths as a vegan athlete?

I think the biggest thing was recovery. My resting heart rate dropped quite a bit over a couple weeks and I always felt fresher immediately after turning vegan. My personal strengths are now in sustained power rather than the peak power that I had when I was 320lbs (145kg).

What is your biggest challenge?

My biggest challenge is trying to get to the Olympics in Long Track Speed Skating. I hit an Olympic qualifying time for a cycling event five years after being over 300lbs (136kg). However my event, the 4km (2.5miles) pursuit on the velodrome, was pulled from the Olympics so I decided to try something new. The Philippines has never had a Winter Olympian and they have very few vegans in the spotlight. The tough thing is that skating is extremely technical and putting on skates for the first time at 27 years of age is a tough thing to do when you're racing people who have been skating since they were 4. I think I have a shot though. I still have a lot to learn but I'm there physically. I just have to learn the technical stuff.

Are the non-vegans in your industry supportive or not?

For the most part they are. They saw it as a bit odd at first but the first doubts they had in regards to my weight made no sense since I normally have a good 20lbs+ (9kg+) on them. I get people asking me questions about veganism all the time, which is a good thing as I'm always eager to answer questions about veganism.

Are your family and friends supportive of your vegan lifestyle?

Mostly everyone in my family is fairly supportive of my being vegan. However I do feel it's difficult to say you support something like veganism without actually attempting to be a vegan.

What is the most common question/comment that people ask/say when they find out that you are a vegan and how do you respond?

I get the protein question as much or more than any other vegan and the first thing I tell them is that pretty much everyone gets too much protein. This definitely includes vegans. I starved myself of protein as much as I could for years while I was cycling - rarely eating over 50g a day for years - and barely lost any weight at all despite training with a severe calorie deficit. Even with my training regiment I eat little more than 70g a day and I weight around 195lbs (88kg) right now. If anything I need to cut back on my protein rather than increase it.

Who or what motivates you?

Time is my number one motivator. There are so many things I can do in my life but being an athlete has a timetable and I definitely have one considering I'm competing in one of the world's most technical sports but I have actually only had less than a year of actual training on the ice.

FOOD & SUPPLEMENTS

What do you eat for Breakfast?

Typically two bowls of cereal with 1-2 bananas.

What do you eat for Lunch?

Maybe a large salad and some soup or a sandwich.

What do you eat for Dinner?

Something hot, maybe some spicy Mexican food or a stir-fry.

What do you eat for Snacks - healthy & not-so healthy?

Typically I snack on carrots or crackers with peanut butter or hummus. I also toss fruits down throughout the day.

What is your favorite source of Protein?

Nuts and seeds.

What is your favorite source of Calcium?

Kale.

What is your favorite source of Iron?

Probably beans.

What foods give you the most energy?

Most definitely fruits, and also sweet stuff, but only for short/high intensity training or on race day.

Do you take any supplements?

Not really. I do consume VEGA and spirulina but nothing I take really falls into the supplement category.

ADVICE

What is your top tip for gaining muscle?

Be willing to really beat yourself up in the gym. If you aren't sore for days you aren't really lifting hard enough. Also eat. I don't believe protein is the key to building muscle - but calories are! You can't work hard enough for your body to require more muscle if you aren't eating enough carbohydrates to fuel you in the gym for more than a few hard sets. Do a lot of volume and if you have any spring in your step when you leave the gym, turn around!

What is your top tip for losing weight?

Self-control. Long/endurance cardio is the key if you're extremely overweight. If you need to only drop a few pounds I suggest interval training (cardio) mixed in with weights through circuit training. Also if you really want to do it 100% only eat enough to get by. Most people (not athletes) have enough muscle that they could afford to lose some, plus they mostly all have too much fat so eat just enough to get through the day without feeling really sluggish.

What is your top tip for maintaining weight?

Stay consistent and never let anything keep you from being active. It's very easy to get complacent with your weight loss and before you know it you're right back where you were.

What is your top tip for improving metabolism?

Just keep working out. I've never been one to believe overweight people generally have low metabolisms compared to thin people – it's just an excuse. Let's say you have an overweight/lazy person and a thin/lazy person with exactly the same diet. The thin person is perceived to have a high metabolism right? Well I bet 99 out of 100 times the thin person will have a lower resting heart rate and blood pressure than the overweight person.

This is just an example but how can the thin person be burning more calories if their heart is doing far less work? It's easy, the overweight person is storing fat as nature intended. However few animals have access to excess food 365 days a year but this is what should happen if you do eat too much every day. The overeating thin person is actually not functioning properly. Basically everyone that wants to improve their metabolism really just needs to eat less or exercise more - their metabolism isn't going anywhere.

What is your top tip for toning up?

I think the best thing for toning is mid-rep lifts with a bit higher speed. Also cycling only seems to get most people only so far and I think running may get you a bit more toned. While I don't do it I also think the CrossFit type of workout is a great way to get toned up.

How do you promote veganism in your daily life?

I promote veganism as much as I can by working my hardest at being the best athlete I can be. I'm a muscular vegan with a lot of vegan tattoos that I never hide so I get a lot of questions from people that would never even think of asking. However I feel my biggest impact will be in the Philippines where people spend big chunks of their money on meat because they think they need it to be healthy when I can eat whatever I want to eat but I chose to eat only vegetables and I'm much better off for it - and it's cheaper.

How would you suggest people get involved with what you do?

Long Track skating is pretty hard to get into. In the United States there are only two indoor rinks that have a 400m track so you've got to move to Milwaukee, Wisconsin (my location) or Salt Lake City, Utah. If you just want to be a good vegan athlete I say pick something you love to do and work hard at it. Don't be afraid to fail but be afraid of letting up because you may quit just short of success.

Jo McKinley
VEGAN DANCER AND INSTRUCTOR

Amaroo, Australian Capital Territory, Australia
Vegan since: 2002

gdance.com.au
SM: *FaceBook*

Jo McKinley is the Founder, Director & Instructor at Gungahlin Dance Academy. She trained from the age of 6 in many styles of dance including classical ballet, jazz, tap, contemporary, Scottish, cabaret and hip-hop and now runs one of Canberra's most successful ballet programs.

Jo has also been a long-time animal rights activist and vegan and has volunteered for many organisations such as Animal Liberation, PETA, Vegan Outreach, Sea Shepherd and Save Japan Dolphins. She has led many campaigns to help stop animal abuse and exploitation the world over. She currently spends her spare time focusing on vegan education as she has come to believe that veganism is the only moral and ethical baseline.

WHY VEGAN?

How and why did you decide to become vegan?
I had been lacto-ovo vegetarian for 4 years prior. I saw some footage on dairy cows and looked further into free-range eggs and discovered how cruel the egg and dairy industries are. I decided to become vegan when I could no longer deny the fact that the animal cruelty involved in these industries is unacceptable, no matter how much I liked the taste of the products. I remember my last vegetarian meal was a cheese pizza when I was 23. I started out as a vegan because of the animals. Along the way I learned about how a vegan diet has the least impact on the planet compared to an animal flesh-based diet, which is environmentally unsustainable, so that further cemented my ethical standpoint on veganism. Lately, I have been fascinated with the health benefits of raw veganism. I discovered the raw vegan movement about 2 years ago and it made perfect sense to me. I have been eating high raw the last 6 months. I will remain a high raw vegan because I have learnt that eating this way gives us health, vitality, prevents disease, cancer and many other poor health conditions.

How long have you been vegan?
Over 13 years.

What has benefited you the most from being vegan?
I have a clear conscience and wonderful health.

What does veganism mean to you?
Veganism to me means living in harmony with nature. It means rejecting speciesism, a form of discrimination of privilege based on species. It means compassion, health and being part of the solution rather than part of the problem.

TRAINING

What sort of training do you do?
I teach dance 6 days a week and I sing and dance in musical theatre. My physical activity varies from dancing a few hours a week to performing vigorously for 12 + hours a week.

How often do you (need to) train?
If I am not dancing, I might go for a run for half an hour. I'll have a day or two off from exercise every week. It's not all about exercise for me. Sometimes you just want to sit on the couch and eat vegan chocolate.

Do you offer your fitness or training services to others?
Yes. I own the Gungahlin Dance Academy in Australia and teach ballet as well as many other styles of dance to students. This is my full-time job, which I enjoy.

What sports do you play?
Tennis and skiing.

STRENGTHS, WEAKNESSES & OUTSIDE INFLUENCES

What do you think is the biggest misconception about vegans and how do you address this?
That we are limited with what we eat and that we must be lacking in some kind of nutrients. I lead by example. I am of excellent health yet I enjoy food too. I take friends and family out to vegan restaurants and cook them vegan treats to show them how easy it is to be cruelty-free and enjoy scrumptious food.

What are your strengths as a vegan athlete?
Stamina; and when performing I generally don't pick up the colds and flus or stomach bugs that can often go through an entire cast.

What is your biggest challenge?
Not enough time in the day to run my business, perform and be an animal activist. It's give and take.

Are the non-vegans in your industry supportive or not?
Yes. I receive a lot of questions on diet and health and I tend to point people in the right direction by sending them articles, web links and documentaries.

Are your family and friends supportive of your vegan lifestyle?
My family and friends are very accepting and it makes getting together easy. My non-vegan friends eat at vegan restaurants whenever we go out. I enjoy showing them how tasty and varied vegan food can be.

What is the most common question/comment that people ask/say when they find out that you are a vegan and how do you respond?
"Where do you get your protein?" When asked about protein I talk about how much protein we really need to be healthy (no one ever died of protein deficiency!) and explain that fruits, vegetables, nuts and seeds all have adequate amounts of protein. I love the quote; "People eat meat and think they will become as strong as an ox, forgetting that the ox eats grass."

Who or what motivates you?
The suffering of animals is my motivation to spread the word as far and wide and as quickly as possible. Strong women also motivate me, and those who have made a difference in the field of animals and women's rights.

FOOD&SUPPLEMENTS

What do you eat for Breakfast?
Fruit or raw buckwheat cereal and almond milk. On a bad day, leftover vegan pizza!

What do you eat for Lunch?
Steamed veggies, raw sushi, rice paper rolls, leftovers or salad.

What do you eat for Dinner?
Usually salad. I also like tofu and vegetable stir-fries. I always overdose on broccoli – it is my favourite food. I'm a big fan of raw chopped crudités with lots of dipping options too! My favourite restaurant in the world is Au Lac, a vegan Vietnamese restaurant in Canberra. I love red wine too.

What do you eat for Snacks - healthy & not-so healthy?
Popcorn, dark chocolate, raw dessert, rice crackers, and the occasional vegan cake or slice.

What is your favourite source of Protein, Calcium and Iron?
Fruits and vegetables have all the protein, calcium and iron we need. I enjoy kale, oyster mushrooms, cabbage and broccoli the most.

What foods give you the most energy?
Raw vegan foods.

Do you take any supplements?
No.

ADVICE

What is your top tip for gaining muscle?
Lift heavy weights.

What is your top tip for losing weight?
Exercise and eat low-fat, raw vegan meals. Maybe do a kick-start juice fast/feast.

What is your top tip for maintaining weight?
Eat well most of the time, and enjoy foods you love too. It is all about balance.

What is your top tip for improving metabolism?
Exercise - get up and move - it doesn't matter what!

What is your top tip for toning up?
Toning up really is just stripping body fat. Expend more energy than you take in and that will happen. Get moving.

How do you promote veganism in your daily life?
In 2013, I ran a program called 'A Vegucation'. It's kind of like being a vegan mentor and coach for people who want to the lifestyle for 6 weeks. They have to read a few books and watch a few documentaries and eat vegan food for 6 weeks. I also talk to people about veganism whenever I have to the opportunity.

How would you suggest people get involved with what you do?
To get involved with dance, just look up your local dance school online. It is a fun way to keep fit, have fun and you don't usually realise that you're working out! To get involved with veganism, saving the planet and getting super healthy, shoot me an email as I'd be more than happy to take you on a Vegucation!

JÜRGEN ANTHONY RIEDELSHEIMER
VEGAN EXERCISE ENTHUSIAST

Costa Mesa, California, USA
Vegan since: 2003

veganathleteperformance.com
themusicfactoryoc.com
SM: *FaceBook, Google+, Instagram, Pinterest, Twitter, YouTube*

Jürgen Anthony Riedelsheimer is the founder of Vegan Athlete Performance and has been a vegan for over a decade. He has helped, trained and inspired many people to adapt to a wholesome plant-based vegan lifestyle. He is a vegan cyclist, triathlete, ultra-runner, musician, environmental and Animal Rights Activist who believes that living a vegan lifestyle will make a difference for the better in all of our lives and the planet Earth. Anthony is also the CEO and Founder of the Music Factory, a school of music in Costa Mesa, California, USA.

WHY VEGAN?

How and why did you decide to become vegan?
I started out as vegetarian and was still experiencing certain health issues. After removing any animal type foods, combined with my active lifestyle I was able to overcome any of my health issues I experienced.

How long have you been vegan?
Over 10 years.

What has benefited you the most from being vegan?
Besides being a healthier and happier version of myself, I got involved with animal rights activism and Sea Shepherd to take on global issues I feel strongly about and which need to be addressed.

What does veganism mean to you?
I believe there are different ways to adapt to a "vegan" lifestyle. Some people try it out for health reasons first, some come from the animal activist corner or perhaps both. For me, I started due to the health issues I experienced, that I couldn't get resolved through a conventional medical approach. I think this was the beginning for me to become a lot more compassionate and aware of animal rights issues and what's really going on. It motivated me to learn and study how we are being deceived and lied to by advertising from our medical society and government.

I started to consume anything and everything to protect and educate others and especially protect my family as a father beyond just bringing home a pay check. It's about questioning the status quo, the system, breaking the chain for one single reason: "Conscious Evolution."

TRAINING

What sort of training do you do?
Cycling, triathlon, and ultra-running.

How often do you (need to) train?
Pretty much every day. Some trainings day are designed for active recovery, which include yoga, light swimming or massage.

Do you offer your fitness or training services to others?
I have trained and nutritionally advised many athletes in the past. Vegan Athlete Performance offers a nutritional and recovery service for athletes. More then 2/3 of your success is based on nutrition and proper recovery. Vegan Athlete Performance and WellSport Systems is based on the "7 Areas to Reconcile to Restore and Optimize Performance & Recovery" which is the most sophisticated recovery principal utilizing:

1. Inflammation and oxidative stress management
2. Metabolic Detoxification
3. Daily Management of Stressors ie nutrition, emotions, mental etc
4. Maintaining cell structure and shape
5. Restore and balance whole body symmetry
6. Implementing appropriate whole body exercise and Training
7. Low caloric and high-density nutrients

STRENGTHS, WEAKNESSES & OUTSIDE INFLUENCES

What are your strengths as a vegan athlete?
Quicker recovery and being able to sustain longer, harder trainings or race efforts.

What is your biggest challenge?
Not to lose sight of what I'm trying to accomplish in this movement. There are a lot of wonderful and passionate people trying to spread this compassionate message about veganism and environmental issues. My goal is it not to constantly preach or try to convince everybody else about what I'm doing or believe in.

Veganism is not this new miracle diet or lifestyle. It's been around for a long time. I believe everyone is on this timeline of perceived consciousness and when the time is right, a person will make a change. All I can do is walk the walk to my best ability and inspire others. If you want to change the world, you've to change yourself first. If I'm mad or angry of someone else's worldview or philosophy or allow myself to think I'm superior, I believe, I'm just as ignorant as that person. L.O.V.E.!

Are the non-vegans in your industry supportive or not?
Overall, yes!

Are your family and friends supportive of your vegan lifestyle?
Yes. They know me and how much passion I have and support it.

What is the most common question/comment that people ask/say when they find out that you are a vegan and how do you respond?
I think everyone who is on a plant-based diet faces the same questions. "Where does your protein come from?" "Isn't it too hard to do?" "What do you eat besides carrots and salad?" and the list goes on. I respond sincere and respectful. A lot of people are trapped in the "Myths of Nutrition" which have been strategically implemented by the food industry and governing bodies. It's a billion dollar industry with a sophisticated marketing team.

Who or what motivates you?
To leave a better world for my children. Successful - Compassionate – Evolution.

FOOD & SUPPLEMENTS

What do you eat for Breakfast?
Green smoothies, salads, quinoa, and oatmeal.

What do you eat for Lunch?
Green smoothies, lentils and bean dishes, fresh green juices.

What do you eat for Dinner?
Green smoothies, salads, soups, and fresh green juices.

What do you eat for Snacks - healthy & not-so healthy?
Gluten-free and alkalizing green bars, and raw nuts.

What is your favourite source of Protein?
Quinoa, beans, lentils, tempeh, tofu, and raw vegan protein powder.

What is your favourite source of Calcium?
A variety of dark leafy vegetables ie broccoli and kale.

What is your favourite source of Iron?
Spinach and legumes.

What foods give you the most energy?
Raw superfoods (e.g. maca powder), green smoothies and juices.

Do you take any supplements?
Yes. Cordyceps mushrooms, Resveratrol and proprietary Ayurvedic recover formula by my company Vegan Athlete Performance, BBAA and L-Glutamine.

ADVICE

What is your top tip for gaining muscle?
Proper wholesome plant-based nutrition, and you've to stress and overload your muscles according to your overall goal. Hydrate with clean alkalized water.

What is your top tip for losing weight?
Detoxing your body with juice cleanses and colonic hydrotherapy. Proper wholesome plant-based nutrition and exercise schedule - depending on your current physical health and goal. Hydrate with clean alkalized water.

What is your top tip for maintaining weight?
Eat for your goals. Eat clean wholesome plant-based nutrition. Hydrate with clean alkalized water.

What is your top tip for improving metabolism?
Green juice cleanses to start out. Get rid of toxins in your body (colonic hydrotherapy) and continue to fuel with clean wholesome plan-based nutrition.

What is your top tip for toning up?
By-product of a healthy lifestyle.

How do you promote veganism in your daily life?
My website and Podcast on iTunes.

How would you suggest people get involved with what you do?
To find more out about my vegan journey and involvement in the vegan movement go to my website.

KARINA INKSTER
VEGAN PERSONAL TRAINER

Vancouver, British Columbia, Canada
Vegan since: 2003

karinainkster.com
SM: *FaceBook, Twitter*

Karina Inkster is the owner and head fitness nut at Karina Inkster Healthy Living Academy, based in Vancouver, BC. With a Masters degree in Gerontology, she specializes in working with adults over 50, she also focuses on vegan and vegetarian clients. Karina has been weight training, swimming, running, cycling, and power yoga-ing her way to fitness since 2003. In 2011, she became a certified personal trainer to share her love for active living with others.

WHY VEGAN?

How and why did you decide to become vegan?
My veganism began with vegetarianism. At the age of 11, I decided I wanted no part in the inhumane treatment of animals, and I aimed to enjoy a diet that had as small an impact on the environment as possible.

How long have you been vegan?
I became vegan in 2003 (had been vegetarian since 1998).

What has benefited you the most from being vegan?
I like knowing that I'm eating a diet that's best for me – physically and psychologically – as well as for the planet.

What does veganism mean to you?
To me, veganism is the respect for and the celebration of all life on Earth. Veganism is a diet, a sense of interconnectedness with the web of life, a form of activism, and a lifestyle.

TRAINING

What sort of training do you do?
I love weight training and swimming most. My training program varies with the seasons, but always involves 6 training days per week. In the spring and summer, I have debilitating pollen allergies and asthma, so I need to train indoors. During these months I weight train 4 days a week (2 upper body days and 2 lower body days) with short cardio and do 2 longer cardio sessions per week, which are usually swimming or running.

After allergy season ends in the fall, I switch to more outdoor training such as running, plyometrics, and rope jumping, with 2 or 3 weight training days per week. When the weather gets too cold for outdoor training, I switch back to a higher volume of weight training and less cardio.

How often do you (need to) train?
6 days per week, 8 hours total per week.

Do you offer your fitness or training services to others?
Most definitely. I offer personal training at an exclusive training studio in Vancouver, along with nutritional counseling and online fitness coaching for vegans and vegetarians.

STRENGTHS, WEAKNESSES & OUTSIDE INFLUENCES

What do you think is the biggest misconception about vegans and how do you address this?
Unfortunately, some people think that veganism and athleticism don't mix. On the contrary! A well-planned and balanced plant-based diet can support an athletic lifestyle very well, whether it's focused on endurance, speed, or strength. The "But where do you get your protein?" question is thankfully becoming old news. I work hard to maintain a high level of fitness, and aim to be a walking billboard for healthy veganism.

What are your strengths as a vegan athlete?
My strengths are in speed and in muscle strength. I'm a fast swimmer but wouldn't last in endurance events, and my love of weight training translates into strong muscles.

What is your biggest challenge?
I deal with a potentially life-threatening condition called food-dependent exercise-induced anaphylaxis, which prohibits me from training after having eaten within 8 hours, in case a food triggers a serious allergic reaction when coupled with exercise. I also face severe seasonal allergies and asthma that limit my activity for 5 months each year, as well as weekly allergy shots after which I can't train - again due to anaphylaxis risk. This means I have to carefully schedule all my workouts, and always train in the mornings (sometimes at 5am so I can get it in before work) after having eaten only oatmeal – a known "safe" food. I also went through full-time graduate school while working 3 jobs and still managed to train 6 days per week. I'm motivated to help others to overcome their barriers, too.

Are the non-vegans in your industry supportive or not?
Generally I encounter support for veganism in the industry, especially considering vegan fitness is a growing trend.

Are your family and friends supportive of your vegan lifestyle?
Most definitely. Two of my best friends are vegans and some of my family members are vegetarian. I cook delicious meals (if I may say so myself) that my non-vegan family and friends always enjoy.

What is the most common question/comment that people ask/say when they find out that you are a vegan and how do you respond?
Q: "So, what do you eat?"
A: "Plants!"

I usually give them a brief list of cuisine types (Thai, Indian, Japanese) as well as some lesser-known foods (amaranth, tempeh, dulce, anyone?) to get them thinking about broadening their food horizons.

Who or what motivates you?
Feeling and seeing the results of my lifestyle are great fuel to keep it going. I feel great, and want to keep it that way. I also want to help others – whether or not they're vegan – to achieve their own results, which is motivation for me to be my best.

"To me, veganism is the respect for and the celebration of all life on Earth. Veganism is a diet, a sense of interconnectedness with the web of life, a form of activism, and a lifestyle."

FOOD & SUPPLEMENTS

What do you eat for Breakfast?
I eat oatmeal for breakfast every single day. Because of my food allergy - and exercise-related condition [see above], I need to eat totally plain oatmeal before workouts. After working out, I eat a second breakfast, which is often flax waffles with peanut butter, or a smoothie.

What do you eat for Lunch?
Salad (e.g. mixed greens, mushrooms, cucumber, red cabbage, hemp hearts, chia seeds) or something heartier such as veggie chili or stew. I also often make tofu scramble with lots of veggies.

What do you eat for Dinner?
Any number of stews, soups, curries, or stir-fries, and sometimes something more fancy such as roasted marinated veggie skewers or lentils and veggies wrapped in spelt phyllo.

What do you eat for Snacks (healthy & not-so healthy)?
I love dark chocolate. I also snack on protein bars, fruit leather, smoothies, crunchy roasted chickpeas, rice crackers with peanut butter or hummus, and much more.

What is your favourite source of Protein?
Tofu, legumes, and chia seeds.

What is your favourite source of Calcium?
Fortified soy or rice milk - I would eat almonds if I could, but I'm allergic to tree nuts.

What is your favourite source of Iron?
Edamame, lentils, quinoa, and spinach.

What foods give you the most energy?
I find matcha green tea to be a long-lasting energy source - given the tea leaves are ingested rather than steeped.

Do you take any supplements?
Protein powder, for muscle building and before bed so I don't wake up ravenous at night.

ADVICE

What is your top tip for gaining muscle?
You need to challenge yourself with the amount of weight you're lifting at the gym. Switch between low rep, high weight days and high rep, low weight days. You must also incorporate lots of recovery time (24 - 48 hours) for muscles to grow.

What is your top tip for losing weight?
Consistency is key. Stick to a regular healthy eating regimen and a regular workout schedule, and results will follow.

What is your top tip for maintaining weight?
It's worth speaking with a dietician to find out approximately how many calories you should be consuming per day, based on your needs and activity level. This number will be different for everyone.

What is your top tip for improving metabolism?
There's a reason everyone says, "Eat smaller meals throughout the day instead of 3 big meals." It works! So, get out there and do it. I eat up to 15 times per day, but small amounts each time.

What is your top tip for toning up?
Don't be afraid to lift heavy at the gym (I'm talking to you, ladies.) You don't need to weight train with heavy weights all the time, but lifting 5lb (2.2kg) "beauty bells" at the gym will do nothing for your physique.

How do you promote veganism in your daily life?
I aim to live by example. I share delicious foods and fitness knowledge, and I incorporate veganism whenever appropriate. It's not about preaching and making veganism overt, but rather providing inspiring examples and using veganism as a background reason and motivation for what I do. Results - things people can see and taste - are more inspiring than statements.

How would you suggest people get involved with what you do?
The first step is getting in touch. In addition to personal training, nutritional counselling, and online fitness coaching, I provide seminars and workshops to suit your organization.

"Don't be afraid to lift heavy at the gym (I'm talking to you, ladies.) You don't need to weight train with heavy weights all the time, but lifting 5lb (2.2kg) "beauty bells" at the gym will do nothing for your physique."

"Every journey begins with a single step."
- Maya Angelou

You will never know your limits unless you push yourself to them.

Kate Strong
Vegan Triathlete

Blackheath, New South Wales, Australia
Vegan since: 2014

strongkate.com
SM: *FaceBook, Instagram, Twitter*

Kate Strong is a Welsh-born international traveller, who has spread her wings far and wide not only geographically but in every aspect of her life. Having graduated with a double Masters in Mechanical Engineering from French and English universities, Kate has had a diverse career path from having a career in fashion in Italy to working as a Divemaster in Mexico.

Until recently, Kate owned and operated a guesthouse and restaurant in the Blue Mountains of Australia. In 2013, she decided to balance her life by taking care of her physical self and committed to the sport of triathlon. Within eleven months of this decision, Kate found herself on Australia's age-group squad competing in the long-distance triathlon World Championship. She won her age group convincingly and is current World Champion for International Triathlon Union (ITU) long-distance triathlon in age group 35-39.

WHY VEGAN?

How and why did you decide to become vegan?
Whilst training, I used to wheeze a lot and some friends recommended I eliminate dairy products to reduce my lung troubles. After following their advice and a big improvement in my breathing thanks to the no-dairy diet, I started to eliminate all other animal products (eggs and meat) and noticed an improvement on many aspects of sport, my overall health and general wellbeing.

How long have you been vegan?
Since mid-2014.

What has benefited you the most from being vegan?
I had always suffered from asthma and this held me back whilst training and competing. By choosing to follow a vegan diet, I now breathe cleaner, deeper and quieter.

What does veganism mean to you?
I have a motto I follow: Live consciously.

I strive to be aware of all aspects of my life: my physical, mental and emotional self, my impact on others and the environment. What I use to fuel my body plays an important part in conscious living and being. Veganism permits me to eat consciously ensuring that I maintain high energy levels sourced from the healthiest, most efficient foods with minimal negative environmental and emotional impact.

TRAINING

What sort of training do you do?
When I'm training for triathlons, I focus on swimming, road cycling and running with some strength, core and stretching thrown in for good measure.

How often do you (need to) train?
I love all outdoor activity, so even when I'm in off-season, it's rare I'm not out doing something. I train 7 days a week.

Do you offer your fitness or training services to others?
I am not a qualified coach, yet I share everything I discover on my blog.

What sports do you play?
I enjoy skiing, snowboarding, scuba diving, rock climbing, surfing, tennis... anything that gets me outdoors and moving.

STRENGTHS, WEAKNESSES & OUTSIDE INFLUENCES

What do you think is the biggest misconception about vegans and how do you address this?
Generally, people perceive vegans as having a very limited choice of food to eat. I love preparing and cooking vegan dishes, snacks and meals for my friends and let them taste how good and varied a vegan diet really is. I also write my vegan recipes and share through social media and with a USA-based column focusing on vegan food.

What are your strengths as a vegan athlete?
By following a vegan diet, I gain all the required vitamins, minerals, amino acids etc. in a cleaner, healthier way. This permits my body to use less energy to break food down to gain the energy and hence recover quicker from an intense workout. I gain more from each workout and my body is less stressed.

What is your biggest challenge?
I compete internationally and also travel extensively for my training. I need to really plan in advance where I can buy my staple food, or know what I have to pack and bring with me. I usually have a little list of vegan friendly cafés in the area saved so I can still enjoy dining out with minimal stress.

Are the non-vegans in your industry supportive or not?
It is great to see more and more triathletes and elite sportspeople turning towards a vegan diet. Unfortunately, we are still the exception and there are still people who don't fully understand nutrition and pass judgment on my diet. Post-race whilst choosing the recovery food on offer is limited. Again, I usually pack some tasty vegan snacks and share with other athletes (and share the information about the ingredients too.)

Are your family and friends supportive of your vegan lifestyle?
My close friends love that I'm a vegan - they enjoy me cooking for them and the variety of dishes I prepare. Also, my knowledge surrounding nutrition is benefiting them and they are altering their eating habits on their own accord. I live far from my family and so we rarely dine together. My good health and success in sport speaks volumes to them and they know that the choice to become vegan is working really well.

What is the most common question/comment that people ask/say when they find out that you are a vegan and how do you respond?
The first question is usually about where I source my protein! I laugh and try to make light of this whilst also sharing that protein is found in green vegetables, chia, lentils, beans - almost everything we already eat!

Athletes only require approximately 1.4g (2.2lb) per kg body weight of protein. For me at 58kg (127lb), I require 82g of protein daily, which is really easy to find through a balanced diet. My goal is to have some protein in every meal I prepare, be it chia seeds at breakfast, a side-salad, or lentils scattered in my pasta sauce.

Who or what motivates you?
I am driven to live a conscious life and ensure that everything I think, do, eat and say is done with positive intention. I often ask myself why I am doing something. Is it being driven by fear or lacking (fear of failing, lacking knowledge...) or driven by love and gratitude? Choosing a vegan diet is a no-brainer when I choose to live by these principles.

"Use how you feel as a gauge, not the number on the scale. If you use a goal weight as a motivator to lose some kgs, once you achieve this target, you've no focus and are more likely to break from your healthy lifestyle and gain the weight you lost. Focus on how you feel and your energy levels. This will ensure you still go to the gym long after you've reached your ideal body look."

FOOD & SUPPLEMENTS

What do you eat for Breakfast?
Homemade muesli with seeds, nuts, chia seeds, goji berries, cranberries and fresh fruit, with a cup of homemade lemon and fresh ginger tea.

What do you eat for Lunch?
Homemade soup made from seasonal vegetables and quinoa.

What do you eat for Dinner?
Sunflower, linseed and buckwheat pizza base with vegetables and 'feta' soy.

What do you eat for Snacks (healthy & not-so healthy)?
I make sesame and chia biscuits; date and goji power balls; and also buckwheat and blueberry energy-bursts as day time snacks. My post-race (unhealthy) cravings usually involve soy ice cream and dark chocolate!

What is your favorite source of Protein?
Quinoa.

What is your favorite source of Calcium?
Chia seeds.

What is your favorite source of Iron?
Kale.

What foods give you the most energy?
My soups always pick me up. Cauliflower, kale and lemon soup is my personal favorite.

Do you take any supplements?
No.

ADVICE

What is your top tip for gaining muscle?
Resting between sessions is key to letting your muscles recover and repair. Carrying out training on tired muscles will reduce the effectiveness of the session.

What is your top tip for losing weight?
Drink more lemon-infused water. Most people confuse hunger with thirst. By regularly drinking lemon-infused water, your body can better absorb water (and you don't have to visit the bathroom as much), your stomach will be alkaline ensuring quicker digestion when you eat and ensure you're not confusing thirst with hunger.

What is your top tip for maintaining weight?
Use how you feel as a gauge, not the number on the scale. If you use a goal weight as a motivator to lose some kgs, once you achieve this target, you've no focus and are more likely to break from your healthy lifestyle and gain the weight you lost. Focus on how you feel and your energy levels. This will ensure you still go to the gym long after you've reached your ideal body look.

What is your top tip for improving metabolism?
Energy attracts energy. If you're feeling tired and lethargic, go outdoors and do some exercise. Even a 15-25 minute walk every morning before breakfast will increase your energy levels for the rest of the day.

What is your top tip for toning up?
Improve your posture. If you slouch and don't activate your core whilst sitting, your body will be trained to hold this poor physical appearance. Get into the habit of 'holding it all together' and you'll look and feel better for it.

How do you promote veganism in your daily life?
I don't push my lifestyle choice on others, but when people show an interest in what I'm eating, I happily share my recipes and food with them. I also have a blog where I share my recipes and lifestyle choices.

How would you suggest people get involved with what you do?
Try a tri! Enter a local triathlon competition for a few months, and start swimming, cycling and running. There are loads of great clubs, coaches and training plans available online for all abilities. Don't use age, time, work etc as an excuse. Go out and have some fun! Contact me and I'll happily assist in helping you get started.

"By following a vegan diet, I gain all the required vitamins, minerals, amino acids etc. in a cleaner, healthier way. This permits my body to use less energy to break food down to gain the energy and hence recover quicker from an intense workout. I gain more from each workout and my body is less stressed."

KATHRYN LORUSSO
VEGAN EXERCISE ENTHUSIAST

Dallas–Fort Worth, Texas, USA
Vegan since: 2000

thankfulfoods.com
SM: *FaceBook, Twitter*

Kathryn Lorusso is a certified Physicians Committee for Responsible Medicine (PCRM) Food for Life teacher, and has a personal passion for plant-based cooking that comes partly from her love of teaching and partly from being a breast cancer survivor. Kathryn sailed through 25 rounds of radiation and two surgeries with no scars or side effects by eating plants, which thrilled her radiologist, surgeon and oncologist. She runs through her neighborhood in the early mornings, practices Bikram yoga within the Dallas/Fort Worth area, and is training for her first competitive body building contest in 2016. Her specialty is new vegans. Kathryn has been an educator for 25 years and owns Thankful Foods, a small plant-based company which provides oatmeal and protein bars online to commercial clients. At 51, she was selected as a fitness icon for O'Neill 365, an athletic clothing line for women.

WHY VEGAN?

How and why did you decide to become vegan?
I became vegan over five years ago when I was diagnosed with stage 1 breast cancer. I was diagnosed on a Wednesday and Thursday I changed my diet. I also threw out five lawn and leaf sized bags of processed food and spent $1000 at Whole Foods and Costco - including a water purifier. My sisters were visiting to help me through my surgery and they thought I lost my mind when I literally started throwing food out the front door!

How long have you been vegan?
I have been vegan for a little more than five years.

What has benefited you the most from being vegan?
The biggest benefit from being vegan has been the self-empowerment I feel from knowing I can help heal myself. I open my refrigerator, which is now my medicine cabinet, and know the food in there is helping my body heal with every bite I take.

What does veganism mean to you?
Veganism, for me, is a way to be the strongest, healthiest version of myself I've ever known and save animal lives in the process. It is the kindest, most compassionate way to exist. Every living thing benefits - including the planet.

"I realize that since I live a very different lifestyle, I need to take the metaphorical high road. I make it a point to keep a good, positive outlook and show vibrant health every day. I am the best example of a vegan diet at 55 when I walk in the room and you can tell I'm in shape and glowing with good health."

TRAINING

What sort of training do you do?

I weight train four times a week with my coach, who is training me for my first fitness competition next year. I'm super excited to be doing this the first time at 55! I also practice Bikram yoga (yoga in a 110F/43C degree room) four times a week and round it off with running through my neighborhood in the early morning (before dawn...Texas is HOT) and have raced successfully and won within my age group. Most days, I will have two workouts.

How often do you (need to) train?

I train every day and usually take one day off per week. It is a priority so everything else gets scheduled around it. That pesky day job is the real problem.

Do you offer your fitness or training services to others?

I invite people to join me at Bikram yoga all the time and have probably brought dozens over the 10 years since I've been practicing. I'm hoping that by bodybuilding competitively, I can show other 50-something women that being strong and muscular is completely possible at any age, and that a plant-based diet is the best fuel to make it happen.

What sports do you play?

I'm not on a team but do play tennis and love it. I am also a brand ambassador for O'Neill 365 (clothing line for women 25 to 35) and wear the clothing when I work out.

STRENGTHS, WEAKNESSES AND & OUTSIDE INFLUENCES

What do you think is the biggest misconception about vegans and how do you address this?

The misconception I run into constantly is that vegans are weak, puny and don't get enough protein. Women particularly think I can't get enough calcium without dairy, too. I offer literature, websites and try to answer questions in the most succinct, least threatening ways that I can so that I don't turn people off. I realize that since I live a very different lifestyle (from mainstream humans), I need to take the metaphorical high road. I make it a point to keep a good, positive outlook and show vibrant health every day. I am the best example of a vegan diet at 55 when I walk in the room and you can tell I'm in shape and glowing with good health. How can you argue with that?

I work in a traditional high school setting during the day as a guidance counselor. I bring veggie burgers to the barbecues and my stir-fried veggies and veggie lasagna to the lunches. Breakfasts will find me eating a tofu burrito, while the others around me are eating eggs, bacon and biscuits with gravy. Not many people challenge my diet anymore because I'm one of the few people on staff that doesn't show up after summer break with an extra 5 to 10 pounds (2.2-4.5kg) on me. Hey, the Parent-Teacher Association (PTA) is finally offering vegan options when they give lunches now! Again, I walk my talk and find that's the best way to show people being vegan works.

What are your strengths as a vegan athlete?

My strengths as a vegan athlete are many! I recover quicker, run and move faster, sleep better, have a clear head (no headaches or fogginess when I'm working out) and have MUCH more energy than I did before. I can also work harder without challenging my immune system so quickly. I don't have all of the blood inflammation that I had as a meat and dairy eater so my "machine runs clean" all the time.

What is your biggest challenge?

My biggest challenge is packing everything into my week. I have really worked on my time management skills, so I shop and cook on Sunday for the week ahead. As long as I have prepared food in the refrigerator and freezer, I can earn a pay check at school, work out in the evenings, make protein bars and oatmeal for Thankful Foods and still have a life. There really is time to do everything if you're organized.

Are the non-vegans in your industry supportive or not?

The non-vegans at school are now supportive but it took 5 years to get there. It's a process of getting comfortable with my differences and knowing that I won't preach to them about what they are eating. If I respect their food choices, they tend to respect mine. I'll still get the "Don't you miss bacon?" comments but I laugh them off. It's important not to take offence at those. It's usually just someone else feeling insecure about their own food choices, not about me.

Are your family and friends supportive of your vegan lifestyle?

My parents passed away years ago and my two sisters are both vegan so that makes things easy. When I was diagnosed with cancer, they changed their diets too, so we can exchange recipes and cook for each other when we all visit. The friends I am closest to are vegan or at least vegan-friendly so that works out well. I have a large network of very supportive, wonderful human beings in my life but the ones I socialize most with are definitely vegan.

What is the most common question/comment that people ask/say when they find out that you are a vegan and how do you respond?

The most common question/comment I hear is: "I just don't have time to cook!" My answer varies (depending on who it is and how well I know them) but it's usually something like, "Sure, you do. It's all about getting organized. I'll show you how" to "Do you have time for chemo and radiation instead?" You definitely have to know your audience before you bust out with that last comment!

Who or what motivates you?

Clearly, I am motivated by my health history and the cancer diagnosis I was given. I am living proof that this diet can get you through treatment and improve your chances of NOT having a recurrence. I barely have a scar from two lumpectomies and never suffered a second of side effects from 25 rounds of radiation. No scars, hardening, redness, peeling or fatigue. I was eating miso soup, sheets of nori seaweed, veggies, fruits, grains and beans and feeling fantastic the whole time. My radiologist called me her miracle girl and used to say, "Whatever you're doing, keep doing it."

I am also motivated by the ethical side of veganism, the horrible factory farms and treatment of animals. I live with two retired greyhounds and am horrified at the cruelty and injustice animals suffer because this planet insists on eating meat. Veganism is better for everyone and everything, including the planet we live on. Rich Roll is a vegan celebrity who I think is amazing. He's in my age group and represents strength, agility, graciousness, and just what we can do with our bodies as we age. He doesn't let his age hold him back at all - I love that!

"Veganism, for me, is a way to be the strongest, healthiest version of myself I've ever known and save animal lives in the process. It is the kindest, most compassionate way to exist. Every living thing benefits – including the planet."

FOOD & SUPPLEMENTS

What do you eat for Breakfast?
Crockpot steel cut oats with almond milk, hemp and chia seeds, fresh fruit and 25g of powdered protein stirred in. I'll drink a green smoothie with more powdered protein around 9:30am for a mid morning snack.

What do you eat for Lunch?
What I call a "goddess bowl" layered with cooked grains on the bottom, some kind of beans or legumes in the middle, and steamed or stir-fried veggies on top with a sauce of some kind. I make a lemon tahini sauce as well as a walnut fruity dressing to dribble on top. I might also have a huge salad with a grain, beans and rice thrown in. I also like to make lentil loaf and veggie lasagna ahead in the freezer to defrost for later. My refrigerator has cooked grains and beans, chopped greens in mason jars and sauces in it at all times so I can just throw things together quickly.

What do you eat for Dinner?
A huge salad with beans, nuts, avocado and lots of greens.

What do you eat for Snacks (healthy & not-so healthy)?
I'll eat leftovers at school mid-morning and mid-afternoon so that means hummus, a veggie burger, some brown rice and beans with sauce on top - even a raw buckwheat cereal I make at home and store at school. I drink two smoothies a day (mid-morning and mid-afternoon) to keep about 150 grams of protein in my day. Desserts are always things I make myself such as a banana dream pie from a Physicians Committee for Responsible Medicine (PCRM) recipe. I love fresh fruit like watermelon, strawberries and apples because I want to enjoy my desserts without guilt. That is key to me. I know if I make them, they're good for me so I can truly enjoy them.

What is your favorite source of Protein?
Tempeh. I love stir-frying it, putting it in loaves and casseroles and making mock tuna. The texture is interesting and it's so wonderfully versatile plus it's a fermented soy product, which is healthy.

What is your favorite source of Calcium?
GREENS, GREENS and more GREENS! I love collards, kale, spinach, radish tops, mustard greens - you name it and I'm steaming, stir-frying, marinating in salads and throwing it in smoothies. Every bone scan I've had in the past 5 years shows me to be normal or above normal and that is true success at 53 when many girlfriends are fighting osteoporosis and falling down and breaking bones. Gotta have my greens.

What is your favorite source of Iron?
Usually the PlantFusion powder in my smoothies, quinoa, pumpkin seeds (I use them toasted with a little Bragg's amino acids) as a condiment; lentils and tomato paste (veggie pizzas on spelt tortillas are quick and easy). I also like dried fruits such as peaches and apricots.

What foods give you the most energy?
The most energy and "clear headedness" for me comes from cruciferous veggies that I steam and have on salads. I just feel clean inside and really "zippy" after I eat a bowl of them. Broccoli, cauliflower, cabbage, and Brussel sprouts rock my world.

Do you take any supplements?
I take a vegan multi-vitamin for women, B-12, D, DHEA, leucine and digestive enzymes.

ADVICE

What is your top tip for gaining muscle?
I gain and maintain muscle by eating at least 150 grams of plant protein per day. I supplement my food with vegan protein powder and 1 teaspoon of leucine each meal so that I can build great muscle at the gym.

What is your top tip for losing weight?
My diet keeps me naturally lean because it is low in fat (no animal products or excessive veggie oils). As far as losing weight, when my students and clients transition over from an animal food diet to a plant-based one, they naturally lose weight. I have a parent from school who went vegan last December and has lost 60 pounds (27kg) since. He's ecstatic!

What is your top tip for Maintaining weight & Improving metabolism?
My body stays at its natural weight between 135-138 pounds (61-61kg) without any problem. I'm 5'10" and wear a size 4 depending on the clothing brand (a small in the O'Neill 365 line) and never worry about portion control. When you're eating plants, little oil, no processed sugar, plus working out consistently with a good amount of weight training, your weight stays low and even, and your metabolism is cookin'! It takes more energy (calories) to maintain muscle and also to repair muscle fibers, so you naturally burn more calories even at rest. It's a great pay off for working out.

What is your top tip for toning up?
Comes from a combination of weight training and eating right. I have found my best reward from lifting weights and watching my body grow stronger and more defined. It's addictive! I feel great, have energy, look good and have strong bones. At 55, that's miraculous!

How do you promote veganism in your daily life?
I promote veganism through my natural foods company, Thankful Foods, and also through the Physicians Committee for Responsible Medicine (PCRM) classes I teach. I post recipes on my Thankful Foods Social Media pages, answer questions from newbies and lecture or teach at the Get Healthy Marshall annual event in Marshall, Texas.

How would you suggest people get involved with what you do?
It's easy for people to find me on any of my Social Media pages. Anyone can send me an email through the sites or even call my cell phone. I welcome contact!

"The biggest benefit from being vegan has been the self-empowerment I feel from knowing I can help heal myself. I open my refrigerator, which is now my medicine cabinet, and know the food in there is helping my body heal with every bite I take."

KIMATNI D. RAWLINS
VEGAN EXERCISE ENTHUSIAST

Silver Spring, Maryland, USA
Vegan since: 2012

fitfathers.com
SM: *FaceBook, Flickr, Instagram, Tumblr, Twitter, YouTube*

Kimatni D. Rawlins is the Founder of Fit Fathers, an inspirational movement encouraging dads to mobilize family values toward healthier eating and daily exercise through various activities. Kimatni's motto is simple, "health, fitness and nutrition are priorities for the extension of life. Stay active, eat well and constantly energize yourself."

WHY VEGAN?

I believe life without animal protein and dairy is the most energizing and life-enhancing diet for humans. More fruits, vegetables, nuts, seeds and whole grains should be inclusive of daily eating to increase energy, control weight and decrease the chances of inheriting a degenerative disease.

How and why did you decide to become vegan?
It was a gradual process beginning in 2011. I've always wanted to become vegan but never had the willpower to do so. The first step was to retrain my brain through various readings, documentaries and vegan friendly travel.

How long have you been vegan?
4 years.

What has benefited you the most from being vegan?
Energy. I ran my first marathon last year fueled by vegan foods. More often than not, I work out twice a day because of the extra levels of energy I sustain.

What does veganism mean to you?
Purity and respect for Mother Nature. A plant-based diet ascertains that my body is operating as efficient as possible.

TRAINING

What sort of training do you do?
A bit of everything from boxing, lifting, yoga, swimming to biking. Yet running is my forte.

How often do you (need to) train?
At least 5 days a week. Unlike an automobile, our bodies improve with usage. Every day we should exercise 30 to 60 minutes.

Do you offer your fitness or training services to others?
Yes, to family, friends and followers of Fit Fathers.

What sports do you play?
Basketball, Football, plus Track & Field.

STRENGTHS, WEAKNESSES & OUTSIDE INFLUENCES

What do you think is the biggest misconception about vegans and how do you address this?
I hear constantly that vegans do not get enough protein. I simply laugh because I can eat just as much protein as an omnivore if I so choose. Yet, we do not need to consume as much protein as the typical American diet calls for. 5%-10% per meal is adequate. Our body's main fuel source is complex carbohydrates, and this is what I center my meals around.

What are your strengths as a vegan athlete?
Since my body is not burdened by digesting heavy meats, I have added energy needed for performance activities. As well, the reduction of an acidic environment increases my pH and alkalizes my body so all organs are operating at their highest capacity.

What is your biggest challenge?
I have not discovered one yet. Maybe eating on the road, as I have to prepare in advance.

Are the non-vegans in your industry supportive or not?
50/50.

Are your family and friends supportive of your vegan lifestyle?
YES. I have them all signed up for Meatless Mondays. They love it!

What is the most common question/comment that people ask/say when they find out that you are vegan and how do you respond?
"You don't look like a vegan!" So I ask them, "What does a vegan look like?"

Who or what motivates you?
I am self-motivated. Once I delve into research and determine my position, I stick with it.

"Unlike an automobile, our bodies improve with usage. Every day we should exercise 30 to 60 minutes."

FOOD & SUPPLEMENTS

What do you eat for Breakfast?
Steel-cut oats with raisins, bananas, almonds, cinnamon and almond milk or a fruit and veggie smoothie.

What do you eat for Lunch?
Salad, brown rice and beans, or a tempeh and avocado sandwich on toasted Ezekiel bread.

What do you eat for Dinner?
Steamed veggies and quinoa.

What do you eat for Snacks (healthy & not-so healthy)?
Kale chips mainly.

What is your favorite source of Protein?
Quinoa and beans.

What is your favorite source of Calcium?
Any green leafy vegetable.

What is your favorite source of Iron?
Pumpkin seeds.

What foods give you the most energy?
Bananas.

Do you take any supplements?
Only a B-12 supplement.

ADVICE

What is your top tip for gaining muscle?
Weight training.

What is your top tip for losing weight?
Running and eating 5 to 6 smaller meals a day with the last meal eaten no later than 6 or 7pm.

What is your top tip for maintaining weight?
Replace one solid meal with a liquid meal and daily exercise.

What is your top tip for improving metabolism?
Assuring the body is fortified with its daily set of nutrients.

What is your top tip for toning up?
Jumping jacks, burpees, sit ups, pushups, pull-ups and dips.

How do you promote veganism in your daily life?
Through social media and all of my blog posts on Fit Fathers.

How would you suggest people get involved with what you do?
Visit my website.

"I hear constantly that vegans do not get enough protein. I simply laugh because I can eat just as much protein as an omnivore if I so choose. Yet, we do not need to consume as much protein as the typical American diet calls for. 5%-10% per meal is adequate. Our body's main fuel source is complex carbohydrates, and this is what I center my meals around."

KYLE KENDALL
VEGAN PERSONAL TRAINER

Hertfordshire, England, UK
Vegan since: 2011

SM: *FaceBook, Instagram, Twitter*

Kyle Kendall is a personal trainer, nutritional advisor, the owner of Veracious Nutrition Ltd, and is currently studying master herbalism.

WHY VEGAN?

Vegan works for me, ethically and physically.

How and why did you decide to become vegan?
Whilst studying for my personal training and nutritional advising exams in 2009/10, it seemed apparent to me that there was a great possibility that I could function at a much higher level, look and feel healthier, and maybe avoid many illnesses if I was practising a plant-based diet.

Therefore, I decided to dive right in and give it a try. Six months into my new vegan diet, I learned about the unethical side of the animal trade, and it affected me strongly - I could not be a part of that, what I learned and watched was not okay with me, and I still feel this way today. The amount of suffering involved in this industry will always be too much for me. I don't push my views onto other people, we all walk our own paths, but I still help many people to become more plant-based and even make the change to a vegan lifestyle by showing them how it can affect you, by being, happy, healthy, strong, positive and full of energy.

How long have you been vegan?
I have been a vegan for 5 years.

What has benefited you the most from being vegan?
ENERGY! A much lighter conscience, and being better connected with nature.

What does veganism mean to you?
Veganism to me, means a large step in the right direction, a much better way of life for all concerned. Animals can live without suffering, and in turn vegans live without so much disease and guilt upon their conscience. A better connection with nature and all living things.

TRAINING

What sort of training do you do?
I love weight training and circuits mainly, but I am also very fond of calisthenics. I enjoy hiking, mountain biking, mountain climbing and pretty much anything that raises the heart rate.

How often do you (need to) train?
My patterns always change but on average, I will train 5-6 times a week. My weights session can be anywhere from 90mins to 180mins depending on the amount of energy

I have built up. Even when weight training, I like to keep the tempo fast, heart rate high and rest times low.

Do you offer your fitness or training services to others?
Yes I do. I offer training programmes, one-on-one tuition, group training, circuit training, diet and nutritional advice, as well as long and short-term plans for all areas of health.

What sports do you play?
When it comes to sports, I am a bit of a 'Jack of all trades.' I love to play nearly all sports but I am never going to be a pro in any specific area. My favourite sports are Thai boxing and mountain biking.

STRENGTHS, WEAKNESSES & OUTSIDE INFLUENCES

What do you think is the biggest misconception about vegans and how do you address this?
For me the biggest misconception about vegans (in my environment) is that vegans are skinny and fragile. I address this by being myself.

What are your strengths as a vegan athlete?
My biggest strength as a vegan athlete is my energy and focus. I drink a lot of green smoothies, these provide me with more than enough energy to power through any type of workout. My recovery time is low, so I have no problem training 7 times per week for months at a time if that's what my goals require.

What is your biggest challenge?
My biggest challenge being a vegan is travelling. Learning what I can and can't eat in a new country, as well as learning to ask for that in the local language can be hard and sometimes I can feel that I am missing out, but it always turns out fine in the end. I have lived in many countries, worked on four continents and managed to eat vegan all the way.

Are the non-vegans in your industry supportive or not?
The non-vegans are very supportive in my industry - they are more interested than anything else. Some cannot believe that I look so well or train so hard on only a plant-based diet. They ask so many questions, but I am always happy to answer them all. Some of my past clients and friends have been so impressed by the vegan lifestyle that they have adopted it for themselves.

Are your family and friends supportive of your vegan lifestyle?
My family and friends are very supportive of my vegan lifestyle, although not all understand it. Since becoming vegan, many of my friends and family have come to accept my decision and even made efforts to try foods, drinks and even home-made natural remedies.

What is the most common question/comment that people ask/say when they find out that you are vegan and how do you respond?
'You don't look like a vegan!' my response - 'Good!' (Even though the idea they carry of a vegan is a stereotype. Germany's strongest man is vegan!)

"Veganism to me, means a large step in the right direction, a much better way of life for all concerned. Animals can live without suffering, and in turn vegans live without so much disease and guilt upon their conscience. A better connection with nature and all living things."

Who or what motivates you?
The thought of being the best I can be motivates me a lot. But not as much as the thought of helping countless others make really positive life changes, and being there to see the results.

Person: Jerhico Sunfire.

Quote: "Our deepest fear is not that we are inadequate; our deepest fear is that we are powerful beyond measure."

FOOD & SUPPLEMENTS

What do you eat for Breakfast?
Green smoothie (my own recipe.) 0.5 litre of filtered water with squeezed lemon juice.

What do you eat for Lunch?
Something light eg hummus, grilled veggies or an Indian dhal with large salad (with more than 51% salad.)

What do you eat for Dinner?
Something filling eg curry or Jacket potato with large salad (with more than 51% salad.)

What do you eat for Snacks (healthy & not-so healthy)?
Raw vegan snack bar, fruit, nuts, seeds, smoothie, rice crackers, berries, banana ice cream, green juice, coconut oil, raw peanut butter (actually any nut butter), raw vegan chocolate.

What is your favourite source of Protein?
Spirulina, quinoa, mushrooms, and chick peas.

What is your favourite source of Calcium & Iron?
Raw greens.

What foods give you the most energy?
My green smoothies, by far.

Do you take any supplements?
Reishi, cordycep, chaga, ashwaganda, MSM, ziolite, vegan A-Z, maca root, açai extract, ginseng, plant oils, probiotics. I listen to my body and take what I feel I need for the amount of time my body tells me. Adaptogens have really worked for me.

"My biggest challenge being a vegan is travelling. Learning what I can and can't eat in a new country, as well as learning to ask for that in the local language can be hard and sometimes I can feel that I am missing out, but it always turns out fine in the end. I have lived in many countries, worked on four continents and managed to eat vegan all the way."

ADVICE

What is your top tip for gaining muscle?
Work hard! Make a solid plan and stick to it, don't make excuses. Make changes!

What is your top tip for losing weight?
Water, chilli, lemon juice, green tea and cinnamon are the first little tips that pop to mind, but personally I use a lot of liquid meals eg fruit smoothies, green smoothies, soups, raw soups. Quick and easy for the body to digest, and keep the stomach un-stretched.

What is your top tip for maintaining weight?

If you're at the weight you are happy with, then keep doing what you are doing - it's obviously working.

What is your top tip for improving metabolism?

This is how I keep mine at a speed I am happy with. Start the day with water (I have been known to put a pinch of Himalayan crystal salt, squeeze of lemon and a pinch of chilli powder if I want an extra boost when I am burning fat) and make sure you get enough throughout the day, drink green teas and nibble on a square or two of dark chocolate (70%+ cocoa solids) in the evening. If extremely fast metabolism is what you are looking for, then I would suggest looking at a ketogenic diet.

What is your top tip for toning up?

First for me is nutrition. This needs to be thought out in advance so you can supply the right amount of fuel for the task at hand. Second is simple: circuits, circuits, circuits, circuits - in the gym, down the park, in your garden or even in your very own home, these bad boys never let you down. Whether you are after losing a little belly flab for a holiday or want to look like Bruce Lee for the summer, good nutrition along with the circuit training will provide all you require. Change your weight routines into a circuit too by super setting muscle groups and throwing in 7-10mins of cardio all throughout your usual sets.

How do you promote veganism in your daily life?

I have a FaceBook page,Twitter and Instagram, where I share information. In addition, every time I step into a gym. And of course, just being myself.

How would you suggest people get involved with what you do?

Try your local college for available courses in nutrition and fitness. You can also look at courses available with open universities, this way you can fit your studying into your own schedule. Get out there and meet others in the positions you wish to be in - most people living this type of happy healthy lifestyle are only too happy to help.

"Six months into my new vegan diet, I learned about the unethical side of the animal trade, and it affected me strongly – I could not be a part of that, what I learned and watched was not okay with me, and I still feel this way today. The amount of suffering involved in this industry will always be too much for me."

Always remember Kindness
Always remember Compassion.

LANI MUELRATH
VEGAN EXERCISE ENTHUSIAST

Magalia, California, USA
Vegan since: 2008

lanimuelrath.com
SM: *FaceBook, Instagram, Twitter, YouTube,*

Lani Muelrath, M.A. is an author, teacher, TV show host, and university kinesiology professor who is certified in Plant-Based Nutrition through Cornell University. She has a Masters degree in Physical Education, is credentialed to teach multiple fitness modalities including yoga and pilates, holds Fitness Nutrition Specialist advanced credential, and is a Certified Behavior Change Specialist. She is celebrity coach and presenter for the Physician's Committee for Responsible Medicine (PCRM) 21-Day Vegan Kickstart and VegRun programs. Lani is the author of "The Plant-Based Journey: A Step-by-Step Guide to Transition to a Healthy Lifestyle and Achieving Your Ideal Weight"; and "Fit Quickies: 5 Minute Targeted Body Shaping Workouts".

WHY VEGAN?

How and why did you decide to become vegan?
As a longtime lacto-vegetarian – for over 40 years – I had intermittently eliminated dairy products. My reasons for adopting a vegetarian diet back then were just as they are now: for health, for humanitarian reasons, for the animals, and for the environmental impact of eating animal products. These same reasons are even more compelling today – and have become ethical considerations in new dimensions. Consider the ethics of monopolizing land, air and water resources to grow plants to feed to animals as livestock – when we could feed far more directly. Consider the ethics of farm subsidies making health-damaging meat and dairy less expensive for the consumer, when those who invest in their health end up paying the disease tab for all. That's just for starters.

How long have you been vegan?
The switch from vegetarian to vegan for me was almost ten years ago.

What has benefited you the most from being vegan?
I've distinctly noted since abandoning animal products: easier weight management, no more ear infections or head congestion. Aside from health benefits, the sense of integrity from making the choice to eat vegan has a profound effect on well-being.

What does veganism mean to you?
It means being a conscious eater who eschews animal products and makes the best choices I can every day to reduce and eliminate harm to other sentient beings – and our planet - with what I choose to eat and wear.

TRAINING

What sort of training do you do?

I run daily and walk just as often, and complete resistance and flexibility training about three times a week. Several times a week I bike ride, when the weather allows. I enjoy hiking and scuba diving as well.

How often do you (need to) train?

Physical activity is essential for proper brain function and well-being, let alone for your health and physical confidence. For that reason I exercise every day, even if it's as simple as long walk.

Do you offer your fitness or training services to others?

I specialize in helping people transition to a whole–food, plant-based diet so that they can realize their ideal weight, have a healthy happy relationship with food, eating and their body – without grueling exercise or excessive hunger – and so that they can live in harmony with their highest ideals. Along with that, I have taught and am credentialed and certified to teach many modalities, including Hatha yoga, pilates, and resistance training. My book "Fit Quickies: 5 Minute Targeted Body-Shaping Workouts" (Penguin/Alpha Books, 2013), provides complete instruction on specific exercises that together form a complete resistance training program. The book has been adopted as required text for a college Kinesiology course. I teach and train groups and clients with these exercises.

"The Plant-Based Journey" has also been adopted as required text and course manual by a growing number of plant-based teachers and coaches. It Is the first plant-based lifestyle transition guide written by a teacher and behavior change specialist, which I am very excited about bringing forward. This forms the foundation of my speaking, writing, and coaching by bringing the focus to plant-based, active, mindful living.

What sports do you play?

Fitness is my focus, so if running and scuba and biking are considered 'sport', I'm in!

"My reasons for adopting a vegetarian diet back then were just as they are now for being vegan: for health, for humanitarian reasons, for the animals, and for the environmental impact of eating animal products. These same reasons are even more compelling today – and have become ethical considerations in new dimensions."

STRENGTHS, WEAKNESSES & OUTSIDE INFLUENCES

What do you think is the biggest misconception about vegans and how do you address this?

Vegans have been perceived as scrawny and weak – this public perception is changing though as we have more athletes and active vegans coming forward and sharing their lifestyles – along with their diets. Veganism has gone mainstream – as evidenced by even large food corporations that are offering vegan alternatives and bringing plant-based living into the conversation.

What are your strengths as a vegan athlete?

Consistency.

What is your biggest challenge?

Getting in pushups and planks! They are my least favorite muscle challenges, yet essential for upper body and overall strength.

Are the non-vegans in your industry supportive or not?
A little bit of each – as people become more educated about 'protein' myths and nutrition in general, consideration and acceptance becomes easier.

Are your family and friends supportive of your vegan lifestyle?
Yes – very! As a matter of fact, decades ago when I first became vegetarian, within a relatively short amount of time so did my parents and sisters. My husband and I were on board at the same time, together.

What is the most common question/comment that people ask/say when they find out that you are a vegan and how do you respond?
The protein question always comes up, which I welcome because it is an opportunity to educate. Other than that, people often say "I could never give up…." I respond differently depending on the person. I respond with positive replacements. The best way to win hearts is through example – and good food!

Who or what motivates you?
All of the above. Making a difference.

FOOD & SUPPLEMENTS

What do you eat for Breakfast?
Fruit and whole grains, sometimes pancakes, waffles or muffins.

What do you eat for Lunch?
Sandwich with hummus, veggies, sometimes cashew cheese, and big slices of tomato and onion with salad or soup.

What do you eat for Dinner?
Whole grain or starchy vegetables with more veggies and salad.

What do you eat for Snacks (healthy & not-so healthy)?
Fruit, toast and nut butter, brown rice with beans and salsa, raw veggies.

What is your favourite source of Protein?
All plant foods. I'm big on beans.

What is your favourite source of Calcium & Iron?
Greens and beans.

What foods give you the most energy?
Whole plant foods in variety – make sure to eat plenty of whole grains and starchy vegetables. We need the calories - you can't get by on just the high water content veggies.

Do you take any supplements?
B-12.

"Aside from the health benefits, the sense of integrity from making the choice to eat vegan has a profound effect on my well-being."

ADVICE

What is your top tip for gaining muscle?
Challenge the muscles and eat enough calories.

What is your top tip for losing weight?
Reduce dietary fat and processed foods – crowd them out with more of the whole plant fare that you like.

What is your top tip for maintaining weight?
Reduce dietary fat and processed foods, and sneak in a little intermittent fasting for improving health.

What is your top tip for improving metabolism?
Stay active and eat enough calories over the course of the week to stay lean yet energized.

What is your top tip for toning up?
Targeted muscle shapers along with comprehensive exercise.

How do you promote veganism in your daily life?
Living by example, writing and authorship, public speaking, teleclasses and webcasts, supporting other authors and speakers by promoting their books, work, and events.

How would you suggest people get involved with what you do?
Start by implementing changes in your diet – keep educating yourself! There are multiple resources on my website and a huge list of books, resources, and websites with information for support, whether you are just getting started, eager to share the joys of vegan nutrition with others, or stuck somewhere along the journey.

"Physical activity is essential for proper brain function and well-being, let alone for your health and physical confidence. For that reason I exercise every day, even if it's as simple as long walk."

Remember:
Positivity
Patience
Persistence

LEILANI MÜNTER
VEGAN RACE CAR DRIVER

Charlotte, North Carolina, USA
Vegan since: 2011

carbonfreegirl.com
SM: *FaceBook, Twitter, YouTube*

Leilani Münter is a biology graduate who eventually became the unusual combination of a race car driver and environmental activist. Leilani has raced from shorts tracks to superspeedways, in both open wheel and stock cars. With years of dedication to environmental issues, she has become a recognized leader in the environmental community.

WHY VEGAN?

I am an ethical vegan, so my main reason is for the well being of animals. It is also a great benefit that being vegan is good for the environment. More greenhouse gas emissions come from raising livestock for the meat industry than the entire transportation sector combined.

How and why did you decide to become vegan?
I have been vegetarian almost my entire life, going vegetarian when I was six. I went vegan in the summer of 2011 as I learned more about the dairy industry.

How long have you been vegan?
Over three years, I went from vegetarian to vegan in July 2011.

What has benefited you the most from being vegan?
I feel healthier, and I am at peace with my ethical choices in my diet - knowing that I am not harming any animals to eat. I have also had a chance to discover so many wonderful vegan restaurants in my travels.

What does veganism mean to you?
It means living your life in a way that does not harm the creatures we share our world with, and taking care of Planet Earth as best we can.

TRAINING

What sort of training do you do?
I do a lot of Bikram yoga. It's very hot in the race car so that helps me stamina-wise to deal with the heat during races. I also like to scuba dive, snowboard, play tennis, and swim.

How often do you (need to) train?
I train much more when I am getting ready for a race. I'm not a work out addict, so my training schedule tends to be more sporadic. When I travel I find it hard to keep up with a workout schedule.

Do you offer your fitness or training services to others?
No, I don't.

What sports do you play?
Outside of racing, I enjoy scuba diving, snowboarding, and tennis.

STRENGTHS, WEAKNESSES & OUTSIDE INFLUENCES

What do you think is the biggest misconception about vegans and how do you address this?
They think we live off of salads. I address it by making amazing vegan meals and feeding it to those who are skeptical!

What are your strengths as a vegan athlete?
With my healthy diet, I don't have to work out as much to fit into my racing suit!

What is your biggest challenge?
Finding good vegan food on the road. Some of the racetracks are in remote places that don't have a lot of vegan food available.

Are the non-vegans in your industry supportive or not?
Both. I would say many of them don't necessarily get it. As a woman in a male-dominated sport, and an environmentalist carrying messages about clean energy and climate change in racing, I am comfortable with the role of oddball or misfit. Once they try some of my vegan food, it tends to change their minds for the most part.

Are your family and friends supportive of your vegan lifestyle?
Yes, they are. Some people give me a hard time, but nothing negative. Facebook and Twitter followers, however is another story.

What is the most common question/comment that people ask/say when they find out that you are a vegan and how do you respond?
"How do you get your protein?" is the most common question. One of my biggest pet peeves is the protein question. I respond by saying, "Have you seen an elephant or a gorilla lately? They are vegan, does it look like they are short on protein?"

Who or what motivates you?
Every day I wake up fighting for a better world for our planet and the animals we share it with.

"I have given over 75 keynote speeches now and eating a vegan diet is my one answer when people ask me what they can do for the environment. Not everyone can buy an electric car or put solar panels on their roof – but everyone can cut back or give up meat in their diet."

FOOD & SUPPLEMENTS

What do you eat for Breakfast?
Coffee, I don't eat breakfast.

What do you eat for Lunch?
My lunch and dinner are different every day. I listen to my body and eat whatever I am craving. I am a big believer in listening to what my body wants.

What do you eat for Dinner?
Same answer as above.

What do you eat for Snacks (healthy & not-so healthy)?
I love making huge salads with garbanzo beans, red onion, pomegranate seeds, walnuts, cucumber, tomatoes, avocado, peas, corn - I put all the veggies on it! Not so healthy snack? I love this brand of frozen vegan macaroni and cheese. There are definitely lots of not so healthy vegan snacks out there!

What is your favourite source of Protein?
Beans, but I also enjoy cooking with the meat substitutes they make now: Beyond Meat, Gardein, Boca, Tofurky, etc.

What is your favourite source of Calcium?
Almond milk.

What is your favourite source of Iron?
Spinach.

What foods give you the most energy?
I think all vegan food gives me energy, I do enjoy a big salad!

Do you take any supplements?
I take a multivitamin and flaxseed.

ADVICE

What is your top tip for gaining muscle?
Exercise, this is not rocket science.

What is your top tip for losing weight?
Juice fast is a quick way to shed some pounds.

What is your top tip for maintaining weight?
Eat healthy, stay away from the junk foods.

What is your top tip for improving metabolism?
Exercise, get sweaty.

What is your top tip for toning up?
Yoga.

How do you promote veganism in your daily life?
I talk about it on my social media channels quite a bit and I always address it in my speeches. I have given over 75 keynote speeches now and eating a vegan diet is my one answer when people ask me what they can do for the environment. Not everyone can buy an electric car or put solar panels on their roof - but everyone can cut back or give up meat in their diet. I am working on a vegan-themed race car to get veganism in front of 75 million race fans. I want to have a booth with a vegan chef giving away free vegan food to the race fans. The way to win over a new audience is to get them to taste it for themselves!

How would you suggest people get involved with what you do?
See my website.

"I am an ethical vegan, so my main reason is for the well being of animals. It is also a great benefit that being vegan is good for the environment. More greenhouse gas emissions come from raising livestock for the meat industry than the entire transportation sector combined."

LUKE TAN
VEGAN STRENGTH AND CONDITIONING COACH

Melbourne, Victoria, Australia
Vegan since: 2011

evolvedgeneration.com
awakemethod.com
SM: *FaceBook, Instagram*

Luke Tan is an author, coach, and vegan athlete for The A.W.A.K.E Method. He is also the founder of Evolved Generation, a brand aimed at spreading the plant-positive message through athleticism and conscious consumption. He is driven to help individuals become stronger, more nourished and and to live their best life through a plant-based lifestyle.

WHY VEGAN?

Veganism is not just another fad diet, it is a way of living. It is a lifestyle that promotes peace, conscious consumption and environmental sustainability. In my case, being vegan has also enhanced my performance as an athlete.

How and why did you decide to become vegan?
My wife first introduced me to the book "The Food Revolution" by John Robbins. The book opened my eyes towards the 'politics' of food consumption and production. It was a great insight into how a plant-based diet is healthier, more ethical and sustainable. Shortly after, I was encouraged to watch the documentary film "Earthlings". The film was an eye opener for me. It showed how animals were exploited as commodities simply to feed the ever-growing demand of meat and their by-products. The film also made me realise my own carninistic belief system (Google it). I literally turned vegan overnight.

Following the switch, I read the book written by Robert Cheeke "Vegan Bodybuilding and Fitness", and realised that not only was it possible to be a vegan and build muscle, but it was optimal. There are many athletes all across the globe thriving on a vegan diet. Through the book the message was clear. The best way to increase awareness is to spread a positive message and lead by example.

I further researched the works of doctors Dean Ornish, Neal Barnard, Caldwell Esselstyn, Colin Campbell, John McDougall, Neal Barnard, Michael Greger, and found that a plant-based diet has also been proven to halt or reverse chronic degenerative diseases (diabetes, cancer, heart disease). To me the choice was crystal clear.

How long have you been vegan?
Since 2011.

What has benefited you the most from being vegan?
I used to eat a high animal protein, low carbohydrate diet (consuming up to 1kg/2.2lbs of meat a day). I used to view carbohydrates (eg fruits, rice, root vegetables) as the limiting factor for getting leaner. I was always watching and controlling my portions to a tee. Always binging on nuts, and craving refined carbohydrates like lollies, cakes, chocolate and having it as my 'cheat' meal.

Since turning vegan, I have changed my relationship with food, and now focus simply on nutrient-dense plant whole foods. Focusing on how foods makes me feel, and how it helps me perform athletically. Since a calorie is not a just a calorie, the focus is how much nutrition I can extract from each calorie. For example, quinoa is more nutritionally dense than white rice; kale more so than iceberg lettuce; activated nuts over roasted varieties; sprouted legumes over canned ones, etc.

As a result of dialing in my nutrition and running on clean fuel, I am now training twice as hard and longer, while recovering twice as fast. Not to mention, I am leaner all year round as compared to my non-vegan days.

I appreciate the sense of community that being part of the vegan movement brings. I've connected with people from all over the world and even had the opportunity to compete alongside Team Plantbuilt with my Evolved Generation team mates in 2015's Naturally Fit Games in Austin, Texas - I came first place for my category.

Being vegan has also given me a deep sense of purpose. It has driven me to spread the plant-positive message through Evolved Generation, become an author of the book "A.W.A.K.E and Alive: Harness your Physical and Mental Potential through a Plant-Based Lifestyle," and further grow my personal coaching brand Awake Method.

What does veganism mean to you?
Being conscious of the choices I make, and the impact I have on the world through each decision that I make.

TRAINING

What sort of training do you do?
I use different training methodologies (kettlebells, crossfit, bodybuilding, isolation style and calisthenics) to optimize athletic performance across all energy systems (ATP, anaerobic and oxidative systems). I work to improve my function through developing better flexibility and mobility, increasing explosive strength and speed whilst improving endurance and conditioning.

I periodize my training into 3 week blocks. I believe in variance with consistency. I am of the belief that you need to progress consistently before changing any variables. A 3-week block works for me and keeps my body progressing without hitting a plateau.

Here's what a weekly cycle looks like for me: Monday - Bodyweight/Calisthenics, Tuesday – Upper body strength, Wednesday – Cardiovascular-based session, Thursday - Olympic lifting, Friday – Lower body strength, Saturday – Flexibility and Mobility, Sunday - Rest or Bodyweight and Calisthenics.

How often do you (need to) train?
Between 6-7 days a week.

Do you offer your fitness or training services to others?
I offer personal coaching as I am passionate about helping individuals become the strongest, most nourished and authentic version of themselves. I do this through my A.W.A.K.E Method coaching philosophy. My plan is to launch personal empowerment seminars, online course and one-on-one coaching when I relocate to Singapore.

STRENGTHS, WEAKNESSES & OUTSIDE INFLUENCES

What do you think is the biggest misconception about vegans and how do you address this?

That a plant-based diet is deficient, and not sustainable for optimal health and enhanced physical performance. I address this by being the best that I can be in all that I say and do, always pushing the boundaries as a plant-fuelled athlete, and showing what can be done if you run on clean, green fuel.

What are your strengths as a vegan athlete?

A relentless drive to be better than I was yesterday, and never, ever giving up if I set my mind towards something. I truly believe that anything and everything is possible if you want it bad enough. Through my past setbacks and injuries, I have come back stronger than I've ever been before. I always try to look at the lessons and the bright side of everything. I've realised that through each perceived negative experience that one encounters, there are many opportunities and hidden lessons that you can choose to take from it. Also, my recovery and energy levels are much higher than they were before.

What is your biggest challenge?

Trying to do too many things at once. I now consciously prioritise my work, and am trying to be more pragmatic and systematic with the way that I approach and complete tasks.

Are your family and friends supportive of your vegan lifestyle?

Yes they are. I know that through my lifestyle, I have inspired them to have a more plant-based approach towards their eating. My parents too have been supportive of my decision and are always checking out new vegan places for us to have family dinners at.

Are the non-vegans in your industry supportive or not?

Yes they are. Just by doing what I do, fellow peers, colleagues and clients are more receptive to veganism. I have also been referred clients through my peers and have been asked for advice on how they should work with vegan and vegetarian individuals.

What is the most common question/comment that people ask/say when they find out that you are a vegan and how do you respond?

Q: "How can I go vegan/more plant-based?"

My answer: Focus on what you are putting in rather than what you are taking out. When the bulk of your calories come from nutrient-dense plant whole foods, there will be less desire to rely on meat and dairy-based foods.

Who or what motivates you?

It is the ideology of creating a community of fit, driven and conscious individuals 'being the change they wish to see in the world'. A thriving culture of passionate and purpose driven individuals living to their fullest. Being at the lowest point of my life a few years ago, now finding health, purpose and a greater sense of spirituality, I want everyone else to believe that life is about living, not simply existing.

FOOD & SUPPLEMENTS

What do you eat for Breakfast?

Steel-cut oats, with a sliced banana, sprinkled with shredded coconut and pumpkin seeds. Drizzled with 'milk' made from a smoothie blend of Prana ON chocolate protein powder, blueberries and almond milk. I then have a green smoothie (a blend of fruits and vegetables) mid-morning to get my daily hit of phytochemicals, fibre, vitamins and minerals.

What do you eat for Lunch?
A large salad with a variety of legumes.

What do you eat for Dinner?
Tofu bake, or stir-fry with veggies eg pumpkin.

What do you eat for Snacks (healthy & not-so healthy)?
Healthy: All sorts of fruits (my favourites are bananas, fuji apples or Valencia oranges)
Not-so healthy: Vegan pizza on the weekends and a raw dessert or two!

What is your favourite source of Protein?
Seasoned tempeh, Prana ON protein shakes, nuts and seeds.

What is your favourite source of Calcium?
Leafy green vegetables.

What is your favourite source of Iron?
Various legumes.

What foods give you the most energy?
My morning green smoothie, and sometimes a good espresso pre-workout.

Do you take any supplements?
Vitamin B12 and Prana ON protein.

ADVICE

What is your top tip for gaining muscle?
Look into bodyweight and calisthenic-type training. Its amazing what you can do with the resistance of your own body. Calisthenics and gymnastics is my one true passion and love. It facilitates strength gains (resulting in muscle growth), increased flexibility, mobility and balance.

What is your top tip for losing weight?
I do not like to focus too much on weight as a point of reference. As muscle weighs more than fat, a person could look leaner or more toned while being heavier on the scales. Since muscles are the only fat burning cells in the body, any form of weight bearing activity will facilitate fat loss and increased muscle tone. Try to keep your diet whole, natural and focus on nutrient-dense plant whole foods.

What is your top tip for maintaining weight?
As above, eating whole, natural, minimally processed and grazing throughout the day.

What is your top tip for improving metabolism?
As above, and keeping active.

What is your top tip for toning up?
Find a sport or activity that you love and just get up and out - make it a lifestyle not a chore.

How do you promote veganism in your daily life?
Through living my life the way I do, and spreading my message to the world through my book and Social Media.

How would you suggest people get involved with what you do?
Contact me through my websites or on Social Media.

LYDIA GROSSOV
VEGAN EXERCISE ENTHUSIAST

Doylestown, Pennsylvania, USA
Vegan since: 2010

fromatovegan.com
expressodesign.com
SM: *FaceBook, Pinterest, Twitter, YouTube*

Lydia Grossov has been a passionate cook since she was 13 years old, a vegetarian since 1991 and now vegan, a graphic designer since 1994, and has been a happily married woman for more years than she can remember. She is the principal of Expresso Design, a co-founder of the Doylestown Food Club and the Doylestown Food Co-op, a supporting member of the Women's Business Forum, an active member of the Bucks County Vegan Supper Club, and co-founder of her blog, From A to Vegan. She's excited to help inform, educate and grow the vegan community.

WHY VEGAN?

For the animals, for my health and for the planet.

How and why did you decide to become vegan?
I became a vegetarian for ethical reasons in 1991 and just stopped at that for many years. With the Internet throwing information at us every day and because my husband and I got involved in a local food movement in our community, we started realizing that being vegetarian wasn't enough. Being vegan was the only way to be true to our ethics. It was the best choice I've made in my life.

How long have you been vegan?
Since 2010.

What has benefited you the most from being a vegan?
My health has improved dramatically. I had serious recurring sinus infections, exercise-induced asthma, adult acne and a severe lactose intolerance that was affecting more than I realized. Had I known that all of these issues would go away just by cutting out dairy, I may have gone vegan a long time ago. I feel fantastic when I get up every morning and that, to me, is priceless.

What does veganism mean to you?
It's a compassionate lifestyle based on doing the least harm possible, which resonates deeply with me and is in harmony with my personal philosophy.

"I encourage others to find their passion, be a positive and inspiring vegan, get involved on a grassroots level and build a strong, local vegan community for support, friendship and fun."

TRAINING

What sort of training do you do?
Weight training and high-intensity interval training (HIIT).

How often do you (need to) train?
5 times a week.

What sports do you play?
I don't practice any sports. I just work out and do yoga occasionally.

STRENGTHS, WEAKNESSES & OUTSIDE INFLUENCES

What do you think is the biggest misconception about vegans and how do you address this?
That we lead a rough lifestyle of deprivation, and generally do not get enough protein or nutrients.

What are your strengths as a vegan athlete?
I'm not an athlete by a long shot, have never been, but I've been going to the gym to work out, off and on, ever since I was a teenager. Now that I'm vegan, I've started taking it a lot more seriously and have found that I'm stronger than I've ever been. Not that simply being vegan has made me stronger, but mostly because I feel empowered by my choices, feel motivated to do more, and take my health and fitness to the next level.

What is your biggest challenge?
I work a full-time job, have an independent business, run a blog, organize activities for a vegan supper club on Meetup.com and do volunteer work for a local co-op my husband and I co-founded, so at times there's a lot going on. I used to find it a challenge to keep a regular workout schedule, but my husband and I found a 90-day online program to train like athletes. It takes 30-40 minutes of our morning, 5 days a week, and we've seen great gains and results. It's always a challenge because we're so busy and we push ourselves, but it's motivating at the same time because we know we'll eventually reach our goals.

Are the non-vegans in your industry supportive or not?
Most of my co-workers are either curious or confused by my choices and a few have even been hostile about it. My closest colleagues don't think much about it and respect me for the work I do, not my personal directive, but they'll proudly share stories of good vegan meals they've had during the week.

Are your family and friends supportive of your vegan lifestyle?
My family is neither supportive nor opposed to me being vegan. They just let me do my own thing. When I first became vegetarian, my mother was mostly concerned about me getting enough nutrients. Years later she started sharing vegetarian recipes with me. My husband is vegan and was the driving force that moved us in this direction. We are members of a vegan supper club on Meetup and have a lot of supportive friends in the group. Our local food community is also supportive, most of our local foodie friends make it a point to always have something vegan for us to eat and have a couple a vegan meals a week themselves.

What is the most common question/comment that people ask/say when they find out that you are a vegan and how do you respond?
"Where do you get your protein?" That question still surprises me, every time. I tell them I get protein from everything I eat, which, in turn, confuses them and leads to

a longer conversation on how much protein we really need and how I/we all get our protein.

Who or what motivates you?
Compassion for all living beings, my husband, my awesome vegan friends and online community. Veganism becoming more mainstream – now you can find more vegan products, menu items and prepared foods at regular grocery stores.

"I became a vegetarian for ethical reasons in 1991 and just stopped at that for many years. With the Internet throwing information at us every day and because my husband and I got involved in a local food movement in our community, we started realizing that being vegetarian wasn't enough. Being vegan was the only way to be true to our ethics. It was the best choice I've made in my life."

FOOD & SUPPLEMENTS

What do you eat for Breakfast?
It varies from day to day, depending on my workout and hunger levels for that day. I workout early in the morning before breakfast. If I've had an intense weight training workout, I'll have a frozen banana blended with protein powder and unsweetened soy milk and half a whole grain bagel with some vegan spreadable cheese. If I've done a high-intensity interval training (HIIT) workout, I'll have some oatmeal with a banana or other fruit.

What do you eat for Lunch?
A variety of whole foods meals that I make from scratch, usually leftovers from the night before - quinoa, beans, veggies galore, sometimes tofu or tempeh, occasionally a store-bought vegan sausage or burger. If I don't have leftovers I'll get an organic frozen meal.

What do you eat for Dinner?
We have community-supported agriculture (CSA) shares all year round so we eat a LOT of seasonal vegetables for dinner. I try to make sure I have some balance between carbohydrates/protein/fat, but I don't count macronutrients. I just make sure I'm getting enough variety of fresh and whole foods.

What do you eat for Snacks (healthy & not-so healthy)?
A lot of fruit, edamame, cherry tomatoes, baby carrots, Primal Strips, chia bars, and some mixed nuts. I've stopped making a lot of baked goods to cut down on added sugar, but occasionally will indulge in some store-bought items or the rare items I make myself. I do, however, still get dessert every time we go out to eat.

What is your favourite source of Protein?
I love tempeh, seitan, also PlantFusion and Nuzest protein powders.

What is your favourite source of Calcium?
Leafy greens and oranges.

What is your favourite source of Iron?
Legumes and beets (I LOVE beets!)

What foods give you the most energy?
Smoothies.

Do you take any supplements?
Vitamin B-12, D3, and protein powder a few times a week.

ADVICE

What is your top tip for Gaining muscle, Losing weight, Maintaining weight, Improving metabolism & Toning up?
Take it at your own pace, do the best that you can and don't be too critical of yourself, but strive to push yourself to the next level if you want serious results. Keep striving to do a little better next time. It's not all or nothing, every little bit you do does count.

How do you promote veganism in your daily life?
I try to lead by example and show people that being vegan can have many benefits. I also talk passionately about how my health has improved after I ditched dairy, because I'm still amazed by it myself, and try to encourage people to learn more about the foods they eat so they can make better choices. I try to keep conversations light and positive. I also share information and experiences via my blog, From A to Vegan, social media, and try to make positive contributions in my local community via Bucks County Vegan Supper Club and the Doylestown Food Co-op.

How would you suggest people get involved with what you do?
I encourage others to find their passion, be a positive and inspiring vegan, get involved on a grassroots level and build a strong, local vegan community for support, friendship and fun.

Be sure to consume the following foods every day:

- 5 or more servings of Grains and Starchy Vegetables
- 3 or more servings of Legumes, Soy foods
- 1-2 servings of Nuts and Seeds
- 4 or more servings of Vegetables
- 2 or more servings of Fruits

(Source: 'Vegan for Life' book by Jack Norris, RD and Virginia Messina, MPH, RD)

"The secret that all empowered activists know is that every day you spend fighting the good fight - no matter how "much" or "little" you achieve - is a good day."
- Hillary Rettig

Mark Hofmann
VEGAN ULTRA-MARATHON RUNNER

Munich, Germany
Vegan since: 2011

laufengegenleiden.de
SM: *FaceBook, Twitter, YouTube*

Mark Hofmann is a vegan ultra-marathon runner from Munich, Germany. He is also founder of "Laufen gegen Leiden" (Running against Suffering), a campaign in which he dedicates his marathons to animal rights organizations and collects donations for them.

In May 2013, Mark organized the world's first ultra-marathon relay: 32 vegan runners in 9 groups ran 450 kilometers (280 miles) alongside Germany's Federal Highway 12 in 54 hours without a break. The Federal Highway local name is "B12" which is a word play and a reference to the vitamin B12, as this is often the focus of nutritionists and critics of veganism. The event was organized in order to disprove the common prejudice that vegans suffer from malnutrition and are therefore unable to achieve peak athletic performance.

WHY VEGAN?

How and why did you decide to become vegan?
It was in 2010 that I sat before my last piece of meat when suddenly I felt I was being watched by a thousand eyes. I stood there totally naked and I could not bring forth a single excuse or even explanation why I was about to eat this. Although I always knew what was going on in the slaughterhouses, although I always knew there were plenty of other options for a man to eat healthfully and live a life without having to force a painful existence and a horrifying death onto other sentient creatures. That was the last time I ever ate meat or fish.

From that day, I started to expose myself to everything I had participated in. I began to understand that being vegan is the logical consequence of being vegetarian. If you consider yourself having respect towards life, nature, morality and healthfulness, there is no other option.

How long have you been vegan?
My evolution from being vegetarian to being vegan was a rather quick one. It was in 2011 when I evolved.

What has benefited you the most from being vegan?
My mind. I know I will never be able to make up for all the horrors that I unleashed upon animal kind - and thus on human kind - but at least I do not participate anymore in these traditions of exploitation. I feel freed and my mind is more at ease.

What does veganism mean to you?
We as humans need to stop the war we declared on the world. We will never be forgiven for what we did, but at least we should not add even more to it. It needs to be stopped. Veganism is the only option we have to make our tortured mother earth a place worth living on for all living creatures.

TRAINING

What sort of training do you do?
I am an (ultra-) marathon runner. This year I started picking up on triathlons with long distances in mind.

How often do you (need to) train?
Six days a week.

Do you offer your fitness or training services to others?
Yes. I offer my services as a vegan running coach.

What sports do you play?
Swimming, biking, running, running, running.

"Just start running. Slowly, steadily, without any pressure. Watch your technique. Read up on what you are doing and why you are doing it. Improve. Make progress. Know your limits and push them farther away from you. Suffer. Excel. And have fun while doing it."

STRENGTHS, WEAKNESSES & OUTSIDE INFLUENCES

What do you think is the biggest misconception about vegans and how do you address this?
"Vegans are (too) extreme!" I think that veganism in fact is the opposite, the renunciation of being extreme. It is extreme is to have animals genetically optimized, forced to live in cramped conditions, drugged, slaughtered alive and eaten. If anything, then vegans are extremely compassionate - that's all.

What are your strengths as a vegan athlete?
Recovery is definitely faster.

What is your biggest challenge?
Adequate calorie consumption to make up for all the calories burned.

Are the non-vegans in your industry supportive or not?
I do not need support. My definition of running is a solitary one. I enjoy being on my own when I train and compete against myself.

Are your family and friends supportive of your vegan lifestyle?
My small family consists of my wife and kid and they are vegan themselves, so there is my solid base of support right there. Just recently I started building up a new friend base consisting of compassionate people who do not kill for fun or out of thoughtlessness.

What is the most common question/comment that people ask/say when they find out that you are a vegan and how do you respond?
"I could never do that." I respond with, "Let's try together. I'll show you how."

Who or what motivates you?
My wife and kid, when it comes to getting up in the morning. My desire to challenge myself, when it comes to sports.

FOOD & SUPPLEMENTS

What do you eat for Breakfast?
A bowl of whole grain organic cornflakes with spelt milk and bananas.

What do you eat for Lunch?
A dish containing a leaf, a grain and a bean.

What do you eat for Dinner?
A dish containing a different leaf, a different grain, a different bean (than I had for lunch).

What do you eat for Snacks (healthy & not-so healthy)?
A lot of fruits and vegetables, nuts, and spelt pretzels sprinkled with sesame seeds.

What is your favourite source of Protein?
Seitan, nuts, beans and lentils.

What is your favourite source of Calcium?
Greens.

What is your favourite source of Iron?
Spinach, millet and oat flakes.

What foods give you the most energy?
Dates and figs.

Do you take any supplements?
Liquid B12 (Methylcobalamin).

ADVICE

What is your top tip for gaining muscle?
Increase workouts, add more protein to your diet, and rest sufficiently.

What is your top tip for losing weight?
Extensive running workouts and completely eliminate saturated fat from your diet.

What is your top tip for maintaining weight?
Go vegan, stay vegan, run vegan.

What is your top tip for improving metabolism?
Extensive running workouts, slow and long.

What is your top tip for toning up?
Weightlifting with more reps, less weight and cardio.

How do you promote veganism in your daily life?
I wear my own merchandise during my workouts thus (hopefully) leading people to my webpage where they can inform themselves more about the cause of what I do. I also (sometimes) answer questions that no one asked.

How would you suggest people get involved with what you do?
Just start running. Slowly, steadily, without any pressure. Watch your technique. Read up on what you are doing and why you are doing it. Improve. Make progress. Know your limits and push them farther away from you. Suffer. Excel. And have fun while doing it.

"We as humans need to stop the war we declared on the world. We will never be forgiven for what we did, but at least we should not add even more to it. It needs to be stopped. Veganism is the only option we have to make our tortured mother earth a place worth living on for all living creatures."

MARY CORNIÈRE
VEGAN PERSONAL TRAINER

Paris, France
Vegan since: 2001

evolvewithfitmarypt.com
SM: *FaceBook, Google+, Twitter*

Mary Cornière's love for health and fitness started 14 years ago. It was then that she saw the benefits that vegan nutrition had in the recovery of a Cancer patient. Because of her desire to live longer and enhance her quality of life, she further learned about the strength and energy gained through the use of vegan nutrition and exercise. This interest for health grew as she furthered her knowledge as a Kinesiology student at Simon Fraser University, Canada and completed her Masters of Physical Therapy in Scotland. Mary is also a National Strength and Conditioning Association (NSCA) Certified Strength and Conditioning Specialist; American Council on Exercise (ACE), Register of Exercise Professionals (REPS) and British Columbia Recreation and Parks Association (BCRPA) Certified Personal Trainer, and Climbing Wall Association (CWA) Climbing Instructor. Mary enjoys rock climbing, hiking, river rafting and running with her vegan dog, Bella. She also loves participating in bouldering competitions and obstacle endurance events like "Tough Mudder".

WHY VEGAN?

How and why did you decide to become vegan?
Fourteen years ago, I was helping a good friend who had cancer in the large intestine. Her doctor recommended to her that she should try a vegan/vegetarian diet because it would be easier on her digestive system and large intestine. As a result, it would help with the healing process. I thought this was very interesting, so I did my research about the health benefits of a vegan diet and from that day forward, I became vegan. My friend no longer has cancer.

How long have you been vegan?
I've been vegan for over 14 years.

What has benefited you the most from being vegan?
My energy levels and health feel like they have skyrocketed.

What does veganism mean to you?
Veganism means the world to me. It's a huge passion of mine. It's important to me to educate those around me who are not vegan and to surround myself with friends who are vegan so that we can share the same values.

TRAINING

What sort of training do you do?
I'm an avid rock climber/boulderer.

How often do you (need to) train?
I climb 3-4 times a week for 4-hour sessions. I lift weights 3 times a week.

Do you offer your fitness or training services to others?
Yes. I've been a Certified Personal Trainer for 10 years. I am also a Registered Physical Therapist.

What sports do you play?
Other than rock climbing, bouldering and training, I also run 10km with my vegan dog, Bella, 5-6 days a week.

STRENGTHS, WEAKNESSES & OUTSIDE INFLUENCES

What do you think is the biggest misconception about vegans and how do you address this?
The biggest misconception is that an athlete can't be successful if they are vegan. Firstly, I educate them about vegan nutrition and how it aids recovery. Then, I show them links to other amazing vegan athletes.

What are your strengths as a vegan athlete?
My recovery is my biggest strength. I can fit more training sessions in a week. Also just feeling clean and energetic - eating an all-natural, vegan diet makes my body feel like a super vegan athlete.

What is your biggest challenge?
Reaching for super small and far holds (the crux!) when I'm climbing outdoors in Fontainebleau, France.

Are the non-vegans in your industry supportive or not?
Most understand my choice of being vegan. Most climbers are very respectful to one another and the environment.

Are your family and friends supportive of your vegan lifestyle?
I have a great vegan community in Paris, France. Most of my close friends are vegan. My mom always supports my vegan diet and makes delicious meals when I visit her. Recently, my husband's family, who are French and not vegan, made me 100% vegan meals - they ate them too!

What is the most common question/comment that people ask/say when they find out that you are a vegan and how do you respond?
Comment: "But you live in France, how can you not eat cheese?" I tell them I love cheese. I eat lots of vegan cheese and I am very addicted to it. Then, I tell them where I get it from and tell them how much healthier it is for me in comparison to dairy cheese. If I have some around, then I offer them to try some.

Question: "Where do you get your protein?" I tell them I get it from many, many plant-based options such as nuts, seeds, legumes, quinoa, soy products, rice, hemp protein, spirulina and vegetables.

Who or what motivates you?
Keeping my body healthy and pure so I can live a long and exciting life to climb and discover boulders all around the world.

FOOD&SUPPLEMENTS

What do you eat for Breakfast?
Usually a kale, berry smoothie with hemp protein, maca and spirulina. Once a week, I make vegan buckwheat pancakes with blueberries and bananas.

What do you eat for Lunch?
This varies every day because I love variety. But, a large organic salad is one of my favourites especially if it has kale and avocado. I usually put some grated ginger and garlic to add a zing. Then I add sunflower seeds, pumpkin seeds, chia seeds and sunflower seeds. For the dressing, I mix fresh lemon juice, sesame oil and a little bit of agave nectar.

What do you eat for Dinner?
This also varies every day. Since I live in France and my husband is French, I like making French recipes, like vegan quiche, ratatouille, crêpes or galettes.

What do you eat for Snacks - healthy & not-so healthy?
Vegan cheese, freshly baked vegan protein cookies, guacamole, raw almonds, apples, bananas and chocolate!

What is your favourite source of Protein?
Quinoa, chia and hemp seeds.

What is your favourite source of Calcium?
Kale and tahini.

What is your favourite source of Iron?
Spirulina and lentils.

What foods give you the most energy?
My morning smoothies.

Do you take any supplements?
Yes. I occasionally take B12 and Vegan Vitamin D.

ADVICE

What is your top tip for gaining muscle?
Weight train at least 3 times a week with low repetitions and heavy weights, then, progress the weight every week if you want to see results.

What is your top tip for losing weight?
Start a calorie intake journal. There has been a lot of scientific evidence that has shown that this is a highly effective method to losing weight.

What is your top tip for maintaining weight?
Keep doing what you are doing - eating well and exercise regularly.

What is your top tip for improving metabolism?
Lifting weights helps build muscle, which in turn helps increase your metabolism at rest.

What is your top tip for toning up?
Lift weights 3 times a week with maximum repetitions of 20.

How do you promote veganism in your daily life?
I tell my clients that I am vegan. Afterwards, they always ask about veganism. I've had several clients become vegan because of me.

How would you suggest people get involved with what you do?
Volunteer with me at an animal sanctuary. Afterwards, I might suggest some easy documentaries like "Vegucated" or "Forks over Knives."

MARY STELLA STABINSKY
VEGAN TRIATHLETE

Wilkes-Barre, Pennsylvania, USA
Vegan since: 2005

cfmarystella.blogspot.com
SM: *FaceBook, Twitter*

Mary Stella Stabinsky is a vegan triathlete and coach who is certified in both CrossFit and CrossFit Endurance training protocols. This methodology is what she uses to train herself as well as her clients. Mary has competing in Ironman NYC as well as various other triathlete events.

WHY VEGAN?

How and why did you decide to become vegan?
I decided to go on a vegan diet in 2005 to address various health issues I was having at the time. Declining health is seen as the norm in the USA these days and I was unhappy with the current state of my life. It has been one of the best decisions I have ever made in my life. I became not only healthier as a result but also a better athlete with this simple change. I can train and recover more than I could in the past. I am also living a better quality of life, as I am not longer using things like caffeine etc. to get through the day. It raised the bar for me and what life can be.

How long have you been vegan?
Over 10 years.

What has benefited you the most from being vegan?
My health. I no longer have any serious health issues that I had in the past like high blood pressure or high cholesterol. In fact, all of my health markers are not only normal, they are very, very good.

What does veganism mean to you?
To me to be vegan is to take your life to a purer level. To eat and live as cleanly as you can and to think about what effects your decisions have on the world. I try to base my decisions on what is the best for the world and me.

TRAINING

What sort of training do you do?
I do CrossFit Endurance training, so I swim, bike and run as well as do CrossFit.

How often do you (need to) train?
I train twice a day most days unless I am tapering, racing, or recovering from racing.

Do you offer your fitness or training services to others?
I do, I train using the CrossFit and CrossFit Endurance protocols both athletes and fitness clients, as well as give virtual coaching.

What sports do you play?
I am a triathlete who races from sprint to Ironman distance events, I also do stand alone events such as racing cyclocross, open water swimming and running races.

STRENGTHS, WEAKNESSES & OUTSIDE INFLUENCES

What do you think is the biggest misconception about vegans and how do you address this?
That the diet cannot support an athlete's training. I put my own training and racing up as proof. To do the amount of training I need to do - in both intensity and volume - and to recover from this is proof enough that it can be done.

What are your strengths as a vegan athlete?
My nutrition. I eat clean and recover well as a result.

What is your biggest challenge?
I often have to put more thought into my packing for racing as I need to have my nutritional bases covered and that sometimes can be more complicated for me. However, it isn't a huge issue. I can pack some of the Vega products and all is well. I've never been to a place that doesn't have a grocery store. I have also never been to a grocery store that doesn't have fruits, vegetables and beans.

Are the non-vegans in your industry supportive or not?
It varies - some people still are not believers. I focus on what I am doing and the results I am getting, and I don't get caught up in the nonsense.

Are your family and friends supportive of your vegan lifestyle?
Again, it varies - some people are more supportive than others. I do what I need to do and I don't expect support from others. If they extend it, wonderful, if not I carry on with what I am doing.

What is the most common question/comment that people ask/say when they find out that you are a vegan and how do you respond?
"What do you eat?" I tell them what I eat.

Who or what motivates you?
Motivation is mostly internal for me. It is a drive that I have to do my best in every situation. As long as I gave all I had to give, I have no regrets. I also find watching and reading about other athlete's lives motivating.

FOOD & SUPPLEMENTS

What do you eat for Breakfast?
Vega whole food optimiser with coconut water; or tofu scramble with veggies or tempeh bacon.

What do you eat for Lunch?
Tofu or tempeh, and veggies with brown rice.

What do you eat for Dinner?
Tofu or tempeh and veggies, sometimes lentils or bean-based meals. I try to avoid seitan.

What do you eat for Snacks (healthy & not-so healthy)?
Vega sport protein powder with coconut water, Vega protein bars, Lara bars, and kale chips.

What is your favourite source of Protein?
Tofu.

What is your favourite source of Calcium?
Broccoli.

What is your favourite source of Iron?
Tofu.

What foods give you the most energy?
Not really an energy source, but staying hydrated with a lot of water is so important to energy levels. Your body just functions better if it hydrated.

Do you take any supplements?
I use Vega products.

ADVICE

What is your top tip for gaining muscle?
Lift heavy weights using power and compound movements - not bodybuilding machines.

What is your top tip for losing weight?
Eat 3 meals and 2-3 snacks a day. Never large portions and always healthy choices.

What is your top tip for maintaining weight?
Weigh yourself daily or every couple of days so you constantly know where you are at before it gets out of control.

What is your top tip for improving metabolism?
Intermittent fasting - I eat dinner and then I do not eat again until after I have trained the following morning. I also take a couple of hours of not eating before my second training session of the day as well.

What is your top tip for toning up?
Moving your body weight around in as many different ways as possible. You don't need a lot of machines etc. Basic body weight movements like squats, push ups, jumping jacks are all highly effective training movements.

How do you promote veganism in your daily life?
I try to be a good role model for others to follow and I am very open to talking about my veganism to others.

How would you suggest people get involved with what you do?
I strongly recommend people get involved with local sporting events such as 5k run/walks, sprint triathlons and larger events to give their training some focus. Having an event to do makes doing the training easier and also you get to use the event as a celebration of your fitness. Most people come away from these events with a huge sense of accomplishment in not only their race but enjoying the process of training and eating and sleeping to recover as well.

"Motivation is mostly internal for me. It is a drive that I have to do my best in every situation. As long as I gave all I had to give, I have no regrets. I also find watching and reading about other athlete's lives motivating."

MATT FRAZIER
VEGAN MARATHONER AND ULTRARUNNER

Asheville, North Carolina, USA
Vegan since: 2011

nomeatathlete.com
SM: *FaceBook, Twitter*

Matt Frazier is a vegan marathoner and ultrarunner who ran his first 100-miler (160m) in 2013. He's the founder of the blog No Meat Athlete, and author of the book "No Meat Athlete: Run on Plants and Discover Your Fittest, Fastest, Happiest Self", where he shares an easy-to-adopt and low-key approach for active people to eat a healthy, plant-based diet.

WHY VEGAN?

How and why did you decide to become vegan?
For me, vegan was a natural progression about two years after I went vegetarian, mainly for ethical reasons. My story of going vegetarian is probably more interesting: I was training to qualify for the Boston Marathon (and had been for about five years), when I started to feel an ethical urge to become vegetarian. I was sure that it would mean not getting enough protein and calories to support marathon training, so I went halfway, and gave up red meat and pork. But, soon my progress plateaued, and since I still felt wrong about eating animals, I decided to go vegetarian, despite what I thought it would do to my training. I was shocked to find out that the exact opposite of what I expected happened: when I went vegetarian, I got faster almost right away, and six months later, I took the last ten minutes off my marathon time and qualified for Boston!

How long have you been vegan?
I went vegan in March 2011, so just over four years.

What has benefited you the most from being vegan?
Wow, it's been such a positive change in so many areas of my life that it's hard to say. My energy levels, my running and fitness, and the congruency I feel now that my diet aligns with my beliefs have all been huge. But, if I'm honest, the biggest benefit for me personally has been that veganism and my way of working it into an active lifestyle is a topic that has resonated with a lot of people. I didn't have a strong voice or a platform or a clue about what I wanted to do with my life before I went vegetarian (and then vegan), and now I do, so that's a huge change.

What does veganism mean to you?
For me, being vegan doesn't feel like a choice. Feeling the way I do about animals and how they're treated in the factory farming industry, there's not really another option for me if I want to sleep at night.

It's a lifestyle that I love too. My version of veganism is a very simple one: my meals are much less complicated than they used to be, and along with the diet, I've embraced minimalism in my running and the rest of my life, too. Veganism, to me, is one aspect of that practice.

TRAINING

What sort of training do you do?

I used to be a marathoner, but recently I've been more interested in ultramarathons and seeing how far I can go, without worrying much about pace. Last summer I did my first 100-miler (160m), and the training for that was 50 or 60 miles (80m or 160m) per week of almost entirely easy-paced running. Really nothing crazy, at least not what I assumed when I used to think about what type of training must be required to run 100 miles.

How often do you (need to) train?

When I'm training for a race, I run five or six days a week, with most runs taking me about an hour, and weekend runs taking anywhere from two to six hours. When I'm not in serious training mode, I'm more relaxed about it and run three to four days a week - more for my mind than my body.

Do you offer your fitness or training services to others?

No, I've really stayed away from private coaching. One-on-one just isn't my thing as I'm an introvert. I've got a lot of digital training programs and guides, plus a new Academy site where I do live video Q&As and things like that.

What sports do you play?

Running is the only sport I actually get out and do these days, but I like skiing and golf when I make the effort to do them. I played golf and baseball in high school, and was a decent golfer back in the day, but rode the bench in baseball.

STRENGTHS, WEAKNESSES & OUTSIDE INFLUENCES

What do you think is the biggest misconception about vegans and how do you address this?

Of course there's the protein thing and "vegans can't be athletes," but one that's more important for me to address is "vegans are preachy." I used to think the same thing, and that actually turned me off for years and was my excuse to keep eating meat. I didn't want to be "one of those people," I told myself. So I'm on a mission now to be the opposite of militant and preachy, to reach all those people like I used to be, who are interested in the personal choice of veganism but not necessarily in becoming an activist.

What are your strengths as a vegan athlete?

I have more energy than I ever used to. I weigh less but haven't lost strength, and that's an advantage in endurance sports. Injuries have become nearly non-existent for me. Is that because of veganism? I can't say for sure, but I didn't dare to dream of running 50 or 100 miles (80m or 160m) before - it was hard enough for me to train for a marathon without injury.

What is your biggest challenge?

Finding the time to do everything I want to do. I've got the energy for it, but with running a business, being a parent, training for ultramarathons, reading, and having a billion other interests that I tend to get obsessed with, it's frustrating to me that there aren't more hours in the day.

Are the non-vegans in your industry supportive or not?

Yes, the people I encounter in the blogosphere are almost all open-minded. I don't see a lot of hate or strong anti-vegan ideas. Maybe my laid-back attitude about my diet, not trying to push it on anyone who isn't interested, doesn't make trolling much fun.

Are your family and friends supportive of your vegan lifestyle?
Absolutely. A few of them have actually become vegetarian or vegan - I like to think as a result of my doing it. Those who haven't, which is most of them, of course, are totally cool with it. I guess we don't really focus on the differences in what we eat and just like to hang out like always. I don't like to make a scene, so I eat ahead of time or bring a dish if there's a party where I know there won't be anything for me.

What is the most common question/comment that people ask/say when they find out that you are a vegan and how do you respond?
They ask what my reason is. What I say is the truth: primarily it was an ethical decision, but I've since discovered the health benefits and they're a big part of it for me too.

Who or what motivates you?
Stories of people who have big, ridiculous dreams, get knocked down over and over, ridiculed and mocked, but for some unknowable reason refuse to give up. You know, like (the movie) "Rudy" - I cry every time I watch that.

"If I'm honest, the biggest benefit for me personally has been that veganism and my way of working it into an active lifestyle is a topic that has resonated with a lot of people. I didn't have a strong voice or a platform or a clue about what I wanted to do with my life before I went vegetarian (and then vegan), and now I do, so that's a huge change."

FOOD & SUPPLEMENTS

What do you eat for Breakfast?
A smoothie, made of berries, a banana, a leafy green, and a bunch of ground up nuts and seeds. Every day.

What do you eat for Lunch?
Leftovers from the previous night's dinner. If for some reason I don't have them, then a huge salad with beans and a nut-based dressing, along with some fruit and a pita with hummus or almond butter spread on it.

What do you eat for Dinner?
A big salad, and then often some combination of a grain + a green + a bean. I love making authentic ethnic food, like Indian, Sri Lankan, and Thai dishes. I'm a sucker for Italian food too, so a lot of pasta dishes with beans in the sauce.

What do you eat for Snacks - healthy & not-so healthy?
Fruit, especially oranges. Whole-wheat pita bread with hummus or almond butter. Mostly raw trail mix (Strider's Snack from Whole Foods). Sometimes cereal with almond milk - recently I've been into Rip's Big Bowl, from Engine 2.

What is your favourite source of Protein?
Lentils, especially red.

What is your favourite source of Calcium?
Broccoli.

What is your favourite source of Iron?
Pumpkin seeds, in my smoothie.

What foods give you the most energy?
Fruits, like in my morning smoothie. Fresh dates when I run, too.

Do you take any supplements?
Yes, a multivitamin and DHA/EPA supplement – both from Dr. Fuhrman.

ADVICE

What is your top tip for gaining muscle?
Stop running and start eating, especially fats. Lift hard at the gym but for just 20-30 minutes, 2-3 times per week.

What is your top tip for losing weight?
Stop eating oil, stop eating between meals, and eat a gigantic salad (with nut-based dressing, not oil) before every meal, or make that your meal if possible. Basically, the Eat to Live plan - I've met so many people who lost 20lbs+ (9kg+) with it.

What is your top tip for maintaining weight?
Base your diet on whole foods, some raw, some cooked. I think a little oil is fine, but don't eat too much of it.

What is your top tip for improving metabolism?
I don't really believe in speeding up metabolism as a healthy goal. From a longevity perspective, I'd prefer to have a slow metabolism, and get by on fewer calories. Just eat whole foods and your body will do what it's supposed to do, in most cases.

What is your top tip for toning up?
Again, eat whole foods, but do some exercise. You don't need to do anything crazy - walking or running for maybe 30 minutes a few times a week, plus some body weight exercises.

How do you promote veganism in your daily life?
Above all, I strive to be an example, and to let people see what I do, read my blog, and hopefully be inspired to give the diet a try. I love when someone in my non-digital life doesn't realize I'm vegan until after we've known each other for a several weeks and hung out several times. I know many vegans feel it's their duty to be as vocal as possible about it, and that's totally cool - some people won't be reached any other way. But, for my part, I like to appeal to another set of people - those who will be pleasantly surprised to learn that you can be both vegan and "normal."

How would you suggest people get involved with what you do?
My No Meat Athlete blog, book, and podcast too. Also on Twitter and FaceBook.

"I'm on a mission now to be the opposite of militant and preachy, to reach all those people like I used to be, who are interested in the personal choice of veganism but not necessarily in becoming an activist."

MATT LETTEN
VEGAN PERSONAL TRAINER

Throughout USA
Vegan since: 2012

veganbros.com
SM: *FaceBook, Google+, Instagram, Pinterest, Twitter, YouTube*

Matt Letten is a renowned fitness coach and serial entrepreneur. He's helped over 3,000 people get closer to reaching their fitness and lifestyle goals. Matt is the Founder of 3 fitness facilities in Michigan. Since launching VeganBros. com, an online community for those interested in getting sexy and living more fulfilling lives, he now resides mostly in Seattle, Washington. Matt spends his days coaching, speaking, traveling, and planning world domination with Vegan Bros Co-founder and brother, Phil. Also his best friend is a pup named Peyton.

WHY VEGAN?

How and why did you decide to become vegan?
My brother, Phil Letten, was a major influence on making the change. For years, I was antagonistic towards vegans and wanted nothing to do with the idea. During a time when I was coming into my own, I began re-examining many of my points of view, and long held beliefs. Around this time, my brother, linked me to a video exposing the cruelty that goes on at factory farms. I remember thinking to myself, while watching it, "I don't think I'm going to be able to eat meat again." I went vegetarian the next day, and vegan a bit further down the road.

How long have you been vegan?
Over 3 years.

What has benefited you the most from being vegan?
I had severe asthma and allergies growing up, which continued into adulthood. When I went vegan, my asthma and allergies literally vanished. I feel vibrant and energetic every day. I never realized how bad I felt on a daily basis, until I went vegan, and feel amazing every day.

My athletic performance has also benefited immensely. I've been able to add clean muscle, move faster and I'm able to power through crazy workouts like they're no big deal.

What does veganism mean to you?
To me, veganism is about living out my values, having a real impact on the world, and showing the fitness community that vegan means strong, fit, and healthy.

"While going vegan is not what propelled my initial weight loss, it is what propels me to be the best I can be, going forward. Since being vegan, I am healthier than at any point prior in my life. The strength from that is being able to relate to others who struggle with their weight and eating habits."

TRAINING

What sort of training do you do?
I train in many different styles, from bodybuilding, to kettlebells, to CrossFit, to circuit training. I get bored easily, and like changing it up. I love tracking my progress, and reaching new Personal Records.

How often do you (need to) train?
I typically train 5-6 days per week.

Do you offer your fitness or training services to others?
I opened my first gym almost 6 years ago, and since have opened 2 others. I was a personal trainer at my facilities. With those now sold, I focus my efforts on Vegan Bros, where we take on clients a couple of times each year.

What sports do you play?
I grew up playing baseball, basketball, and soccer. As an adult, I like to stay active, with group CrossFit-style workouts, and recreational league softball. I also will play soccer and volleyball whenever I catch word of a game I can get involved with.

STRENGTHS, WEAKNESSES & OUTSIDE INFLUENCES

What do you think is the biggest misconception about vegans and how do you address this?
I believe there is just a lack of solid information for the public, about what vegan is, and what it means. Typically, I get a couple of responses when people find out I'm vegan. First off, sheer disbelief, as they assume all vegans are skinny and weak. I really enjoy being a person's first introduction to what a vegan is. I will keep working hard, just for that reason alone. And then - of course, "Where do you get your protein from?"

One of the awesome things I've noticed of late, is the tide seems to be changing. When I get into a conversation about plant-based eating, many people I speak with, refer to a vegan diet as a superior, healthy diet, that they simply haven't attained yet. It's then great speaking with people about simple changes they can began making, to work toward reducing their animal consumption.

What are your strengths as a vegan athlete?
One of my main strengths comes from prior weakness. I was extremely unhealthy and obese growing up. This carried into my college years, when I got fed up. I began to attend the gym and make nutritional changes, and through hard work and determination, I was able to lose nearly 100lbs (45kg), and it transformed my life from the inside out.

While going vegan is not what propelled my initial weight loss, it is what propels me to be the best I can be, going forward. Since being vegan, I am healthier than at any point prior in my life. The strength from that is being able to relate to others who struggle with their weight and eating habits.

My physical strengths as a vegan athlete, I believe, would be my overall fitness. I work hard to meet strength with endurance. This allows me to be strong, while also agile, and able to work hard and fast for long periods of time.

What is your biggest challenge?
My biggest challenge is myself. I'm constantly trying to better myself so that I can be at my best for my clients, in helping them reach their fitness goals, and ultimately to reduce and hopefully eliminate their animal consumption.

Are the non-vegans in your industry supportive or not?
I talk about this with many close friends. I believe it's really a mixed bag. While the world at large is growing more and more supportive of veganism each and every day, there are some in the fitness industry trying their best to hold on to animal proteins as an essential part of the diet. Thankfully, research on the immense health benefits of a vegan diet, are putting the final nail in the coffin of the shrinking "we must eat animals" crowd.

Are your family and friends supportive of your vegan lifestyle?
I have an incredible group around me. My brother and both parents are vegan, along with many friends. New friends are asking me about it each and every week. It's exciting to see people wake up, just like I did!

What is the most common question/comment that people ask/say when they find out that you are a vegan and how do you respond?
People ask where I get my protein, how difficult it must be and ultimately disbelieve that someone healthy and strong can be vegan. I truly enjoy being an advocate for animals. I am by no means perfect, but I have worked hard to get where I am, and view my career as working to save animals, by way of showing how easy, beneficial, and healthy a vegan diet is. I always let people know how easy it is to be vegan and how great I feel every day. Not to mention how amazing it feels to know that I have fully opted out of an industry of torture and death.

Who or what motivates you?
I am motivated by many of my friends and family, who work tirelessly on behalf of animals, volunteering and working with organizations such as Mercy For Animals, Vegan Outreach and The Humane League. I have amazing friends who doing amazing things. I am also motivated to help others undergo the same transformation I have had the privilege of going through. I simply want everyone to feel the way I do.

FOOD & SUPPLEMENTS

What do you eat for Breakfast?
Sun Warrior Protein shake with oatmeal added.

What do you eat for Lunch?
Either a protein or fruit smoothie, a loaded salad, or Thai stir-fry in a low calorie white sauce, with loads of veggies and tofu.

What do you eat for Dinner?
Tempeh stir-fry with plenty of spices.

What do you eat for Snacks (healthy & not-so healthy)?
I'll bite at the not so healthy here. I have a weakness for Double Stuf Oreos. NO, not regular Oreos. DOUBLE STUFF or bust!

What is your favourite source of Protein?
Sun Warrior Protein powder and spinach.

What is your favourite source of Calcium?
Broccoli.

What is your favourite source of Iron?
Spinach and kale.

What foods give you the most energy?
Sun Warrior and bananas are my staples for energy.

Do you take any supplements?
I do take Sun Warrior Protein Powder, along with BCAA's, and Creatine. I also take B-12, Vitamin C, and Vitamin-D.

ADVICE

What is your top tip for gaining muscle?
Nutrition is key. Be sure to get a good combination of protein and carbohydrates PRE and POST workout. Also, work in hypertrophy range, lifting heavy in sets of 8-12 repetitions.

What is your top tip for losing weight?
Monitor your calories. Be sure to eat a higher protein diet, moderate fats and moderately lower carbohydrates. Find what works for you. Do not be afraid to lift heavy, fat loss will come faster.

What is your top tip for maintaining weight?
Simply work on eating mostly whole foods. Stick to fruits and veggies and you're going to be in great shape.

What is your top tip for improving metabolism?
High protein, high fiber, faster cardio in the morning, sprint training occasionally and ultimately build muscle mass.

What is your top tip for toning up?
Stick with mostly high repetition range days of 15-25, with occasional 8-12 repetition sessions, along with high-intensity interval training (HIIT) cardio after your strength session.

How do you promote veganism in your daily life?
At Vegan Bros, we blog, post videos on YouTube, and occasionally throw sold out events benefitting animal advocacy groups. Also, we recently launched our exclusive high end course, The Ultimate Vegan Fat Loss Course, to vegans who want to lose weight. We walk our clients through a total body transformation using the most effective fat loss exercises and scientifically proven nutrition habits.

How would you suggest people get involved with what you do?
Head over to our website, and download a free digital copy of our book, "The Top 6 Mistakes Preventing You From Losing Belly Fat." Also, check get involved in our Facebook community and our YouTube Channel.

"I am motivated by many of my friends and family, who work tirelessly on behalf of animals, volunteering and working with organizations such as Mercy For Animals, Vegan Outreach and The Humane League. I have amazing friends who doing amazing things. I am also motivated to help others undergo the same transformation I have had the privilege of going through. I simply want everyone to feel the way I do."

MATT RUSCIGNO
VEGAN ENDURANCE ATHLETE

Los Angeles, California, USA
Vegan since: 1996

truelovehealth.com
strongesthearts.org
SM: *FaceBook, Instagram, Twitter*

Matt Ruscigno is a vegan of nearly two decades, with nutritional degrees from Pennsylvania State and Loma Linda Universities, as well as certification as a Registered Dietitian – one of the only professional nutrition credentials available. In addition to working with vegetarian clients and athletes, Matt is the Past-Chair of the Vegetarian Nutrition Group of the Academy of Nutrition and Dietetics, and he co-authored the "No Meat Athlete" book with Matt Frazier, and "Appetite for Reduction" with Isa Moskowitz.

An athlete himself, Matt has raced the World's Hardest Ironman in Eidfjord, Norway, numerous ultra-marathons, 24-hour mountain bike races and is a 3x solo finisher of The Furnace Creek 508, a 500-mile (804m) non-stop bike race through Death Valley, USA that National Geographic Adventure calls the 8th hardest race in the world.

WHY VEGAN?

How and why did you decide to become vegan?
I have loved animals since a very young age and after a few failed attempts at vegetarianism I went vegan in 1996 at the age of 17. As a teenager, I was part of the hardcore punk music scene and influence by bands like Earth Crisis and Chokehold who espoused ethical veganism as part of a bigger commitment to social justice.

What has benefited you the most from being vegan?
The compassionate, motivated, driven people I have met who turn their anger about injustice into passionate activism. It is a unified struggle - in veganism you are never alone.

What does veganism mean to you?
Vegan means I'm trying to suck less, as Food Fight! Grocery says. There's a lot we can do to make the world a better place and being vegan is an important part of the solution to end injustice.

"Many vegans think that what works for them should work for everyone, but that's not the case. We need to think beyond our own habits, culture, etc to understand how other people can eat more vegan foods. It's a privilege to purposefully restrict your food and sometimes vegans forget this. We have to meet people where they are at and recognize social inequalities."

TRAINING

What sort of training do you do?

My main focus is endurance cycling so I spend a lot of time on the bike. I ride road, mountain, cyclocross and track, so it never gets old! I also do some ultra-running, and mix up my training with yoga, pilates and some free weight work.

How often do you (need to) train?

Between cycling, running, surfing, pilates, yoga and the gym I probably train every day. I do what's fun and whatever I'm feeling into - I don't follow a strict regiment - never have, even when training for something like Ironman. I like fun more than strict rules.

Do you offer your fitness or training services to others?

As a Registered Dietitian I take clients who want to eat healthier and understand nutrition. My goal is to help them make the best choices for them. Sometimes this includes tips for training and working out.

What sports do you play?

I don't really play any "sports".

STRENGTHS, WEAKNESSES & OUTSIDE INFLUENCES

What do you think is the biggest misconception about vegans and how do you address this?

That vegans are privileged and one-dimensional. I approach this by having an open mind and not always talking about veganism. I let my actions speak for themselves, and when it comes up I discuss it passionately, in a non-judgmental way. I often hear, "I didn't know you were vegan because you don't talk about it all of the time." People are then amazed at how much I do and that I've been vegan more than half of my life. The best way to influence people is to be a positive example.

What are your strengths as a vegan athlete?

Most of my foods are superfoods - eating all of those leafy greens, cruciferous vegetables, bad-ass legumes and whole grains is a huge strength. Fruits are hydrating and all those antioxidants help with my recovery so I can train more often.

What is your biggest challenge?

I've bike toured through Central America, Alaska, rural Montana, to name a few, and finding healthy vegan meals can be challenging. But, I've always found a way - veganism forces you to be creative. As a professional it is a challenge to change people's behaviors - it's not an easy task!

Are the non-vegans in your industry supportive or not?

As a Registered Dietitian, I am sometimes seen as radical, but most RD's are more supportive than the general public realizes. I'm part of a Vegetarian Group of the Academy of Nutrition and Dietetics and we have over 1500 members that are RD's and Diet Techs. Sure, not all of them are vegan, but they are interested enough in plant-based diets to be a part of our group. The world is starting to lean toward eating more plants- it's a great time to be a nutrition professional.

Are your family and friends supportive of your vegan lifestyle?

I have many vegan and vegan-ish friends and my family is very supportive - they know I work hard at what I do, not for myself, but for the animals and for other people. Many of my non-vegan friends have a great respect for my work and now eat more vegan meals.

What is the most common question/comment that people ask/say when they find out that you are a vegan and how do you respond?
Most people are genuinely curious about what I eat all day. Everyone imagines their own plates but with the meat and cheese missing; they can't even comprehend what an entirely plant-based meal looks like. I reach them by learning about what they eat and discussing similar vegan options. Many vegans think that what works for them should work for everyone, but that's not the case. We need to think beyond our own habits, culture, etc to understand how other people can eat more vegan foods. It's a privilege to purposefully restrict your food and sometimes vegans forget this. We have to meet people where they are at and recognize social inequalities.

Who or what motivates you?
The world is a screwed up place, but I'm fortunate to know many hardworking activists who have dedicated their life to making it better. It takes more than a vegan food blog to make real change. There are environmental and animal rights activists in prison right now because of what they believe in! We cannot forget them and all of the people who came before us. Their sacrifices motivate me to work harder and be the best activist I can be.

FOOD & SUPPLEMENTS

What do you eat for Breakfast?
I love: mashed bananas with almond butter, diced apples and blueberries.

What do you eat for Lunch?
Burritos, burritos, burritos, burritos. Rice, beans, salsa, and avocado in a tortilla is possibly the tastiest human invention of all time.

What do you eat for Dinner?
Stir-fry with a lot of broccoli and purple cabbage with peanut sauce over brown rice or noodles. YUM.

What do you eat for Snacks (healthy & not-so healthy)?
Fortunately I love fruit and snack on it all of the time, especially citrus. Pretzels and hummus are a classic vegan snack I've been eating since day one. I've been known to eat a vegan doughnut or two in my time as well. And chocolate!

What is your favourite source of Protein?
Peanut butter and pinto beans. Well, not together. But as in both of them are my favorite. I think.

What is your favourite source of Calcium?
KALE and corn tortillas.

What is your favourite source of Iron?
Blackstrap molasses. Just kidding. Does anyone actually eat that stuff?! Beans is my final answer.

What foods give you the most energy?
Fruit or burritos, but not together.

Do you take any supplements?
I take B-12, as every vegan should. Also, nutritional yeast and flax oil are kind of like supplements.

"I have loved animals since a very young age and after a few failed attempts at vegetarianism I went vegan in 1996 at the age of 17. As a teenager, I was part of the hardcore punk music scene and influence by bands like Earth Crisis and Chokehold who espoused ethical veganism as part of a bigger commitment to social justice."

ADVICE

What is your top tip for gaining muscle?
Work hard, smart, and consistently. Gotta rest. And eat carbohydrates post-workout, not just protein.

What is your top tip for losing weight?
Eat more vegetables. Eat slower. If you love eating why rush it?

What is your top tip for maintaining weight?
Pay close attention to your body. Know you are going to fluctuate and that's okay.

How do you promote veganism in your daily life?
As a nutrition professional, I'm constantly writing or talking about veganism. Plus I believe strongly in intersectional politics and building inclusive communities beyond veganism. I'm also co-creator of Strongest Hearts, a web series on vegan athletes. I work with Sasha Perry, a professional filmmaker, so they are high-quality videos, each with a strong message about how vegans can kick ass!

How would you suggest people get involved with what you do?
Becoming an RD is very hard work, but if you love science I say go for it.

"The world is a screwed up place, but I'm fortunate to know many hardworking activists who have dedicated their life to making it better. It takes more than a vegan food blog to make real change. There are environmental and animal rights activists in prison right now because of what they believe in! We cannot forget them and all of the people who came before us. Their sacrifices motivate me to work harder and be the best activist I can be."

Accept Every Challenge That Comes Your Way

MAURO REIS
VEGAN EXERCISE ENTHUSIAST

Bucks County, Pennsylvania, USA
Vegan since: 2010

fromatovegan.com
SM: *FaceBook, Pinterest, Twitter, YouTube*

Mauro Reis is a recent (since 2013) fitness enthusiast, trying to balance his very physical day job as a farrier, a second job as web developer for his wife's business, and other social obligations and hobbies, while still saving up some energy for a regular exercise routine. Sometimes it even works out.

WHY VEGAN?

Because I can't morally justify what nowadays is an unnecessary and detrimental practice. We don't need to use or kill animals anymore.

How and why did you decide to become vegan?
I was a vegetarian for over 17 years, but for many years had been slowly learning about what is really involved in animal agriculture. After awhile I couldn't ignore it any longer.

How long have you been vegan?
Since 2010.

What has benefited you the most from being vegan?
I've lost some extra weight I'd been carrying around and had other health improvements like lowered cholesterol and better skin condition. Plus, now I eat a lot better - as a vegetarian my diet was not really that great.

What does veganism mean to you?
It's an ethical framework, one of trying not to cause unnecessary harm.

TRAINING

What sort of training do you do?
Weight/bodyweight training mostly, with some high-intensity interval training (HIIT).

How often do you (need to) train?
I train 5 days a week for about 20 to 30 minutes.

What sports do you play?
Are board games a sport?! I used to practice Aikido, but because my work is too physically demanding, I had to stop some years ago.

"My biggest fitness-related challenge is being able to maintain a regular exercise schedule on top of a physically demanding profession. I have a good rhythm, but it's hard some days. I don't think I have any big vegan-related challenges anymore, my life is pretty well organized around being vegan nowadays."

STRENGTHS, WEAKNESSES & OUTSIDE INFLUENCES

What do you think is the biggest misconception about vegans and how do you address this?
That we only eat salad. I try to talk about the food we eat and depending on the person, even go to a vegan restaurant with them.

What is your biggest challenge?
My biggest fitness-related challenge is being able to maintain a regular exercise schedule on top of a physically demanding profession. I have a good rhythm, but it's hard some days. I don't think I have any big vegan-related challenges anymore, my life is pretty well organized around being vegan nowadays.

Are the non-vegans in your industry supportive or not?
Most of the people I deal with are indifferent, but at least are not hostile to veganism. When I started, they told me I wouldn't be able to handle my work because I didn't eat meat, but after all these years they realized that was not true at all.

Are your family and friends supportive of your vegan lifestyle?
My sisters - who are the people in my family I'm most close to - are. I have a number of friends that, while not vegans, see veganism as a good thing. I'm also part of a vegan supper club so I do have a lot of supportive friends. The friends that were hostile to veganism, well, are not friends anymore.

What is the most common question/comment that people ask/say when they find out that you are a vegan and how do you respond?
"How do you get your protein?" I usually respond "The same way you do. Pretty much everything I eat has protein in it."

Who or what motivates you?
Compassion for the animals.

FOOD & SUPPLEMENTS

What do you eat for Breakfast?
Most days is a bagel with vegan cream cheese, either instant coffee mixed on a cup of soy milk – or a protein shake, depending on how hard my workout was – and a banana.

What do you eat for Lunch?
It's a variety of different foods, there's really no fixed menu. Sometimes it's sandwiches, sometimes it's leftovers from the night before.

What do you eat for Dinner?
I have a Community-Supported Agriculture (CSA) share so we eat a LOT of vegetables, especially during the growing season. I try to make sure I have some balance between carbohydrates, protein and fat, but again, there's no fixed menu.

What do you eat for Snacks - healthy & not-so healthy?
Carrots and fruit, edamame, cherry tomatoes, primal strips, granola bars, I also keep a bag of whole wheat pretzels for emergencies in my truck. If my wife bakes a cake or pie, I'll eat that too.

What is your favourite source of Protein, Calcium, Iron?
I don't worry about that too much, I just eat a variety of whole and fresh foods. So far it has worked out okay.

Do you take any supplements?
B-12 vitamins.

ADVICE

What is your top tip for Gaining muscle, Losing weight, Maintaining weight, Improving metabolism, Toning up?
For me, what really worked was finding a good workout program that we could stick to. My wife and I found one last year and it worked wonders, in a very short amount of time. I'm in the best shape of my life, working out only 20-30 minutes, 5 days a week, at home with minimal equipment. The program gave us structure and a schedule to stick to, and it took the guesswork out of the equation for us.

How do you promote veganism in your daily life?
I work with animals, and at some point or another everybody learns I'm vegan. So I let my general ethics and the way I work with the animals speak for themselves.

How would you suggest people get involved with what you do?
With veganism, try finding a vegan group around where you live – Meetup.com is a good option, or FaceBook. If there isn't a group, start one yourself. For fitness, there are tons of online resources where you can find workout programs to get started.

"I am vegan because I can't morally justify what nowadays is an unnecessary and detrimental practice. We don't need to use or kill animals anymore."

Whatever you do today gets you closer to where you want to be tomorrow.

Meagan Duhamel
VEGAN PROFESSIONAL FIGURE SKATER

Montreal, Quebec, Canada
Vegan since: 2009

twitter.com/mhjd_85

Meagan Duhamel is a Canadian pair skater. With current partner Eric Radford, she is the four-time Canadian national champion (2012-2015), 2011 Four Continents silver medalist, 2011 Canadian national silver medalist two-time World Bronze medalist (2013 & 2014). She is also an Olympic silver medalist in the team figure skating event and 2015 world champion. Megan has previously skated with Craig Buntin, with whom she is the 2010 Four Continents bronze medalist, 2009 Canadian national silver medalist, and 2008 & 2010 Canadian bronze medalist.

WHY VEGAN?

The vegan diet is healthy and leads to a compassionate lifestyle.

How and why did you decide to become vegan?
I went vegan after reading the book "Skinny Bitch". I had no intention of becoming vegan but that book was a real eye opener and I decided I wanted to change my life.

How long have you been vegan?
I've been vegan for over 5 years.

What has benefited you the most from being vegan?
I've gotten so many benefits. My weight is easily maintained, my skin glows, I sleep better and I feel more energized.

What does veganism mean to you?
Veganism means living compassionately. It's not only a diet but also a lifestyle. Being a vegan is life changing, not only for oneself but also for the people around you. You'll lead a more positive, patient and gracious life.

TRAINING

What sort of training do you do?
I am training for the 2018 Olympics as a pairs figure skater.

How often do you (need to) train?
I train Monday-Friday, 3 hours daily spent on the ice, training elements and our routine. I spend 2 hours off the ice everyday training as well, doing Pilates, yoga, running and stretching.

Do you offer your fitness or training services to others?
I coach in my spare time as well as help the other skaters at my rink with their flexibility and off-ice training.

What sports do you play?
I mostly only have time to figure skate. However, this summer I'm playing on a baseball team.

STRENGTHS, WEAKNESSES & OUTSIDE INFLUENCES

What do you think is the biggest misconception about vegans and how do you address this?
That we are malnourished hippies! It's not true. We are just individuals who want to live a healthy lifestyle without harming anything or anyone is in process.

What are your strengths as a vegan athlete?
I feel I have become stronger since I started a vegan diet and I have more energy to train harder and longer.

What is your biggest challenge?
My biggest challenge comes when I travel. We have meals supplied to us through the organizing committee of competitions and it's very rare that they include meals for me. Usually it's just lots of meat, cheese and pasta.

Are the non-vegans in your industry supportive or not?
Everyone is supportive. The other athletes love the treats I bring with me to competitions and often ask me for recipes.

Are your family and friends supportive of your vegan lifestyle?
Yes, my family and friends are very supportive and never judgmental.

What is the most common question/comment that people ask/say when they find out that you are a vegan and how do you respond?
They ask me what I eat – haha! It surprises a lot of people when they hear my answer. They assume I only eat fruits and vegetables.

Who or what motivates you?
I am easily motivated. I am always looking for ways to improve myself and it's a never-ending process.

FOOD & SUPPLEMENTS

What do you eat for Breakfast?
A green smoothie with spinach, beets, banana, mango, almond milk, chia seeds and cacao bits. Or I will make myself a breakfast bowl. I chop up kale, and put grapefruit juice on it (to get extra vitamin C), then add blueberries, banana, goji berries and cacao bits, and I add in some homemade granola. Or cereal with almond milk.

What do you eat for Lunch?
I make homemade muffins - my carrot muffins are my favourite - trail mix, granola bars (Krono bar) and fruits is my go-to lunch when I'm on the road.

What do you eat for Dinner?
Quinoa salads, kale salads, brown rice tempeh bowls. Basically a whole grain with veggies and a simple protein, tempeh, tofu or beans. I eat very clean foods, nothing fancy.

What do you eat for Snacks - healthy & not-so healthy?
I make some pretty amazing chocolate cupcakes. I love to bake so anything from muffins to cookies to trail mix.

What is your favourite source of Protein?
Beans.

What is your favourite source of Calcium?
Broccoli, kale and other green vegetables.

What is your favourite source of Iron?
My iron supplement!

What foods give you the most energy?
Mostly anything. I make some super-charge-me cookies filled with seeds and dried fruits and those usually do the trick.

Do you take any supplements?
I take an iron supplement and B12 vitamin along with a multi vitamin and Omega 3-6-9 vitamin.

ADVICE

What is your top tip for gaining muscle?
Pilates or yoga. It is not hard on the body and you can do it at home by yourself or in the studio with a trainer.

What is your top tip for losing weight?
Move! Don't stop eating; just add exercise to your daily routine.

What is your top tip for maintaining weight?
Eat a balanced diet.

What is your top tip for improving metabolism?
Eat a balanced diet.

What is your top tip for toning up?
Again, Pilates or yoga.

How do you promote veganism in your daily life?
I try to talk to anyone who is interested. I am not surrounded by any other vegans in my life so I'm advocating alone for veganism.

How would you suggest people get involved with what you do?
This I don't have an answer because I'm not involved in much because like I said, I don't really associate with other vegans, I don't personally know any.

"Veganism means living compassionately. It's not only a diet but also a lifestyle. Being a vegan is life changing, not only for oneself but also for the people around you. You'll lead a more positive, patient and gracious life."

I expect to pass through this world by once; any good thing therefore that I can do, any kindness that I can show to any fellow creature, let me do it now; let me not defer to neglect it, for I shall not pass this way again

- Etienne De Grellet

MICHAEL PERRY
VEGAN TRIATHLETE

Gold Coast, Queensland, Australia
Vegan since: 2007

taonutrition.com.au
SM: *FaceBook, Instagram, Twitter, YouTube*

Michael Perry is a passionate tri and endurance athlete spending a great deal of his spare time outdoors, and enjoying competitive level swim, bike and run. Discovering that athletes could benefit significantly from high quality fuel, his curiosity for optimising athletic performance through nutrition became a passion. Michael is also co-founder of Tao Nutrition, a premium natural protein and superfood. He is proud to provide a genuine and authentic nutritional tool that many can use in their own pursuit of personal greatness.

WHY VEGAN?

How and why did you decide to become vegan?
My first realisation that something was not right with my current lifestyle came when I was reading an environmental ethics book. It highlighted that animals as sentient beings had rights too. It catalysed a thought process that gained momentum and supported an underlying knowing since I was young, that producing animals as a resource for human gain and the way they were treated was not right. The second issue that was significant for me was the environmental cost of 'producing' animals.

Realising that I could make a change in my world to impact what was going on, I went vegetarian. Over a number of years I learned more and more about the environmental, social, ethical and health benefits which lead to going plant-based (vegan). I am so happy with my journey, the choices I have and continue to make, and the place that I am at right now.

How long have you been vegan?
Eight years now.

What has benefited you the most from being vegan?
Being conscious of how things are produced, what goes into them and having that awareness around their lifecycle gives me the opportunity to make choices everyday that make a difference. I love putting conscious awareness into day-to-day actions and decisions. I think that this simple task or action, if done by everyone would make a huge difference in the world as we know it. I feel the outcome of these decisions (especially in my space) aligns with my intentions, goals and aspirations. Healthy mind, body and soul.

What does veganism mean to you?
Living a life full of conscious experience in harmony and symbiosis with the earth.

TRAINING

What sort of training do you do?
I am a passionate triathlete, and love it.

How often do you (need to) train?
Two to three sessions per day, up to 20+hrs per week. Luckily I love it!

Do you offer your fitness or training services to others?
I help friends and family on a one-on-one basis but also made a conscious choice about 2 years ago to provide service in a different way. I co-founded a natural protein and superfood powder Tao Nutrition. Our vision is to share and inspire health in the community through healthy nutrition. We have focused our product on providing a healthy and super nutritious, convenient snack option rich in healthy proteins and superfood ingredients for nutrients – 100% plant-based and vegan of course.

We also put a huge amount of effort into educating our passionate community as we think that awareness and positive behaviour change is one the most effective ways to make a difference. We love putting out high quality articles on health, wellbeing, performance and of course delicious recipes.

STRENGTHS, WEAKNESSES & OUTSIDE INFLUENCES

What do you think is the biggest misconception about vegans and how do you address this?
That we are i) doing something extreme; and ii) our diet is lacking in proper nutrients. For some people who live the standard Australian lifestyle, living consciously is extreme and I can see their perspective and why they would be threatened by a group of people that cause self-reflection. That doesn't mean I agree with it though.

I respectfully address these misconceptions with educated responses about what I have learnt and my personal experiences. I am pushing my mind and body to the limits day in and day out. If my nutrition was inadequate in any way, I simply wouldn't be able to do the things I do. My lifestyle and the way I live it speaks for itself.

In the past, I have tried arguing with people, sighting this study and that health concern, appealing to how their behaviour affect the animals and the environment, but have found the most effective option is being a positive role model for a plant-based healthy lifestyle.

What are your strengths as a vegan athlete?
I recover fast and have stable energy levels throughout the day. I never get colds or the flu, which means less down time and more training. Also bringing meditation into my lifestyle has allowed me to shed physical and most importantly mental fatigue meaning that I am sharper, can deal with life situations rationally and make better decisions.

I was unfortunately hit by a car whilst training on my bike in November 2013. I broke both of my legs and sustained heaps of lower limb injuries. My doctors were shocked at how quickly I healed! I had a lot of large skin grazes that had healed within 2-3 weeks and they said my physical recovery was about 2-3 times faster than a normal person.

I couldn't have done it without a high quality lifestyle, being plant-based and the inclusion of high quality nutrition like Tao Nutrition.

Are your family and friends supportive of your vegan lifestyle?
I think some are still waiting for my wheels to fall off, or some major negative health event to happen. Even after 15 years of being vegetarian and over 5 years being vegan. I quietly keep achieving my goals and reaching new levels of health and performance, and I think my actions and who I 'am' speak loudly enough.

The occasional joke is thrown my way, but when you see a training buddy using the raw balls recipe you let them try the week before or see them making a change in a way I have passively inspired, I can see their support in that way too. They are generally tolerant of a vegan lifestyle and try to choose somewhere when eating out that serves 'our type' of food.

What is the most common question/comment that people ask/say when they find out that you are a vegan and how do you respond?
"Where do you get your protein, iron, calcium from?" I used to say, "Where do you get your protein from?" and then walk them through where and how their animal derived sources arrive conveniently in the supermarket, but found that to not be a very successful conversation.

I now approach the question a little more respectively and it's not what they are asking but why. They come from a position where society has marketed them into thinking they must eat x, y and z to live, or else. Explaining to them how much protein humans actually need and that plant-based sources of the nutrients are where it's at. I go through some awesome recipes that we make at home for meals and if I have anything on hand will give them a try of whatever I am eating - I am usually eating something. Again, I think people take more from what they see than what you say. If you are thriving, it's hard to argue against that.

Who or what motivates you?
I am inspired by people who become aware of their situation and make a conscious change for the better. That is the catalyst for a life changing behaviour or situation, and can lead to experiences that would not have come about otherwise.

The second thing that inspires me is walking through the supermarket and seeing all of the toxic food moving from the shelves into people trolleys. I see unhappy people walking around the aisles putting low quality food into their trolleys wondering why they feel so bad. I am motivated to give the community products and information that build health - from a company that is genuine and whose vision is authentic.

FOOD & SUPPLEMENTS

What do you eat for Breakfast?
Smoothies are a staple breakfast for me as they are convenient, portable and I can get heaps of nutrients in there, Tao Nutrition is a key ingredient of course. One of our smoothies, or a sugar-free, whole food, gluten-free, superfood muesli with Tao Nutrition on top with rice or coconut milk.

What do you eat for Lunch?
A huge salad - you would love to see the size of my salads - with heaps of fresh veggies and avocados. Yum.

What do you eat for Dinner?
Roasted vegetables on bed of salad, homemade pizza (gluten-free dough), homemade veggie burgers, laksa, curries, and stir-fries.

What do you eat for Snacks - healthy & not-so healthy?
Tao Power Balls, Choc Mint Smoothie, organic vegan fair-trade dark chocolate, Fruit – Yum!

What is your favourite source of Protein?
Tao Nutrition.

What is your favourite source of Calcium?
Sesame seeds, kale and coconut water.

What is your favourite source of Iron?
Leafy greens and amaranth.

What foods give you the most energy?
Long burn energy in between sessions – salads with avocado, coconut milk and Tao Nutrition smoothies. During sessions – big juicy organic medjool dates will keep me going for 6hr+ sessions.

Do you take any supplements?
B12, Tao Nutrition, Omega 3 DHA and K2 - all vegan sources.

ADVICE

What is your top tip for gaining muscle?
Lift weights, low reps, high recovery, don't skimp on eating a whole food plant-based diet rich in healthy protein, carbohydrates and fat. Ensure recovery before you work each muscle again that week, might be 2-3 days between workouts.

What is your top tip for losing weight?
I feel that weight gain is a by-product of malnutrition and storing toxins by making bad food choices. To rectify these focus on: fresh whole foods ie veggies and fruits that don't come in packets, plant-based foods and organic if possible.

The closer you get to achieving 100% of your diet with these things, your life will transform to a place of endless energy, mental clarity and joyous experience. I think gaining health should be the focus and the weight loss will be a by-product of that. It's like marching for peace instead of against war.

What is your top tip for maintaining weight?
Eat health-building foods until you are satiated and full and your body will reach its natural healthy weight. Be honest and don't starve yourself, the world is an abundant place.

What is your top tip for improving metabolism?
Be active every day. Standing workstation, squats in the toilet stalls, pushups, taking the stairs, riding to work, join your friends on that lunchtime walk or run or make new ones doing something fun. Lots of fresh veggies especially leafy greens – high nutrient density, bigger volume gets the digestive fire burning.

What is your top tip for toning up?
High quality nutrition, and being active. No secrets here, you want to look athletic, be athletic. That includes cardio, strength and fun.

How do you promote veganism in your daily life?
By being the change I want to see in the world, and by being the co-founder of a plant-based premium protein superfood.

How would you suggest people get involved with what you do?
Visit my website.

MIKE PORTMAN
VEGAN TRIATHLETE

San Francisco, California, USA
Vegan since: 2009

portmancoaching.com
SM: *FaceBook, Twitter*

Mike Portman had a typical childhood of school and sports. Over the years he became more of a couch potato, and he never felt energetic or happy and he always tried to find to magical pill or food that would solve all his woes. Over the college years, Mike started running and then became a triathlete. He has become a winner of multiple races and it is common to see him on the podium whether overall or his age group. Attributing much of his gains to his positive mental outlook to training and vegan diet, Mike also coaches athletes in endurance sports to help them get the results they desire.

WHY VEGAN?

How and why did you decide to become vegan?
I become vegan after I learned about the environmental impact a person's diet has on the planet. After I learned this, I slowly made changes to my diet and lifestyle. Went lacto-ovo vegetarian for 2 years and then thought if I was really serious about what I stand for, then I should become fully vegan. Since the process for me was rather slow compared to most, it wasn't too hard of a shift to be 100% animal-free when I made the commitment.

How long have you been vegan?
It's been over 5 years. Didn't really have a start date, it just happened.

What has benefited you the most from being vegan?
Hard to say, as so many things in my life have improved. I'd probably say my quality of life has benefited most overall. The way I feel mentally and physically almost always stays constant. That way of feeling keeps me motivated on tackling the day whether it's training, coaching, or something else.

What does veganism mean to you?
To me veganism means a lifestyle that is not limiting the way you live your life, but embracing ways that are healthy for yourself, others, animals, and the planet.

"All endurance athletes thrive on roughly the same macronutrient percentages of carbohydrates, proteins, and fats. The downside of animal foods is that they give the human body no carbohydrates. Plant foods are the only foods that have carbohydrates, which is the macronutrient that endurance athletes need the most of before, during, and after a workout. The great thing about being vegan is that I never need to worry that my body doesn't have enough carbs in my system to perform optimally."

TRAINING

What sort of training do you do?
I am a triathlete. Which means I perform in races that are swimming, biking, and running all in one day. Back to back... to back.

How often do you (need to) train?
It depends on the time of year and what I am training for, but on average, it's 3-4 hours a day. Some days more, some days less. This includes swimming, biking, running, and cross training (functional strength and core work). I spread out the workload so it's usually swim and run one day, then bike and core work another. Layers upon layers is what makes an athlete great.

Do you offer your fitness or training services to others?
Yes. With USA Triathlon certification, I coach people in person or globally in building training plans for endurance athletes to meet their goals. It's a great line of work and very rewarding.

STRENGTHS, WEAKNESSES & OUTSIDE INFLUENCES

What do you think is the biggest misconception about vegans and how do you address this?
That we are weak and malnourished. Plant-based whole foods have no competition when it comes to the amount of nutrients they bring to an individual, per calorie. If you are a vegan and eat enough calories from whole fruits, veggies, nuts, seeds, and beans then you are a nutrient powerhouse!

What are your strengths as a vegan athlete?
All endurance athletes thrive on roughly the same macronutrient percentages of carbohydrates, proteins, and fats. The downside of animal foods is that they give the human body no carbohydrates. Plant foods are the only foods that have carbohydrates, which is the macronutrient that endurance athletes need the most of before, during, and after a workout. The great thing about being vegan is that I never need to worry that my body doesn't have enough carbs in my system to perform optimally.

What is your biggest challenge?
Traveling can be tough. Living in California makes it easy as we have such a great supply of fresh produce, but travelling can sometimes be difficult. It's easy to stay vegan, at least in the United States, but sometimes the choices of good high quality food can be limited.

Are the non-vegans in your industry supportive or not?
It varies from athlete to athlete. Usually the more experienced athletes are more supportive as they know the value of lots of fruits and vegetables in their own diet. The concerns usually come from people who are new and/or aren't as knowledgeable. Leading by example is the best educator around.

Are your family and friends supportive of your vegan lifestyle?
At first, many were concerned as it was something that they didn't know much about. But over time as they realized not only am I surviving, but thriving this way - they understood more about the lifestyle being more than sustainable.

What is the most common question/comment that people ask/say when they find out that you are a vegan and how do you respond?
I've accepted that I will probably live the rest of my life answering the protein concerns. I do not roll my eyes, as before I made the switch I had the same questions and concerns. I answer by saying that the only way a vegan who eats fruits, veggies, nuts, and seeds will be protein-deficient is by really under-eating their calorie needs. By people observing what I eat, they understand that I definitely eat enough.

Who or what motivates you?
One of the biggest motivators for me is actually negative energy. People who say I cannot do something due to what I don't eat or do. Many people work well with positive encouragement. I like it from time to time but for me I don't need someone to encourage me to work harder. Perhaps that is why I enjoy doing triathlons as it's a sport in which you spend a lot of time alone training. To do well a person really needs to 'enjoy' working hard and being alone with their thoughts.

"To me veganism means a lifestyle that is not limiting the way you live your life, but embracing ways that are healthy for yourself, others, animals, and the planet."

FOOD & SUPPLEMENTS

What do you eat for Breakfast?
Usually some type of smoothie. I really enjoy frozen bananas, mangoes, and dates blended into an 'ice cream'.

What do you eat for Lunch?
By this time I've done at least one workout, so I usually have a bowl of whole grains (brown rice or quinoa) topped with veggies, herbs, and avocado.

What do you eat for Dinner?
Usually some type of green smoothie. A common one I make is 2 bananas, berries, hemp seeds, and a leafy green (usually kale, spinach, or collard greens.)

What do you eat for Snacks - healthy & not-so healthy?
I'm a sucker for dates or bananas with peanut butter. It's a good source of protein and fiber which is what I try to eat in all my meals or snacks. I suggest the peanut butter without sugar, oil, and salt.

What is your favorite source of Protein?
Hemp seeds or leafy greens.

What is your favorite source of Calcium?
Kale.

What is your favorite source of Iron?
Kale - you can never go wrong with kale.

What foods give you the most energy?
Fruit as it's easy to absorb the sugars to give me good energy throughout my day. That plus the fiber, prevents me from having sugar spikes and crashing an hour later.

Do you take any supplements?
I take B-12 a few times a year as well as protein powder as insurance to make sure I have enough protein to recover from workouts.

ADVICE

What is your top tip for gaining muscle?
Work out! No food, supplement, or powder that promises muscle gains will make you gain muscle. If they did bulk people up and make them ripped then there would be no point in going to the gym.

What is your top tip for losing weight?
Concentrate on eating better. More foods from the produce aisle and try to limit the oils you eat. Once a person eats better then the pounds will go away on their own. It's not about diet, it's about your lifestyle.

What is your top tip for maintaining weight?
Count your calories and make sure you are eating enough. If you are vegan who eats minimally processed plant-based whole foods you'd be surprised on how much you have to eat to maintain weight.

What is your top tip for improving metabolism?
Protein and fiber. Those together help keep a person's metabolic efficiency constant. Some examples – fruit with peanut butter, green smoothie, blended frozen bananas with hemp seeds. Also, have your breakfast be the largest meal of the day. That helps curb off cravings throughout the day to stay lean.

What is your top tip for toning up?
Use it or lose it!

How do you promote veganism in your daily life?
Leading by example. No one will ever believe what you say about the benefits of eating a plant-based diet unless you can back up your claims with real life examples. There's no better real life example than yourself so work hard, eat well, and enjoy whatever you do.

How would you suggest people get involved with what you do?
Feel free to check out my coaching website, like my FaceBook page, or shoot me an email.

"I become vegan after I learned about the environmental impact a person's diet has on the planet. After I learned this, I slowly made changes to my diet and lifestyle. Went lacto-ovo vegetarian for 2 years and then thought if I was really serious about what I stand for, then I should become fully vegan. Since the process for me was rather slow compared to most, it wasn't too hard of a shift to be 100% animal-free when I made the commitment."

Less Meat = Less Heat

MINDY COLLETTE
VEGAN FITNESS MODEL

New York City, New York, USA
Vegan since: 2010

mindycollette.com
SM: *FaceBook, Instagram, Twitter*

Mindy Collette is a female vegan athlete residing in New York City, who wants to change the world exemplifying love by living vegan. Mindy is an actress, singer, songwriter, dancer and freelance journalist, currently writing articles for Vegan Health & Fitness Magazine. She works hard to find ways to promote a vegan lifestyle and animal liberation to those around her, living to promote and fight for human rights and liberation as well. She has dreams of writing books, performing, and living abroad to help human and non-human animals globally.

WHY VEGAN?

Initially, it was for health benefits. Quickly it became about the animals, equality, and compassion. With more knowledge, I realized being vegan is not merely healthy for our bodies and our environment's healing, but so much more! I've come to understand it is the only loving, compassionate, cruelty-free way to live. If I can't eat plant-based, I'd rather suffer than contribute to the suffering, neglect, abuse, and rape of animals. The facts are heart-wrenching, I wish I'd known from day one.

How and why did you decide to become vegan?
I first met Robert Cheeke at a bodybuilding competition in May 2009. He was super friendly to everyone, and had the most genuine smile. We became connected on FaceBook and within months, I was in progress to my life change. I ordered his book, got involved online, and the rest is history - in the making.

The initial draw was honestly for my health, as I had been ill. Though quickly that focus adjusted to animal welfare and environmental care. I identify with feminism, all human rights, and animal rights, those are my passions, which, as vegans, we stand for the equality of these three activisms combined. A vegan lifestyle assures saving animals inadvertently, which makes it easily the perfect, harmonious way to make positive changes. I believe it is my responsibility to gently share and educate others without judgment, in the same gentle way I was first "vegucated".

How long have you been vegan?
Since 2010 - and will be forever!

What has benefited you the most from being vegan?
If this question was asked three years ago, I would've immediately said "my health." Not now. Genuinely, my heart. I truly feel like I love deeper, feel more compassionately, and am able to be changed by real issues. It has completely changed my life. I deem it one of the greatest gifts to have been blessed with. Being vegan is not just a diet, it is a way of life - to live compassionately with unconditional, passionate love. I am not perfect, nor do I expect to reach perfection, but being vegan has encouraged me to learn to love much more freely.

What does veganism mean to you?

Veganism is the acknowledgement that we are not more worthy, nor should one ever value oneself more, than any other living being. By eating a plant-based diet and adhering to a cruelty-free, vegan lifestyle, we promote equality, love, and compassion. Being vegan is much more than food, and I will do all within my power to initiate positive change. Furthermore, veganism is better for the planet, and without a vegan lifestyle our planet will continually be degraded and deteriorate all the more, which hurts all walks of life. Besides, who doesn't want to live with an open mind and heart, with a clearer conscience?

From as far back as I can remember – when I was around 5 years old – I wanted to save all the orphaned babies around the globe. So, when I adopted a cruelty-free lifestyle it was heartfelt, and was a seamless transition. My passion was already there. All I've ever wanted is to save lives from pain and suffering."

TRAINING

What sort of training do you do?

Typically, mostly weight training and yoga. I love to mix it up, and keep my training life interesting.

How often do you (need to) train?

I train 5-6 days a week, and that day off usually drives me a bit batty - so, I tend to still find a way to be physically active. Need and want are simultaneous for me because of my high-energy.

Do you offer your fitness or training services to others?

I did for a while, and may again in the future, but not at this time. Never say never though, right?

What sports do you play?

I'm not necessarily an athletic type by way of organized sports, though I do enjoy softball, soccer, and football. My favorite ways to be physically active are dance, yoga and weight lifting.

STRENGTHS, WEAKNESSES & OUTSIDE INFLUENCES

Strengths: I'm usually very positive, self-motivated, driven, and able to achieve the tone or look I'm going for. I am very passionate and straight forward - but that can at times be misconstrued and taken the wrong way. Something I am working on finding balance in.

Weaknesses: Sweets, and wanting to be social can be weaknesses at times. I'm really hard on myself too so that is also something I work on - staying positive and focusing on others instead of my mistakes or flaws.

Outside Influences: Robert Cheeke and veganbodybuilding.com, the PlantBuilt team, and a ton of amazing people on Social Media.

What do you think is the biggest misconception about vegans and how do you address this?

A) That we're militant. Which, some may be, but I'd like to think that militance is for ourselves and compassion toward others is a fair mix and that's the balance I work to achieve.

B) That we are weak, emaciated, and sickly. I think that is slowly being overturned!

C) That we only eat salads. I eat veggies but not a lot of salads, I think that surprises people.

D) Vegans are hippies. Just like carnivores, we are all different. I may be a bit of a hippie, but not everyone is.

What are your strengths as a vegan athlete?
People tend to know my personality and notice I'm into fitness before they know I'm vegan. I enjoy casually mentioning not using whey protein or eggs which prompts questions, instead of pushing it right out the gate. I've found that if others get to know you and can visibly see results they are more likely to listen to your advice than the other way around.

What is your biggest challenge?
Sleeping! I have so much energy that it can be a struggle to get six hours of sleep a night.

Are the non-vegans in your industry supportive or not?
Some are, some aren't. For the most part, people are really understanding, excited, and even impressed.

Are your family and friends supportive of your vegan lifestyle?
Yes. Even if they don't understand it, they've all come to love and accept me through it.

What is the most common question/comment that people ask/say when they find out that you are a vegan and how do you respond?
"Whoa! How do you do that? You eat eggs and yogurt though, right? Oh! And chicken?"
Me: no, actually, no eggs, dairy, fish, meat.
"Wow, so you eat a lot of salads then?"
Me: nah, I just eat. Pretty much everything you eat as a carnivore, I can eat plant-based. I eat fruit, veggies, nuts, and desserts and tacos and pizza. Usually the conversation just progresses from there, with a lot of questions and sharing images of other vegan friends etc.

Who or what motivates you?
I am motivated by lives that are jeopardized or aren't shown equality and fairness in our society. Animals, women, transgendered, inter-sexed, gay, lesbian, orphaned children, anyone who has been abused, raped, attacked, and the misunderstood, rejected, and used. Every day I am grateful to have lived through the experiences I have, and am driven to help others who have been or are going through inequality in any way shape or form. From as far back as I can remember - when I was around 5 years old - I wanted to save all the orphaned babies around the globe. So, when I adopted a cruelty-free lifestyle it was heartfelt, and was a seamless transition. My passion was already there. All I've ever wanted is to save lives from pain and suffering.

FOOD & SUPPLEMENTS

What do you eat for Breakfast?
Lately it's my protein paste with oats: 1/4 cup oats, 1.5 scoop plant protein, almond or soy milk (unsweetened), cinnamon, truvia, and cocoa powder.

What do you eat for Lunch?
I like tofu scrambles in a tortilla, or a beast burger from Beyond Meat with veggies.

What do you eat for Dinner?
Similar to lunch, protein, veggies, and carbs.

What do you eat for Snacks (healthy & not-so healthy)?

Fruit, protein pudding, hummus with veggies or crackers, smoothies, or a "fun" coffee (like a soy green tea latte, chai, or a non-dairy mocha.) Confession: cupcakes, ice cream (sweets in general) are my weakness.

What is your favourite source of Protein?

Vega Sport chocolate, SunWarrior Brown Rice protein-chocolate, and Plant Fusion natural for smoothies, and cookies n creme is my number one again now.

What is your favourite source of Calcium?

Soy milk (non-GMO, organic), molasses, tempeh, and broccoli.

What is your favourite source of Iron?

Lentils, tofu, molasses, cashews, and leafy greens (collard and kale are my two faves.)

What foods give you the most energy?

Fruit and kale - and coffee!

Do you take any supplements?

Currently: Clean Machine Cell Block 80, Plant Fusion Cookies n Creme protein, Rainbow Light once a day, and Adreset (mushroom based supplement for adrenal fatigue - due to a really busy & stressful season of life.)

"If I was asked about the benefits three years ago, I would've immediately said "my health." Not now. Genuinely, my heart. I truly feel like I love deeper, feel more compassionately, and am able to be changed by real issues. It has completely changed my life. I deem it one of the greatest gifts to have been blessed with. Being vegan is not just a diet, it is a way of life – to live compassionately with unconditional, passionate love. I am not perfect, nor do I expect to reach perfection, but being vegan has encouraged me to learn to love much more freely."

ADVICE

What is your top tip for gaining muscle?

Eat! Lift Heavy! Sleep! Drink your water! In order to gain muscle we must feed our body the right foods to gain.

What is your top tip for losing weight?

Eat! Lift weights! And make wise diet decisions. Meaning that the food you eat is carefully selected and is purely fuel for your body. The best advice I have for losing weight and trying to tone, at least for me, is: drink lots of water, eat primarily fruits and veggies, sleep, lift weights, and get outdoors (uneven terrain) for cardio or walks. If someone wants to just lose weight, it's about portion control in conjunction with physical activity. I personally haven't been in a place where I have needed major weight loss, but I would refer those looking to lose to follow people like my dear friend Tricia Kelly in Austin, Texas. She lost incredible amounts of weight, is vegan, extremely knowledgeable, and is a sweet and inspiring soul.

What is your top tip for maintaining weight?

For me, maintaining my weight is the easiest of these three - gaining muscle, losing weight, or maintaining. I have maintained my weight for the past three+ years by eating consistently mostly clean, plant-based foods, lifting weights 4-6 days a week, drinking plenty of water, and trying to get the same amount of sleep on average every night. To be honest, it is actually pretty difficult for me to gain or lose more than 5-7lbs (2.26-3.17kg) or so, which can be really frustrating when it comes to competing and so forth.

What is your top tip for improving metabolism?

Lift weights, build muscle, drink water and sleep! Do I sound a bit redundant? GOOD! These are the main keys to a healthy body. The more muscle we have the more our bodies use the fuel (food) we give it, and in turn we are less likely to store it (fat). This is why we often hear trainers summarize the science behind it all with: muscle burns fat, because really that is what a more muscular body does. So, for me, the more muscle I put on by lifting heavier, the hungrier I am.

What is your top tip for toning up?

Toning comes from eating clean, but not necessarily a super strict (no sweets ever, etc) diet, combined with consistent workouts. When I first started working out, I didn't really know much about health or fitness. So, I hopped online and found women who, at that time, had more muscle than me. A lot of what I read said: light weights, high repetition, water, sleep, and clean food. That's what I did. I lost body fat and gained some muscle tone, which was what I was going for. What did my clean eating consist of? A lot of veggies and fruit for snacks, protein and veggies with half the amount of potatoes or rice as usual, etc. That worked for me for toning. My workouts were minimal then, pretty light weights for arms and legs, really high reps, and 20-30 min of cardio after. Though, again, I wasn't necessarily trying to lose weight, I just wanted to "tone" at that time.

How do you promote veganism in your daily life?

By wearing it via veganbodybuilding.com sweatshirts, tees, and shorts, or SunWarrior, veganproteins.com, Plant Fusion, Plant Built, or Herbivore tees and tanks, and I promote it through Social Media or online through veganbodybuilding.com, as well as my personal website. I live, breathe, eat, and speak veganism every day. For me, this is so much more than a diet, it's about promoting a lifestyle - a lifestyle of honesty, compassion, and love - I want to share that with others and hopefully leave this world a much better place than I found it.

How would you suggest people get involved with what you do?

I try to post regularly on Social Media and have recently revised my website, I hope to see you there!

"I am motivated by lives that are jeopardized or aren't shown equality and fairness in our society. Animals, women, transgendered, inter-sexed, gay, lesbian, orphaned children, anyone who has been abused, raped, attacked, and the misunderstood, rejected, and used. Every day I am grateful to have lived through the experiences I have, and am driven to help others who have been or are going through inequality in any way shape or form.

Mirko Buchwald
VEGAN GOJU-RYU KARATE-DO CHAMPION

San Francisco, California, USA
Vegan since: 1984

sfgoju.com
sfzanshin.com
SM: *FaceBook*

Mirko Buchwald is a 5th degree black belt in Goju Ryu, a hard style of Japanese martial arts. He has been practicing for close to 30 years, is a two-time British champion and a former world International Okinawan Goju-Ryu Karate-do Federation (IOGKF) champion, and also a former Kanazawa Cup men's grand champion. Mirko was a member of the British karate team and after moving to the USA became captain of the USA IOGKF karate team. He splits his time teaching internationally and running his own martial arts gym Zanshin Martial Arts Center in San Francisco, California, USA.

WHY VEGAN?

How and why did you decide to become vegan?
I became vegan out of respect for animals. I was born into a vegetarian family. My grandfather stopped eating meat following training as a veterinary surgeon, and my mother was therefore raised as a veggie. So, I was raised as a third generation veggie. I have fond memories of helping a neighbor feed local wild foxes near my home. I learnt that people hunted these creatures for fun and was upset by it, so I got involved in direct action against fox hunting. I joined a Hunt Saboteurs group and became active around age 14. Contact with older activists led me to become vegan.

How long have you been vegan?
Over 30 years.

What has benefited you most from being vegan?
The ability to feel compassion for all species, my great health, and the opportunity to travel the world and use my voice to spread the word of how good it is to be a vegan athlete.

What does veganism mean to you?
It means seeing the world as it really is, through the veil of the carnistic world we live in. It means compassion for all life. It means standing up for something bigger. It means making a choice everyday to not conform to the violent ideology the permeates every aspect of life. It means love.

"People think it's hard to be vegan. People think that you have to be really strict and that it's really difficult to eat. As we all know it's really not hard at all, is it?"

TRAINING

What sort of training do you do?
I do a combination of weight training and cardio, and I practice karate, judo, ju jitsui and kickboxing.

How often do you train?
I train 3 times a day, early morning cardio, rest, then weight training followed by an evening martial arts session.

Do you offer your fitness or training services to others?
Yes anyone interested can come train directly with me at my martial arts gym Zanshin Martial Arts Center in San Francisco, California. They can also train with me at many international events.

What sports do you play?
I have never been into playing sports - I just never got into playing with balls. I was very focused on martial arts from an early age. I do enjoy weight training and riding a bicycle on top of martial arts.

STRENGTHS, WEAKNESSES AND OUTSIDE INFLUENCE

What do you think are the biggest misconceptions about vegans and how do you address this?
The biggest misconception I think is people think it's hard to be vegan. People think that you have to be really strict and that it's really difficult to eat. As we all know it's really not hard at all, is it? I address this by explaining the kind of foods I eat and more specifically all the things that I - or they - could use as vegan substitute foods eg non-dairy milks.

What are your strengths as a vegan athlete?
As a vegan athlete, my biggest strength is the knowledge I have inside from a lifetime of healthy eating, which I share with anyone who asks questions about my diet or life style. Also the broken stereotype that I feel I represent.

What is your biggest challenge?
My biggest challenge is living in a world of speciesm and carnism and the daily challenge of dealing with all that entails.

Are the non-vegans in your industry supportive of your lifestyle?
Many of my own students have become vegan from training with me and reading my monthly nutritional articles on my student website. Many of my peers - once they get to know me and know that I'm vegan, are interested - especially as I am 6'3 and 240lbs (108kg) - but I think they are still living inside the "meat matrix" as I like to call it. So they are mostly filled with the same misinformation and propaganda they have grown up with.

Are your family and friend supportive of your vegan lifestyle?
My family is nearly all vegan - including my grandparents, mother and siblings. My friends are 50/50 - half enjoy going to vegan restaurants and half don't care.

What is the most common question people ask you when they find out you are vegan and how do you respond?
I get a combination of the protein question along with "What do you eat?" "How do you keep weight on?" "Isn't it hard to be vegan?" I answer by explaining what protein is and

where it comes from, I list the variety of foods I eat, I explain it's about quality calories and I explain how easy veganism is once you educate yourself on diet and nutrition.

Who or what motivates you?
I am inspired by my love for all Earthlings, anyone on this planet who either simply makes a choice to eat vegan, or by people who feel the need to break open cages and take direct action. I am also personally inspired my many vegan friends. Alex Pacheco specifically of 600milliondogs.org is a great man who has done so much for the Animal Rights movement and who is currently working on a pill that will sterilize the current 600 million stray dogs worldwide.

"Being vegan means seeing the world as it really is, through the veil of the carnistic world we live in. It means compassion for all life. It means standing up for something bigger. It means making a choice everyday to not conform to the violent ideology the permeates every aspect of life. It means love."

FOOD AND SUPPLEMENTS

What do you eat for Breakfast?
Oatmeal with flax and chia seeds, fruit, water and a protein shake.

What do you eat for Lunch?
Large salad, protein shake, fruit or Vitamix smoothie.

What do you eat for Dinner?
Large salad or pasta (whole wheat), protein shake, black beans and brown rice.

What do you eat for Snacks - healthy & not-so healthy?
Protein bars, with the occasional vegan cookie or popcorn.

What is your favorite source of Protein?
On top of getting as much as I can from actual whole foods I make a blend of protein powders with almond milk, hemp, soy, pea, potato and the Plant Fusion brand I like.

What is your favorite source of Calcium?
I get it from a balanced whole food diet, mainly dark leafy greens.

What is your favorite source of Iron?
I eat kale every day.

What food gives you the most energy?
Carbohydrates and foods with a low glycemic index. I also like the Vega sports pre and post work drinks.

Do you take any supplements?
I take 40 to 50 grams or a protein shake 4-5 times a day. I also use Creatine, B12 under the tongue supplement, a multi vitamin, MSN, Glutamine, ZMA and protein bars.

ADVICE

What is your top tip for gaining muscle?
Lift weights with less repetitions and more weight. Understand which exercises are better to build bulk and which are better for definition. For example, close grip bench press will do more for your triceps that a finishing movement like dumbbell kickbacks. Eat more and supplement your diet with more protein daily equal to your body weight (if you weigh

200lbs then consume 200 grams of protein daily) 4 or 5 shakes a day should do it.

What is your top tip for losing weight?
Less calories, cut out the sugars and processed foods, cardio daily.

What is your top tip for maintaining weight?
Once you figure out the right nutritional and exercise balance and reach a weight you're comfortable with, be consistent with your diet and training.

What is your top tip for improving metabolism?
Learn about your active and resting heart rate and your aerobic threshold, make sure your diet is alkaline, read "Thrive" - a great book on vegan fitness.

What is your top tip for toning up?
Diet, cut the sugars and fats, do a combination of cardio and strength training and plenty of abs work.

How do you promote veganism in your daily life?
As a vegan, everything we do and say is a reflection of each other. I personally try daily whenever the opportunity arises to engage people to make them think and question why I do and say the things I say. I think that every time someone ask a question or even makes a stupid question it's an opportunity to give them something to think about. It's learning how best to respond that takes time, but once you are able to, you may someday help them see through the matrix of carnism and help them see that all species deserve a life just like you and I.

How would you suggest people get involved in what you do?
Feel free to contact me and I can connect you with someone in your area, or if you live in the San Francisco Bay area come see me.

"I became vegan out of respect for animals. I was born into a vegetarian family. My grandfather stopped eating meat following training as a veterinary surgeon, and my mother was therefore raised as a veggie. So, I was raised as a third generation veggie. I have fond memories of helping a neighbor feed local wild foxes near my home. I learnt that people hunted these creatures for fun and was upset by it, so I got involved in direct action against fox hunting. I joined a Hunt Saboteurs group and became active around age 14. Contact with older activists led me to become vegan."

MOLLY CAMERON
VEGAN CYCLOCROSS RACER

Portland, Oregon, USA
Vegan since: 1999

mollycameron.pro
portlandbicyclestudio.com
SM: *FaceBook, Instagram, Twitter*

A World Cup veteran and local superstar, Molly Cameron is a world traveling cyclocross racer. Founder of both a bicycle shop and custom bicycle studio in Portland, Oregon, Molly brings passion and energy to her racing, business and life.

WHY VEGAN?

How and why did you decide to become vegan?
I never liked meat. Even as a kid, I never wanted to touch the stuff. I went vegetarian in my teens, almost by accident. My family did not have a particularly healthy diet; fast food was all we could seem to afford. When I was able to make my own decisions about what I ate, I chose to eat veg.

How long have you been vegan?
Since 1999.

What has benefited you the most from being vegan?
Not eating crap. My lifestyle is pretty minimal. Just doing my part to make the planet a better place.

What does veganism mean to you?
Taking responsibility for and being conscious of what I put into my body.

TRAINING

What sort of training do you do?
Like all bicycle racers, lots and lots of hours spent on the bike. I'll include strength/core work, weight lifting and running in the off-season and pre-season. On-the-bike workouts vary during a race season from long unstructured rides to short and intense interval sessions.

How often do you (need to) train?
Daily! A PRO rides their bicycle every day, whether for active recovery or challenging workouts. 20-30 hours a week on the bike.

Do you offer your fitness or training services to others?
I do! I am a cycling coach and work with a range of clients from beginners to elite athletes. Writing up training plans, working on a daily one-on-one basis with athletes, teaching clinics and leading workouts and classes.

What sports do you play?
My speciality is Cyclocross racing. I also race on the road, track and do a little mountain bike racing when I can.

STRENGTHS, WEAKNESSES & OUTSIDE INFLUENCES

What do you think is the biggest misconception about vegans and how do you address this?

That the diet will hinder athletic performance, aka "where do you get your protein and Iron?"

What are your strengths as a vegan athlete?

My ability to consume lots and lots of food and not take myself too seriously.

What is your biggest challenge?

Finding the energy to cook really good meals when I am too exhausted to stand after hard rides.

Are the non-vegans in your industry supportive or not?

Cycling is a pretty big "industry." For the most part, sure. Veganism is nothing new to the bicycle-racing scene. If anything, my shortcomings get attributed to my vegan diet and my successes are viewed as "in spite of" my vegan diet. Annoying, but I can't win everything.

Are your family and friends supportive of your vegan lifestyle?

Friends and family? Absolutely.

What is the most common question/comment that people ask/say when they find out that you are a vegan and how do you respond?

"Where do you get your protein?" My answer: "From food."

Who or what motivates you?

Intense, driven people, that can still crack a smile and enjoy life. They motivate me.

> "I never liked meat. Even as a kid, I never wanted to touch the stuff. I went vegetarian in my teens, almost by accident. My family did not have a particularly healthy diet; fast food was all we could seem to afford. When I was able to make my own decisions about what I ate, I chose to eat veg."

FOOD & SUPPLEMENTS

What do you eat for Breakfast?

Oatmeal, toast or pasta on race days. Coffee.

What do you eat for Lunch?

Usually on the bike food like bananas and PROBARS.

What do you eat for Dinner?

Quinoa, Kale, beans, more greens.

What do you eat for Snacks - healthy & not-so healthy?

Chocolate. Love chocolate.

I don't eat in a typical three meals a day style. I'll eat food all day long in smaller portions to keep my blood sugar and energy levels consistent.

What is your favourite source of Protein, Calcium and Iron?

I don't know if I have favourites. I eat a lot of quinoa, rice and kale, beans, veggies, veggies, veggies and I'll eat a little fake meat stuff once in a while for fun. Though, I don't eat any soy. I try to stay away from heavily processed and manufactured food.

What foods give you the most energy?
I love veggies, broccoli, kale, I can't get enough of it. I should mention PROBARS. I love them, they are balanced, vegan, whole food bars with a lot of calories and great, simple ingredients in them. When training, I'll take a bunch of bananas and a few PROBARS to fuel me through a 6-hour ride.

Do you take any supplements?
I have taken iron and a multivitamin in the past. Not really taking any supplements in the last year. I just kind of stopped last season, no reason. I try to keep the processed food to a minimum. I get my blood tested regularly to make sure I am getting everything I need.

ADVICE

For other cyclists and bicycle racers, this is general advice:

What is your top tip for gaining muscle?
Lifting weights and cross training in the gym is a start.

What is your top tip for losing weight?
Ride your bike. Ride your bike. Ride your bike. Eat a couple hundred calories every hour you are on the bike. Never finish a ride hungry as that might make you overeat later.

What is your top tip for maintaining weight?
Eat regularly. Small meals several times a day.

What is your top tip for improving metabolism?
Exercise daily. Even a 30 minute easy spin on the bike will keep the metabolism going.

What is your top tip for toning up?
Eat your veggies. Skip the processed carbs.

How do you promote veganism in your daily life?
By riding the best and hardest I can.

How would you suggest people get involved with what you do?
Shoot me an email, visit me at Portland Bicycle Studio or, come say hello at a bicycle race.

"Cycling is a pretty big "industry." For the most part, the non-vegans are supportive. Veganism is nothing new to the bicycle-racing scene. If anything, my shortcomings get attributed to my vegan diet and my successes are viewed as "in spite of" my vegan diet. Annoying, but I can't win everything."

NICK PENDERGAST
VEGAN ICE-HOCKEY PLAYER

Perth, Western Australia, Australia
Vegan since: 2007

progressivepodcastaustralia.com
ara.org.au
SM: *FaceBook, Twitter*

Nick Pendergast has been vegan and also played ice-hockey competitively for many years. He has represented the Western Australian ice-hockey team and plays ice-hockey at the top level (Super League) in Western Australia. He has completed his PhD thesis on human/non-human relations and the animal advocacy movement, teaches Sociology and Anthropology at Curtin University, co-hosts the podcast Progressive Podcast Australia and volunteers with Animal Rights Advocates (ARA), assisting with the Vegan Perth website.

WHY VEGAN?

How and why did you decide to become vegan?
I became interested in animal rights after visiting an Animal Rights Advocates (ARA) stall promoting veganism. After deciding that veganism was too difficult, I became a vegetarian. After years as a vegetarian, I became vegan after reading the following quote from the book "The Ethics of What We Eat" by Peter Singer and Jim Mason:

'Suppose, however, that you object to the idea of killing young, healthy animals so you can eat them. That ethical view leads many people to become vegetarian, while continuing to eat eggs and dairy products. However, it is not possible to produce laying hens without also producing male chickens, and since these male chicks have no commercial value, they are invariably killed as soon as they have been sexed. The laying hens themselves will be killed once their rate of laying declines. In the dairy industry much the same thing happens – the male calves are killed immediately or raised for veal, and the cows are turned into hamburger long before normal old age. So rejecting the killing of animals points to a vegan, rather than a vegetarian, diet'.

How long have you been vegan?
Since 2007.

What has benefited you the most from being vegan?
I think being more aware of and comfortable with my choices towards other animals. I believe that veganism has put ideas that I already had - such as not wanting other animals to be harmed - into practice in all of my choices.

What does veganism mean to you?
To me, veganism means a commitment to animal rights, the idea that other animals are sentient beings with inherent value rather than just "things" for us to use and kill as we like, and putting this philosophy into practice in all of my choices.

TRAINING

How often do you (need to) train?

I play ice-hockey twice a week at the moment – one game and one training session, which involves shooting and passing drills, skating etc. Beyond hockey, I exercise every day. I go walking with my dog twice a day and most days I also do stretching for flexibility and some form of exercise for strength, whether it's a few pushups or sit ups, or some weights.

Do you offer your fitness or training services to others?

No - I have coached ice-hockey before, but am not currently coaching.

What sports do you play?

Ice-hockey.

STRENGTHS, WEAKNESSES & OUTSIDE INFLUENCES

What do you think is the biggest misconception about vegans and how do you address this?

I think the biggest misconception is that veganism is likely to mean deprivation in terms of nutrients and energy. I believe I address this by living a very active lifestyle, which I'd want to do anyway. But I believe that the more active, energetic vegans there are out there, the more we can show that veganism is no obstacle to achieving whatever we want to achieve, and is actually likely to be beneficial in terms of our health and energy.

What are your strengths as a vegan athlete?

I think animal products really slow people down, especially when eaten directly before sport. Well before I had even thought about the ethical issues associated with animal products, I stopped eating animal flesh in my meal before playing hockey, because I really felt it weighed me down and slowed me down – I didn't feel at my best after eating flesh before I skated. Vegan food is generally much "lighter" and I feel that I can be quicker and more energetic by leaving out animal products.

What is your biggest challenge?

No challenges that I can think of!

Are the non-vegans in your industry supportive or not?

I did play hockey with a guy from New York who used to be vegan when he was in the US, but generally, my veganism doesn't come up very often. I remember when I became vegetarian years ago, one guy I played hockey with congratulated me, but said I shouldn't go vegan because life's too short. Looking back now, I should have responded with a lyric from the band Propagandhi: 'life's too short to make another's shorter'.

Are your family and friends supportive of your vegan lifestyle?

Definitely! My family is always happy to make and eat vegan food when I come over, and many of my friends who weren't vegan before have now become vegan – which is very encouraging!

What is the most common question/comment that people ask/say when they find out that you are a vegan and how do you respond?

The most common comment I get is that veganism must be so difficult. I reply that it is actually very easy after an initial adjustment, and I give them a card for our Vegan Perth website which I always have in my wallet.

Who or what motivates you?

The people around me who become vegan and constantly show that people can and do make this positive change. In addition, my dog constantly reminds me that other animals are very unique, perceptive individuals whose interests we should consider.

In terms of fitness and exercising, music is a good motivator. One CD I've recently bought which I like to listen to while exercising is "The Workout" by "Stic" from the hip hop group Dead Prez.

FOOD & SUPPLEMENTS

What do you eat for Breakfast?

As soon as I get up, I have a green smoothie every morning. I rotate between a bunch of different recipes, but here is one that I use (makes 2 serves, blend all ingredients until smooth): 200ml orange juice, 100ml cold water, 1 apple, 1/2 a banana (I chop them up and put them in the freezer for a cooler smoothie), 5-6 strawberries (I buy them fresh, wash them and then freeze them), greens eg kale, silverbeet, bok choy, lettuce etc (rotate between different greens).

When I get back from exercising in the morning, I'll generally rotate between a couple of different high-protein meals. This includes having 3 Weet-bix with Table of Plenty 'Nicely Nutty' Muesli, Pura Veda and soy milk, or a peanut butter and banana smoothie. This smoothie recipe is slightly adapted from a recipe in "Living Vegan" magazine because I don't use protein powder. Here are the ingredients for 1 serve – blend all ingredients until smooth: 250ml soy milk (or another vegan milk of your choice), a little bit of sweetener (I use Natvia), 1/3 cup rolled oats, 2 tablespoons peanut butter, 1 banana (I chop them up and put them in the freezer for a cooler smoothie).

What do you eat for Lunch?

Generally I'll just have leftovers from dinner the night before or, if I don't have any, I'll usually make something quick like baked beans and toast with some salad – I've often got a salad made and "ready to go" in the fridge.

What do you eat for Dinner?

Some of my favourites are Cheesy Bean and Cheese Enchiladas, Grilled Tortillas with Sour Cream from "Veganomicon" and Autumn Pasta from "Now Vegan!" My partner and I have recently made a list of 30 of our favourite meals that have 30 minutes or less preparation time, and we generally rotate amongst those 30 recipes – although I'm sure this will be an ever-growing list!

What do you eat for Snacks - healthy & not-so healthy?

Chocolate raw balls – I make choc hazelnut, choc peanut, choc mint, choc goji berry etc and raw ice-cream. To make raw ice-cream, I cut up bananas and freeze them, then put the frozen banana in a food processor with a little bit of vegan milk and sweetener, and process until smooth. Also peanut butter to this for peanut butter ice-cream, strawberries for strawberry ice-cream, cocoa/cacao for chocolate ice-cream etc.

What is your favourite source of Protein?

My peanut butter and banana smoothie described above.

What is your favourite source of Calcium?

Kale.

What is your favourite source of Iron?

Kidney beans in Mexican food like Cheesy Bean and Cheese Enchilladas, and Grilled Tortillas.

What foods give you the most energy?
Definitely green smoothies!

Do you take any supplements?
No – I get my B12 through my Vitasoy milk, which is fortified with B12. Many other brands are also fortified with B12.

ADVICE

What is your top tip for gaining muscle?
Noah Hannibal from Uproar is probably a good person to go to on this one – he recommends (on veganstrength.org) consuming 20-30 grams of protein after working out. The foods I have post-exercise (described above) all have an amount of protein that is in this range. Regarding the workout itself: heavier weights with fewer repetitions – 6-10 per "set".

What is your top tip for losing weight?
I haven't tried this myself, but I'd imagine it would be best to avoid "fad" diets like low carb diets etc. It would probably be better to stick to a healthy, balanced diet you can sustain in the long-term and increase the amount of exercise you do.

What is your top tip for maintaining weight?
Eat a healthy, balanced diet, and stay active.

What is your top tip for toning up?
Same answer as for 'Maintaining weight' – although there would be specific exercises for this goal, such as lighter weights with more repetitions – 20/30 per "set".

How do you promote veganism in your daily life?
I think the most important way people can promote veganism is just by "living by example" and showing how easy and healthy veganism can be. I try to do that. Beyond that, I try to use my academic research to promote veganism. My conference presentations often focus on veganism, so I generally end up talking to other academics about veganism. I also give lectures on animal rights and veganism, which puts veganism "on the radar" for students.

I am also involved with Animal Rights Advocates (ARA) where I live in Perth, Western Australia. With ARA, I promote veganism in a number of ways, sometimes using my PhD research and lectures. For example: I give public talks and promote veganism in other public forums such as on the radio or on panels; hold vegan information stalls at universities and public events; promote veganism online through the ARA FaceBook page and also through our new Vegan Perth website; write articles promoting veganism (including non-academic ones which reach more people), as well as flyers for ARA and content for the ARA website.

I also co-host the political podcast Progressive Podcast Australia that promotes veganism and other social justice causes.

How would you suggest people get involved with what you do?
You can listen to my podcast Progressive Podcast Australia. To get updates on what ARA is doing, you can follow ARA on social media and sign up to receive email updates on our site.

NOEL POLANCO
VEGAN FITNESS ATHLETE

New York City, New York, USA
Vegan since: 2009

getfitordietrying1.blogspot.com.au
SM: *FaceBook, Google+, Instagram, Twitter, YouTube*

Noel Polanco is a vegan fitness athlete and print model from New York City. Growing up as a chubby kid in Washington Heights, Noel lost weight through jumping rope. Little Noel was an animal lover so he soon adapted to a vegetarian diet and later went completely vegan. Now he is a vegan health and fitness advocate, defender of animal rights and protector of women who have been victims of domestic violence. Noel focuses on inspiring younger kids who are now affected with diabetes and obesity. He makes inspiring videos to motivate other people into living a healthier lifestyle.

WHY VEGAN?

I am vegan because I love animals. After seeing so many people suffering with diseases such as diabetes, obesity and cancer, I asked myself if the Standard American Diet (SAD) was in fact so healthy, then why are people getting sick? All of these diseases could be prevented though a vegan diet. As we have now seen, even Bill Clinton went vegan to reverse his own heart disease. I am vegan because I love animals and want to prevent sickness.

How long have you been vegan?
For over 5 years. Was mainly vegetarian before.

What has benefited you the most from being vegan?
I have more energy. I haven't had a cold, or flu. I love it.

What does veganism mean to you?
Veganism to me means living in peace with the animals that share this planet with us. As well as living without causing any harm to our bodies, planet and animals.

TRAINING

What sort of training do you do?
I do all kinds of training from bodyweight exercises, to exercises with a weighted vest. I am always doing different stuff - whatever my body feels like doing on the day.

How often do you (need to) train?
I train every day.

Do you offer your fitness or training services to others?
Yes, I offer fitness advice and help people lose weight, and also make inspiring workout videos that you can see on my YouTube channel.

What sports do you play?
I play basketball, football, and track.

STRENGTHS, WEAKNESSES & OUTSIDE INFLUENCES

What do you think is the biggest misconception about vegans and how do you address this?
Biggest misconception about vegans is that vegans are weak. When they see me workout, I prove them wrong.

What are your strengths as a vegan athlete?
My strengths as a vegan athlete are that I have mastered my own bodyweight. I can do human flags, one arm pull ups, one arm pushups, one legged squats. Basically, every difficult exercise with your own bodyweight I am able to do. I still train hard every day because you can always find harder stuff and exercises to do.

Are the non-vegans in your industry supportive or not?
Not every non-vegan person is supportive. When people can't do something themselves they want to tell you that you can't do it.

Are your family and friends supportive of your vegan lifestyle?
Most of them are, they are open-minded and give it a try. I have inspired and helped many people become vegan.

What is the most common question/comment that people ask/say when they find out that you are a vegan and how do you respond?
"Where do you get your protein?" I think every person who is vegan gets asked that same question over and over again. I answer it in a friendly way and tell them the truth about the protein myth. People should be worrying about NOT consuming too much protein to stay healthy.

Who or what motivates you?
It's kind of sad but my motivation is my family, the people around me, and my results. By seeing my family, friends etc suffering with diseases and being overweight, it motivates me to work out every day, to keep following a vegan diet to not end up like them. My main goal in life is to prevent sickness, and be healthy. I want to inspire the younger kids because I once was chubby and not healthy when I was little. Also, seeing my results, my energy and the way I feel and look. That keeps me motivated.

FOOD & SUPPLEMENTS

Every day is not the same I don't eat the same thing over and over again. I wrote down what I ate today.

What do you eat for Breakfast?
Quinoa with tofu and 1 cup of vanilla soymilk.

What do you eat for Lunch?
Ezekiel cereal with chia seeds and raw oats.

What do you eat for Dinner?
Brown rice and beans, raw cucumbers, tomatoes and hummus.

What do you eat for Snacks - healthy & not-so healthy?
Snacks that I like to eat are Clif bars, Larabars, any fruits, any nuts or seeds, raisins, and fruit smoothies.

What is your favourite source of Protein?
Quinoa.

What is your favourite source of Calcium?
Broccoli.

What is your favourite source of Iron?
Broccoli.

What foods give you the most energy?
Fruit smoothies.

Do you take any supplements?
I don't take any supplements. I believe don't believe in artificial or powder stuff. I get all my nutrients from the food that grows on the planet.

ADVICE

What is your top tip for gaining muscle?
My tip for gaining muscle would be TRAIN HARD. When you feel you don't want to train, that's the day that you need to train the most. Get enough sleep and just train every day. Make training a daily routine in your lifestyle. Don't rush into getting big muscles, just train to be healthy and fit. Then when you look at yourself after 5 years you will be like: WOW hard work pays off. Never rush into trying to get results. Have fun when working out and train every day. Don't follow the rules in magazines etc.

What is your top tip for losing weight?
My tip for losing weight is that if you own or use a treadmill throw it out the window. Go outside and run or walk. That's how you lose weight. Stop focusing on using all these machines and fake equipment. Run, sprint, walk or climb up and down the stairs. Eat non-processed food, more fruits and veggies. Also following a plant-based diet will help you lose weight.

What is your top tip for maintaining weight?
My tip for maintaining weight would be to eat enough calories. Never starve, and don't be afraid of consuming avocados, nuts, and coconut milk.

What is your top tip for improving metabolism?
My tip for improving your metabolism would be simple: just eat more fruit.

What is your top tip for toning up?
My tip for toning up would be to exercise EVERY DAY.

How do you promote veganism in your daily life?
I promote veganism everyday either in person or online via websites and social networks. I also make videos where I talk about the benefits of a vegan diet, and show people how to exercise like I do. I also share disturbing images of what the meat is like before it gets to your plate.

How would you suggest people get involved with what you do?
If you want to get involved in what I do, follow me on FaceBook and YouTube.

"Veganism to me means living in peace with the animals that share this planet with us. As well as living without causing any harm to our bodies, planet and animals."

ORVEL DOUGLAS
VEGAN EXERCISE ENTHUSIAST

New York City, New York, USA
Vegan since: 2001

E: nutritionspecialist26@gmail.com

Orvel Douglas has lived in New York City for 18 years, originally coming from Birmingham, England. He is a nutrition and diet coach who works for the non-profit organization BodySculpt. Orvel aims to educate the masses on the importance and value of nutrition as a vehicle to a better lifestyle.

WHY VEGAN?

How long have you been vegan?
I have been a vegan for over 12 years.

What has benefited you the most from being vegan?
More energy, never get sick, better body composition, just feeling great every single day.

What does veganism mean to you?
We could feed all the starving people in the world and save the rainforest from destruction.

TRAINING

What sort of training do you do?
I do a combination of weight training and high intensity interval training.

How often do you (need to) train?
Six days a week. I alternate the weight training days and cardio days.

Do you offer your fitness or training services to others?
I do offer fitness advice to others but not fitness services

STRENGTHS, WEAKNESSES & OUTSIDE INFLUENCES

What do you think is the biggest misconception about vegans and how do you address this?
The biggest misconception I find is people think we are all stick thin and weak and we only eat tofu and salads. I explain to them that being a vegan does not equal to being stick thin, you have meat eaters who are stick thin, and we are all different physically. It depends on what you eat and how you exercise, and that applies to vegans and non-vegans.

What are your strengths as a vegan athlete?
Eating the right foods, knowing that what I eat will fuel my body for the rest of the day.

What is your biggest challenge?
I don't have any challenges being a vegan. I make sure I am always prepared for every situation.

Are the non-vegans in your industry supportive or not?
The non-vegans in my industry are supportive towards me. Because they tell me I blow away the myth of what a vegan is supposed to look like.

Are your family and friends supportive of your vegan lifestyle?
My family are very supportive of my vegan lifestyle, One of my sisters is a vegan and my mother eats animal protein maybe once every month or so. They all love vegan dishes.

What is the most common question/comment that people ask/say when they find out that you are a vegan and how do you respond?
"Where do you get your protein from?" My answer is, "The same place the animals you are eating get theirs." A common comment I get when I tell people I am a vegan is "I couldn't give up meat."

Who or what motivates you?
Waking up day in day out and feeling full of life and energy. I see so many people who are the same age as me and younger who have all these chronic diseases, low energy, always tired all the time. I tell them I can't identify with what they are going through, I basically put it down to my lifestyle choices.

> "Food is fuel. You have to treat your body the same way as you treat a car. If you put the wrong fuel in a car it's going to break down, and that's exactly how the human body works."

FOOD & SUPPLEMENTS

What do you eat for Breakfast?
Green smoothie made with coconut water, kale, parsley, watercress, celery, piece of apple, orange, banana, ginger, hemp seeds, flaxseeds and chia seeds.

What do you eat for Lunch?
Herb salad with ½ avocado, yellow and red peppers diced, red onions, cauliflower hummus and raw braised mushrooms.

What do you eat for Dinner?
Raw sweet potato soup.

What do you eat for Snacks - healthy & not-so healthy?
Almonds and dates.

What is your favourite source of Protein?
Shelled raw hemp seeds.

What is your favourite source of Calcium?
Dark green leafy vegetables.

What is your favourite source of Iron?
Spinach and dates.

What foods give you the most energy?
Green smoothies gives me the most energy.

Do you take any supplements?
I do not take supplements.

People ask me, "Where do you get your protein from?"
I answer, "The same place the animals you are eating get theirs."

ADVICE

What is your top tip for gaining muscle?
Include essential fats into your diet like nuts and avocados, also hemp is a great source of protein.

What is your top tip for losing weight?
Exercise first thing in the morning on an empty stomach, when your body is still in a fasting stage from the night before. If you work out first thing in the morning, your body will tap into its fats stores.

What is your top tip for maintaining weight?
When your body reaches its ideal weight, weight will be maintained naturally.

What is your top tip for improving metabolism?
Eating enough fruits and veggies, and less grains.

What is your top tip for toning up?
I recommend high intensity interval training high-intensity interval training (HIIT). Doing high intensity exercise will torch fat well after your workout is over, compared to traditional cardio.

How do you promote veganism in your daily life?
When I do my nutrition workshops, I talk about how you can save your own life by becoming vegan. Eating all that animal protein puts you at risk for all degenerative diseases, compared to a plant-based diet that is going to promote good health and vitality.

How would you suggest people get involved with what you do?
To get people involved in what I do, I try to change their mindset about food. I tell them that food is fuel. You have to treat your body the same way as you treat a car. If you put the wrong fuel in a car it's going to break down, and that's exactly how the human body works. I live by example and people do listen to me when I talk, I think it's because of my age and my physical appearance.

"The biggest misconception I find is people think we are all stick thin and weak, and we only eat tofu and salads. I explain to them that being a vegan does not equal to being stick thin, you have meat eaters who are stick thin, and we are all different physically. It depends on what you eat and how you exercise, and that applies to vegans and non-vegans."

PAM BOTELER
VEGAN PIONEERING CANOEIST

Washington, DC, USA
Vegan since: 2007

womencanintl.com
SM: *FaceBook*

Pam Boteler is a pioneering canoeist, former U.S. National Team paddler and President of WomenCAN International, a global voice for equality in Olympic canoeing. She helps open doors for women and girls around the world to compete equally in Olympic Canoeing, and was the first woman in the U.S. to race in Sprint Canoeing at the U.S. National Championships in 2000. Through her efforts, in 2002, USA Canoe/Kayak changed their bylaws to give women events of their own, equal to the men. She was undefeated in the U.S. from 2000-2008 and still holds several American records. Pam retired from Sprint Canoeing in 2010 at age 42, adding more national records to her resume and finishing her career with 32 national championship medals and 11 international medals. She continues to race in Hawaiian Outrigger canoes and other paddling disciplines.

WHY VEGAN?

How and why did you decide to become vegan?
They say change doesn't happen until it is more painful not to change. I got to a place in my life in early 2007 where too many things seemed to be going wrong and right all at the same time. I was mostly vegetarian by this time, still consuming some dairy-based products and the occasional fish, with little processed foods. I felt like I was moving at 100 mph in some areas of my life and 1 mph in others. Essentially, I learned the hard way that even a decently clean diet could not prevent a physical, mental, emotional, spiritual breakdown, nor prevent alarming health issues that needed immediate attention and reversal.

A lot of what was missing is that I had not fully comprehended the power of holistic nutrition and holistic (mind/body/spirit) living and being, nor had I fully comprehended the other reasons why choosing plant-based nutrition was so powerful. I continued to study health and nutrition and was fortunate to become friends with the "NotMilk Man" Robert Cohen. His information and support were the tipping points for me regarding going fully vegan in 2007 and having more awareness about compassion toward animals. The switch regarding food for healing and high performance didn't flip until August 2007 when Cohen wrote an article about me. From that I was introduced to Dr. Doug Graham and began working with him on a low-fat raw vegan diet. He also helped me work on my mental and emotional game. From there, I began rebuilding in earnest and things were changing for the better on the water and in the gym. I felt like I found a magic formula for healing and high performance to help me raise my game as an "aging" athlete.

As I studied more about compassion for self and compassion for animals and the environment, I was at a point where even the thought of an animal product crossing my lips was repulsive – and saddening. The images, sounds and stories of violence, pain, stress and suffering would flash through my mind. As I was working to move away from negative things in my life (the way I was treating myself and allowing others to treat me) and striving to be more compassionate to myself and others, I could no longer justify contributing to this. I could find no peace there.

'Brutality to animals is cruelty to mankind - it is only the difference in the victim.'
- Alphonse de Lamartine, 1847

How long have you been vegan?
8 years.

What has benefited you the most from being vegan?
Eating a whole foods, high fruit, plant-based diet, I have raised my game physically, mentally, emotionally and spiritually and it has paid off in sports and in life. By being more compassionate toward myself, I've fostered an environment within which I could heal, and thrive. I am able to be more compassionate toward others, and conscious of how my choices affect animals and the environment. I am focused outward rather than inward, and, feeling more at peace with life. I'm becoming a better person.

What does veganism mean to you?
Compassion for self, animals and the environment. Peace.

TRAINING

What sort of training do you do?
I am a paddler and train and race in canoes and kayaks. I also run and do strength training. During winter months I will do more indoor training and add the rowing ergometer and/or spin bike for cardio.

How often do you (need to) train?
6 days per week, 8-12 hours per week.

Do you offer your fitness or training services to others?
If others are interested, I will give my two cents, but I am not a paid fitness or personal trainer. If and when I do engage, I offer my two cents with a holistic (physical/mental/emotional/spiritual) focus in mind.

What sports do you play?
I race and train in canoes and kayaks: Hawaiian outrigger canoes, marathon canoes, Olympic-style canoes and kayaks, and surf skis. Individual and team boats.

STRENGTHS, WEAKNESSES & OUTSIDE INFLUENCES

What do you think is the biggest misconception about vegans and how do you address this?
That we are all judgmental, militant, skinny and unhealthy animal rights activist nut bags, who eat un-tasty food which lacks protein. We can address this by stopping using labels like "vegan," "vegetarian," "paleo," "raw," etc. My name is Pam and I eat what I want and what makes me happy and strong. You eat what you want and what makes you happy and strong.

I struggle with those who commit crimes in the name of animal rights, though, I also admit I applaud their bravery for seeking to end horrific practices against animals and efforts to save animals. These tasks seem overwhelming and insurmountable but we can all make a difference by not feeding the industries responsible for this violence and abuse.

All diet "communities" have a sense of arrogance and judgment - a sense of being in a "higher order." Religious fanatics do this. It is unnecessary. Thrive in your own way and people will be drawn to your positive energy. Do less of shoving one's lifestyle in the face of others. It feels religious at times and it does not need to be. Extend grace and compassion to yourself and to others.

Education must continue. Plant food is quite tasty, particularly in its natural state e.g. raw fruits and greens. I have yet to suffer from a protein deficiency and I continue to raise my athletic game at age 47. I try to just do more and talk less. If people are interested in my story or ideas, I will certainly share and I hope they will share too.

What are your strengths as a vegan athlete?
My mental and emotional strength and poise have by far been the greatest improvement. By removing mental and emotional barriers in all areas of my life and becoming even more convicted about my "Why" (why do I exist?), I am unlocking strength and endurance that I never thought I had, but always wanted. I also have great SECS every day - Sleep, Exercise, Clean Food, Study. It is really that simple. The window of possibilities is limitless.

What is your biggest challenge?
Not eating enough fruit to get that clean, easy to digest base of calories.

Are the non-vegans in your industry supportive or not?
For the most part, yes. And I am playfully the butt of jokes, but come race day, they know I am going to deliver the goods to help our team do well. Almost all gladly take fruit that I share.

Are your family and friends supportive of your vegan lifestyle?
Yes. My boyfriend is vegan, and my Washington Canoe Club teammates go to great lengths to accommodate everyone.

What is the most common question/comment that people ask/say when they find out that you are a vegan and how do you respond?
"Where do you get your protein?" Same place gorillas and elephants get their protein – plants.

Who or what motivates you?
People doing grander things than I am. People who are stronger than me. People thriving on a primarily or all-raw diet. People thriving on a whole-food or real-food plant-strong diet. Writing and doing sports herstory. Being a voice for others for positive change. Helping others who can't help themselves. Waking up every morning and seeing a map of the world, knowing that is my playground. Making myself better, stronger, smarter and more at peace with the world every day – more than I was yesterday.

"Ask yourself: What is my goal? What do I want to accomplish? Why do I want this? Until you have your "Why?" you will never achieve your "What?" You must take a holistic approach to everything. Many factors affect one's ability to gain or lose weight and it's not just diet."

FOOD & SUPPLEMENTS

What do you eat for Breakfast?
I eat when I'm hungry, but start the day with seasonal fruit – usually more juicy fruit (fresh squeezed orange juice, grapes, watermelon, other melons, some sort of citrus-based smoothie.) Sometimes during heavy training, banana smoothies with young coconut water, and possibly dates and other fruit blended with young coconut water. If I'm feeling really wild, some raw cacao powder and almond milk. Over the last year I have added more greens in my smoothies and if I need added density, nut butters and chia seeds.

What do you eat for Lunch?
I try to eat as much fruit until mid-afternoon as a goal. Sometimes, I'll have big salads, hummus with vegetables or rice with vegetables. I'll also have pre-made vegetable wraps, with just romaine lettuce, cucumbers, and cilantro, and use a Thai peanut dressing to dip.

What do you eat for Dinner?
Dinners vary. Usually more cooked: sweet potatoes, quinoa, curry lentils, rice, brown rice noodles (for pasta) vegetables and salads. I have had success making curry lentils and blending with spinach and cilantro, eaten over rice. Also, Vietnamese brown rice noodles with organic marinara sauce, spinach and any other vegetable I like in the sauce, topped with nutritional yeast. This is a fun dish, particularly as my paddling mileage gets higher.

What do you eat for Snacks - healthy & not-so healthy?
I have a weakness for chips and salsa.

What is your favourite source of Protein, Calcium and Iron?
Vegetables and greens for sure and some nuts and seeds. My goal is the highest quality calories – highest nutrient to calorie ratio and I seem to be getting what I need with this. I don't eat food for isolated nutrients because nothing works in isolation. And I don't eat food for a particular macro nutrient. If I have to think about protein, adding greens or celery to smoothies and/or vegetables to other meals is a good way to get more raw protein and calcium and electrolytes.

What foods give you the most energy?
Food does not give me energy. I feel that food gives me the fuel I need to do what I want to do. I try to eat foods that do not require a lot of energy to digest, absorb and assimilate and eliminate. I have more energy because I don't feel weighted down. My top choices for this are raw fruits, mostly low fat but I don't avoid fats.

Do you take any supplements?
I have occasionally used Vega Protein powder - my favorite is Chai-Vanilla. I have also used Hammer Perpetuem vegan sports drink for supplemental calories. In 2013, I raced in the Adirondack 90 miler and I used Perpetuem. The race was a 3-day, 90-mile (144m) canoe race with running portages (running with a 90lb/40kg boat). I was racing with 3 pro male canoeists. This race was 70 miles (112m) longer than I had ever paddled and my longest race prior to that was 3.5 hours. This race was 5, 4 and 3 hours per day, respectively, and I wanted to ensure I got my calories in. I did NOT want to bonk and let my teammates down. I have also used Perpetuem in the General Clinton 70 miler, which I did in 2014 and 2015. That race lasts 8-9 hours depending on water conditions. In the 90 miler, our team finished 3rd in our division and 4th out of 70 4-person canoes. In 2015, my partner and I won the women's Amateur division and were the 2nd women's crew overall, finishing mid-pack of the mixed gender crews.

I ate bananas, dates, and grapes during these races, cut up pieces of Eli Earth Bars vegan bars and made banana and peanut butter and peanut butter and jelly sandwiches. I had my necessary food with me, but felt I needed some extra caloric security as sometimes I couldn't reach for the food. It worked and I felt strong each race. I also use Scratch powder in water for longer training sessions and races which are less than 3 hours.

ADVICE

What is your top tip for gaining muscle?
Eat more real food, lift big and sleep more! Ask yourself: What is my goal? Gaining muscle or getting stronger? And why do I want this? Stronger = stronger. Bigger muscles does not necessarily mean stronger. In my sport, bigger muscles doesn't mean faster in the boat. I've beaten people with bigger/leaner muscles and have lost to people with less muscle and more fat. Strength, efficiency, mental toughness, resiliency in rough conditions, and technical skills – these are things I must prepare for. Big/cut muscles are nice and I'm as vain as the next person, but I like winning more than I like big muscles.

What is your top tip for Losing weight, Maintaining weight, Improving metabolism & Toning up?
Ask yourself: What is my goal? What do I want to accomplish? Why do I want this? Until you have your "Why?" – you will never achieve your "What?" You must take a holistic approach to everything. Many factors affect one's ability to gain or lose weight and it's not just diet. A good first step is to increase whole fresh fruits, greens and vegetables and eliminate processed foods. Drink adequate water and get adequate sleep. Lack of sleep and unmanaged stress can disrupt hormones and contribute to weight gain. Get off the scale and stop looking in the mirror every 5 seconds. Close your eyes and go within and feel what it's like to breathe and work hard physically and mentally. Focus on DOING great things and BEING a good human being and help others – not a number on the scale.

How do you promote veganism in your daily life?
I live my life and work hard, on and off the water. I am noticeably "different" socially, but my performances speak for themselves. If people are interested in what I do and why I do it, I tell them.

How would you suggest people get involved with what you do?
If people ask me for advice, suggestions, or my opinion, I'll offer it based on the research I have done and my personal experience. And I'll offer my support and references and places they can go to do their own research. Others offered resources, support and extended me grace during my journey. I so appreciate that. I seek only to continue to improve myself – my whole game. To continue to learn and grow and give where I can.

"All diet "communities" have a sense of arrogance and judgment – a sense of being in a "higher order." Religious fanatics do this. It is unnecessary. Thrive in your own way and people will be drawn to your positive energy. Do less of shoving one's lifestyle in the face of others. It feels religious at times and it does not need to be. Extend grace and compassion to yourself and to others."

PAT REEVES
VEGAN POWERLIFTER

Kingswinford, West Midlands, England, UK
Vegan since: 1967

foodalive.org
SM: *FaceBook*

Pat Reeves is a practitioner of Nutritional and Functional medicine, full member of the British Association for Applied Nutrition and Nutritional Therapy (BANT) and Complementary and Natural Healthcare Council (CNHC), qualified in nutritional medicine, advanced biochemical medicine, phytotherapy, kinesiology and other allied techniques. Pat has worked with hundreds of patients, resolving all manner of health challenges – including her own genetically-fuelled osteosarcoma, stemming from original meningioma thirty years ago. All fourteen bone tumours remain inactive.

Pat has won many marathons and triathlons, and switched from competitive bodybuilding to power-lifting. She has been the British champion for almost twenty consecutive years and for the past seven years has remained World champion.

WHY VEGAN?

How and why did you decide to become vegan?
To address a genetic cancer situation of mine, osteosarcoma stemming from original meningioma.

How long have you been vegan?
48 years.

What has benefited you the most from being vegan?
Control of 14 bone tumours, recovery from required power-lifting training, and fantastic energy!

What does veganism mean to you?
My use of a plant-based regime initially was purely for health improvements - now obviously I acknowledge the cruelty issues and am happy I do not add to those.

TRAINING

What sort of training do you do?
Strength work, plus cardiovascular and high-intensity interval training (HIIT).

How often do you (need to) train?
Daily.

Do you offer your fitness or training services to others?
Yes.

What sports do you play?
Play is an incorrect description for myself!

STRENGTHS, WEAKNESSES & OUTSIDE INFLUENCES

What do you think is the biggest misconception about vegans and how do you address this?
Not sure how to answer that. I see extremely poor people who follow a plant-based diet and I also have patients who are relatively wealthy, though perhaps some semblance of 'hippy' still exists.

What are your strengths as a vegan athlete?
My excellent recovery and energy.

What is your biggest challenge?
Maintaining a cancer-free status.

Are the non-vegans in your industry supportive or not?
Not in the 'industry' - though most nutritionists are extremely supportive of plant-based eating.

Are your family and friends supportive of your vegan lifestyle?
Absolutely!

What is the most common question/comment that people ask/say when they find out that you are a vegan and how do you respond?
Because I'm in the media a lot, most of my patients are already aware about being vegan and my successes. With many great compliments, I respond by encouraging them to follow a plant-based and living food regime.

Who or what motivates you?
Me! Challenges! Increasing my World-records!

FOOD & SUPPLEMENTS

What do you eat for Breakfast?
Different every day, but likely miso soup, sprouted quinoa, and fruit.

What do you eat for Lunch?
Different every day, handfuls of sprouted greens, seed 'cheese' and almond yoghurt.

What do you eat for Dinner?
Different every day, sprouted pulses, occasional tempeh or tofu, sprouted buckwheat and amaranth, seaweeds, sprouted broccoli, sunflower, buckwheat, and lettuce.

What do you eat for Snacks - healthy & not-so healthy?
Raw hummus in celery, soaked or sprouted seeds with berries, always green juices using spelt wheatgrass or barley grass.

What is your favourite source of Protein?
Sprouted pulses, raw rice and hemp protein powder.

What is your favourite source of Calcium?
Green leaves, almonds, sesame seeds and sea vegetables.

What is your favourite source of Iron?
Asparagus, green juices, parsley and oat grouts.

What foods give you the most energy?
Living foods.

Do you take any supplements?
I make my own from living foods - mainly anti-oxidants, probiotics, serrapeptase, curcumin, astaxanthin.

ADVICE

What is your top tip for gaining muscle?
Optimal resistance training.

What is your top tip for losing weight?
Supporting blood sugar via eating natural foods every three hours, and always including protein with meals.

What is your top tip for maintaining weight?
As above, slightly higher caloric intake to suit.

What is your top tip for improving metabolism?
As under losing weight, plus activation of 'brown fat' via cold water intake, cold showers or baths, if applicable.

What is your top tip for toning up?
Optimal exercise and eating regime specific to personal goals.

How do you promote veganism in your daily life?
By walking my talk, along with my website, book "A Living Miracle" and seminars.

How would you suggest people get involved with what you do?
What is important is not so much what I do personally, but what I can do for others as a practitioner.

"How wonderful is it that nobody need wait a single moment before starting to improve the world."
- Anne Frank

What are you willing to do to get what you want?

PHIL LETTEN
VEGAN FITNESS COACH

Throughout USA
Vegan since: 2007

veganbros.com
SM: *FaceBook, Google+, Instagram, Pinterest*

Phil Letten is an experienced animal advocate and leading fitness coach. He has completed 9 nationwide tours on behalf of the nation's foremost animal protection organizations including Mercy For Animals, Vegan Outreach, and the Humane League; and has been featured on hundreds of mainstream media outlets all across the USA. Having been immersed in the fitness industry for over 8 years he has had the opportunity to help countless people reach their fitness goals.

WHY VEGAN?

How and why did you decide to become vegan?
I am opposed to animal abuse. Meat producers confine animals in cages so small they can barely move, mutilate them without painkillers, and brutally slaughter them. I want no part in that.

How long have you been vegan?
I stopped eating meat 11 years ago, and went vegan 8 years ago.

What has benefited you the most from being vegan?
I know that I'm not paying others to abuse and exploit animals for profit.

What does veganism mean to you?
To me veganism means doing your best to lessen the amount of suffering in the world.

"Yes, there is a lot of suffering in the world. If we let this cause us to be angry, then we are just adding to the amount of misery in the world. When we are joyful, people not only want to be around us, but they are more likely to want to be like us as well."

TRAINING

What sort of training do you do?
I primarily focus on big compound lifts such as the dead lift, squats, presses, rows etc. For conditioning, I enjoy doing sprints and circuit-style training.

How often do you (need to) train?
I think it varies by person. The minimum I allow myself to train is 3 times per week. 4 times per week is the norm. When I get crazy, I up it to 5 or 6 days per week.

Do you offer your fitness or training services to others?
My brother and I are the head coaches over at VeganBros.com where we are raising up an army of fit, sexy vegan soldiers to spread the delicious, cruelty-free Gospel of peace and compassion to a lost and dying world.

What sports do you play?

When I was younger, I did everything from soccer, baseball, and basketball to snowboarding and skateboarding. Although I'm not nearly as competitive as I was when I was younger, I still enjoy playing various sports on community leagues.

STRENGTHS, WEAKNESSES & OUTSIDE INFLUENCES

What do you think is the biggest misconception about vegans and how do you address this?

The obvious is that you can't build muscle etc. My least favorite misconception is that we are all angry. I address this by being positive and happy. Yes, there is a lot of suffering in the world. If we let this cause us to be angry, then we are just adding to the amount of misery in the world. When we are joyful, people not only want to be around us, but they are more likely to want to be like us as well.

What are your strengths as a vegan athlete?

Although I only weigh 167 pounds (75kg), I can dead lift 455 pounds (206kg).

What is your biggest challenge?

There are no specific crazy challenges that I can think of.

Are the non-vegans in your industry supportive or not?

More and more professional athletes are going vegan every day, proving that you can be vegan and an elite athlete at the same time. We are reaching a point where it is hard to be successful in this industry if you are still saying, "You can't be vegan and an athlete at the same time."

Are your family and friends supportive of your vegan lifestyle?

Definitely. Since going vegan, I've seen my brother, Mom, and Dad go vegan as well as aunts, uncles, cousins, and even my grandparents have begun dabbling in it. I've seen so many friends go vegan. I love it!

What is the most common question/comment that people ask/say when they find out that you are a vegan and how do you respond?

"Where do you get your protein?" From vegan meats, beans, nuts, seeds, kale, spinach, and protein powder.

Who or what motivates you?

The animals are my main motivation, they need me to counter the stereotype of what a vegan looks like.

"My fitness tip is to not transform your diet overnight, but rather focus on one habit at a time for 1-2 weeks. Once you have mastered the habit, move onto the next habit. Such as eating protein with every meal, or eating 5 servings of vegetables per day."

FOOD & SUPPLEMENTS

What do you eat for Breakfast?

Super shake with berries, banana, kale, nuts, steel-cut oats, protein powder, and GreensPlus.

What do you eat for Lunch?

Stir-fry with various veggies, yams, tofu or some sort of vegan meat, and quinoa.

What do you eat for Dinner?
Salad loaded with veggies, spinach, tofu, and quinoa.

What is your favourite source of Protein?
Any of the vegan meats.

What is your favourite source of Calcium?
Kale.

What is your favourite source of Iron?
Spinach.

What foods give you the most energy?
Quinoa, brown rice and sweet potatoes.

Do you take any supplements?
I take protein powder, creatine, GreensPlus and B-12.

ADVICE

What is your top tip for gaining muscle, losing weight, maintaining weight, improving metabolism and toning up?
My advice for all of these is to not transform your diet overnight, but rather focus on one habit at a time for 1-2 weeks. Once you have mastered the habit, move onto the next habit. Such as eating protein with every meal, or eating 5 servings of vegetables per day.

How do you promote veganism in your daily life?
I am not preachy about it in normal life. I only talk about it when asked. I am also involved in activism as well. One activity I do a lot is leafleting on college campuses to educate the kids on the horrific cruelties involved in factory farming. I am consistently amazed at how effective this is.

My brother and I have also recently started Seattle Veg Connect, a new way for vegans, vegetarians, and those interested in meatless eating to come together, hang out, and plan world domination. Our first event sold out of all 70 tickets in less than 4-days. And, we've got big plans for the future of it.

How would you suggest people get involved with what you do?
Head to our website, download our free eBook, and check out the articles.

"More and more professional athletes are going vegan every day, proving that you can be vegan and an elite athlete at the same time. We are reaching a point where it is hard to be successful in this industry if you are still saying, "You can't be vegan and an athlete at the same time.""

RAMONA CADOGAN
VEGAN PERSONAL TRAINER

Long Island, New York, USA
Vegan since: 2006

fitveganchef.weebly.com
academictutor.weebly.com
SM: *FaceBook, Instagram, Twitter, YouTube*

Ramona Cadogan is a science educator, who has a tutoring service, and has competed in Olympic weightlifting. She is a vegan/raw vegan chef, Pilates instructor, hula hooper, the NY Ambassador to Team Green, and was featured in the August 2014 edition of Vegan Health and Fitness Magazine.

WHY VEGAN?

I became raw vegan in 2006 and have been off meat since 2000. I did it to protect the animals.

How and why did you decide to become vegan?
I decided to go vegan because I wanted to protect the animals and for a cleaner diet. I became vegan based on influence from my friends who had opened the first raw vegan restaurant in Queens, NY called Exotic Super Foods.

How long have you been vegan?
9 years.

What has benefited you the most from being vegan?
The benefits are protecting the environment, not harming animals, eating a plant-based diet, and following the lifestyle.

What does veganism mean to you?
Veganism means respecting animals - not just about the diet.

TRAINING

What sort of training do you do?
Olympic weightlifting and powerlifting.

How often do you (need to) train?
I train 5 to 6 days a week.

Do you offer your fitness or training services to others?
Yes as a personal trainer, vegan and raw vegan chef, Pilates teacher and a hula hooper. I provide meal plans and work with athletes and non-athletes to lose weight, build muscle, prepare for competitions.

What sports do you play?
Tennis.

STRENGTHS, WEAKNESSES & OUTSIDE INFLUENCES

What do you think is the biggest misconception about vegans and how do you address this?
The biggest misconception is about where I get my protein. I do not let misconceptions get to me. I consume protein by eating nuts, seeds but mainly tons of greens.

What are your strengths as a vegan athlete?
My strength as a vegan athlete is my power and strength.

What is your biggest challenge?
My biggest challenge is to realize that I must not overtrain.

Are the non-vegans in your industry supportive or not?
50/50.

Are your family and friends supportive of your vegan lifestyle?
Yes, I have supportive friends and family.

What is the most common question/comment that people ask/say when they find out that you are a vegan and how do you respond?
The most common question is, "How do you get all your nutrients?" I tell them I get all my nutrients from greens, fruits, nuts, seeds and taking raw vitamin B12 and D3.

Who or what motivates you?
I motivate myself by my daily affirmations.

FOOD & SUPPLEMENTS

What do you eat for Breakfast?
Smoothie with chia seeds, almond butter, spinach, bananas, protein powder from LOVE by Purium or UmniSuperfoods with coconut water or alkaline water.

What do you eat for Lunch?
Large green salad with dulse, pine nuts, lemon, tomatoes, sprouts, avocado, and goji berries.

What do you eat for Dinner?
Raw zucchini pasta.

What do you eat for Snacks - healthy & not-so healthy?
Berries, dates, apple or a raw vegan sprouted trail mix.

What is your favourite source of Protein?
Tons of greens and Beyond Meat.

What is your favourite source of Calcium?
Again tons of greens, and bananas.

What is your favourite source of Iron?
Even more greens.

What foods give you the most energy?
Dates, bananas, oatmeal, chia seeds, vegan pancakes, branch chain amino acids by Geoff Palmer from Clean Machine.

Do you take any supplements?
B12 and D3.

ADVICE

What is your top tip for gaining muscle?
Post workout: Beyond Meat, vegan glutamine with Omnisuperfoods or with LOVE by Purium and Branch Chain Amino Acids by Geoff Palmer. Plus 8 to 10 hours of sleep, vegan nutrition, meditation and water.

What is your top tip for losing weight?
Exercise your large muscle groups like back and legs using resistant and aerobic combo training.

What is your top tip for maintaining weight?
Based on current weight, know how much protein and carbohydrates are needed - probably would need more or less depending on your metabolism and fitness level.

What is your top tip for improving metabolism?
Lemon juice in warm water first thing in the morning.

What is your top tip for toning up?
Use light weights with more reps and plenty of squats.

How do you promote veganism in your daily life?
Through the group, Friends of the Animals.

How would you suggest people get involved with what you do?
Connect with me online, send me an email, and find me on Social Media.

Get Involved with Activism:

- Attend events organised by Animal Rights and Vegan groups in your area
- Volunteer at events, sanctuaries and tables
- Wear your Veganism proudly e.g. t-shirts
- Include a quote or link about veganism in your email signature
- Write Letters to newspapers, Members of Parliament, stores and companies
- Create and hand out vegan information and literature
- Make great vegan food for others
- Share links and information on your Social Media channels
- Use your skills, know what you like to do, and do it!

RAUL RAMIREZ
VEGAN MARTIAL ARTIST AND CATCH WRESTLER

Culver City, California, USA
Vegan since: 2006

kungfukulture.com
catchwrestlingalliance.com
SM: *FaceBook, Instagram, Twitter, YouTube*

Raul Ramirez was born and raised in southern California, and is now a licensed acupuncturist working at his clinic, Nei Jing Eastern Medicine in Culver City, California. He's been training seriously in many styles of martial arts since the 1990's. Along the way he passed the American Council on Exercise personal trainer exam and became a trainer for University of California, Los Angeles (UCLA).

Raul has had the privilege of training with the top martial arts instructors at the best schools in the world. He trained with the best professional Sanda (Chinese Kickboxing which allows takedowns and slams), and wrestling coaches while at Beijing University of Physical Education. For Catch Wrestling, he trained with the two best coaches in the world, Billy Robinson and Roy Wood. Raul also trained in non-sport, self-defence martial arts in Indonesia and in Los Angeles. He won two national championships in Sanda, a silver medal in international Sumo wrestling, and is currently undefeated in the International Catch Wrestling competition.

WHY VEGAN?

Veganism makes the most sense to me. We have all the evidence to prove that this is the best lifestyle for our health and the ecosystem.

How and why did you decide to become vegan?
I was at the mall waiting for a movie to start in 2005. I stepped into the bookstore to kill time, and I saw a book called "The China Study". I bought it, was blown away by the research, checked out other research then switched. I never looked back. I was more interested in the health benefits at first, but the environmental and animal rights issues are hard to ignore. I have since joined the Physicians Committee for Responsible Medicine (PCRM) in order to take a more active role in supporting such issues.

How long have you been vegan?
I don't remember an exact date when I went vegan, but I'm over the 9 year mark now. I'm really happy and proud to be vegan.

What has benefited you the most from being vegan?
The major benefit that I noticed was faster repair after hard workouts. I can also adapt quicker to increases in intensity - like when preparing for competition I increase the intensity and duration of workouts in the weeks before the competition. I feel that my body adapts quickly to such increases.

What does veganism mean to you?

Since my son was born, veganism has meant more to me than ever. Veganism means that my son will have less of a chance of developing the common childhood diseases. It means that I have a greater chance of being healthy enough to keep up with him as he grows and gets involved with many different activities. I hope he wants to learn catch wrestling from me, and I want to be fit enough to train him.

The life saving aspect of veganism is also very real to me. I see the effects almost daily in my clinic. I've seen people overcome serious medical conditions with the plant-based diet. They have been able to stop taking some serious medications.

TRAINING

What sort of training do you do?

I mainly focus on catch wrestling, Chinese kickboxing, and meditative kung fu styles, like Qi Gong. I also work on strength and conditioning by keeping a regular weight lifting routine, cardio training which can vary from running, stairs, or even cycling. And last but certainly one of the most important things that I do that keeps injuries to a minimum, is stretching after each workout. I also try to make yoga part of my routine when I have the time.

I know many people don't like stretching, or don't know how to stretch properly. Many people come to my clinic because of injuries that could have been prevented by stretching. Flexibility has nothing to do with age. I have seen young and old patients who have suffered from flexibility related injuries. We just have to make sure that we don't forget to stretch.

How often do you (need to) train?

I usually workout six days a week, but the intensity varies depending on if I'll be competing soon. I think I've gotten used to this schedule. I might not need to train so many days out of the week, but I actually enjoy working out and being active.

Do you offer your fitness or training services to others?

I worked as a personal trainer for many years at the University of California, Los Angeles, (UCLA), recently I have shifted most of my extra time to training people in catch wrestling, kickboxing or self-defence.

What sports do you play?

Nowadays, I mainly practice catch wrestling, because I still compete in this sport. It is one of the most physically demanding and painful sports there is. It was extremely popular around the world in the early 1900's and I'm now helping to bring it back into the spotlight. One wins by pin or submission. A wide variety of submissions are legal, like wrist-locks and face locks, neck cranks, etc. It is a very exciting sport.

I believe that this sport will make a comeback, so I created a promotion called the Catch Wrestling Alliance. I was able to get the support of the main catch wrestling schools in the world. We are all working together to put on exciting catch wrestling events, where the highest-level catch wrestlers from around the world compete. We held our first show in June 2014 and we also had women's matches. Many of the wrestlers were inspired by me to go on a plant-based diet while training for the event.

STRENGTHS, WEAKNESSES & OUTSIDE INFLUENCES

What do you think is the biggest misconception about vegans and how do you address this?
I think the biggest misconception is that we are weak and fatigue easily. I address this by not getting tired during workouts. I've gone through weeks of intensive martial arts training, and had people comment on how fresh I looked after training hard for so long where others seemed to be wearing out.

What are your strengths as a vegan athlete?
Quick recovery and adaptation are the strengths that come to mind first. It is nice to know that I'm helping my body by eating the right foods and not taxing my body while it is trying to recover from a hard workout.

What is your biggest challenge?
I don't feel like being a vegan is challenging at all. The only thing I have to remember is to pack some food if I travel to a new place, but I can usually find vegan food anywhere.

Are the non-vegans in your industry supportive or not?
In the combat sports no one seems to care what I eat, but in medicine, I have seen many uneducated doctors promoting fad diets. It is sad to see so many physicians in the dark about nutrition. It is understandable, because nutrition is not really covered in medical schools, but it is still a real shame.

Are your family and friends supportive of your vegan lifestyle?
Yes, everyone is very supportive. I am also lucky to live in LA where vegan restaurants are sprouting up everywhere. The idea of veganism isn't too strange or scary to my non-vegan friends and family. I wish more of them would take the plunge and just be vegans too.

What is the most common question/comment that people ask/say when they find out that you are a vegan and how do you respond?
People often say that it must be difficult to be vegan because they wouldn't know what to eat. I tell them that there are already many foods that they eat that are vegan, like guacamole, hummus, salsa, corn tortillas, etc. I tell them that cooking is about knowing your ingredients, and that the flavor comes from the natural compounds in the food as well as the spices you add to the food you cook.

Who or what motivates you?
I am motivated by the Bluezones research. It is amazing that we have evidence showing the fact that the longest-lived people on the planet eat very little to no meat. I'm thankful for every day I get to spend with my son. I hope to have a long life supporting him as he grows into adulthood. Perhaps he will have kids. I want to be a healthy grandpa for them too.

FOOD & SUPPLEMENTS

What do you eat for Breakfast?
Usually some sort of grain like oatmeal, black rice, etc., with fruit, or a fruit and vegetable smoothie.

What do you eat for Lunch?
It can be any dish from Asian, Mexican, Indian, Middle Eastern cuisines.

What do you eat for Dinner?
Can be similar to lunch. Sometimes my family eats raw, sometimes not.

What do you eat for Snacks - healthy & not-so healthy?
My son loves blueberries and goji berries, so we always have those around. I also love chips and spicy salsa, guacamole, garlic aioli, and hummus.

What is your favourite source of Protein?
I like tempeh, seitan, tofu, and most any kind of bean.

What is your favourite source of Calcium?
Veggies.

What is your favourite source of Iron?
Beans.

What foods give you the most energy?
I feel a real increase in energy with proper hydration and eating a lot of fruit. I never feel at a loss of energy while training when I'm getting large amounts of fruit and water.

Do you take any supplements?
I will take some Eastern medical herbs from time to time in the weeks leading up to a competition, like curcumin, or some that help wound healing, but I don't supplement most of the year.

ADVICE

What is your top tip for gaining muscle?
Consistency and patience. Make sure you hit the same muscle group more than once a week.

What is your top tip for losing weight?
It is more important to focus on losing fat. I like having strong muscles and having a healthy body fat percentage. So, I don't care about my weight if my body fat percentage is in the healthy range. If the percentage creeps up, then I know that I have probably overindulged in salty and fatty foods. It also means to me that I've probably gotten used to the intensity of my workout and it's time to kick it up a notch.

What is your top tip for maintaining weight?
Try to minimize the junk foods and keep a consistent workout routine.

What is your top tip for improving metabolism?
Move your body and strength train.

How do you promote veganism in your daily life?
I am not shy about the nutrition advice I give to my patients. I also subscribe to several vegan magazines that I put in the waiting room. Many patients have commented that they found some of the articles very interesting. It is also nice when I actually appear in the magazine like Vegan Health and Fitness. My patients and martial arts students like seeing stuff like that. Many of them have incorporated more plants into their diet.

How would you suggest people get involved with what you do?
For more info on the martial arts and eastern medicine please visit my website and send me an email.

"Since my son was born, veganism has meant more to me than ever. Veganism means that my son will have less of a chance of developing the common childhood diseases. It means that I have a greater chance of being healthy enough to keep up with him as he grows and gets involved with many different activities. I hope he wants to learn catch wrestling from me, and I want to be fit enough to train him."

Regan Smith
VEGAN EXERCISE ENTHUSIAST

Brisbane, Queensland, Australia
Vegan since: 2012

otherwaysoflife.com
SM: *FaceBook, Instagram, Twitter, YouTube*

Regan Smith is a gym instructor who lives in Brisbane, Australia. He has been vegan for almost 3 years, with health and fitness his initial driving force to explore the diet - it has evolved from there.

WHY VEGAN?

How and why did you decide to become vegan?
About 3 years ago, I was starting to gain weight and wasn't feeling healthy despite exercising so I decided to look into fixing my diet. At first, I just cut out added sugar, then I started eating organic, went vegetarian for a week then made the switch to a vegan diet. At first, I became vegan for health reasons and I was still eating honey, but I was getting more and more into meditation and wanting to live a peaceful lifestyle. A friend posted on FaceBook 'Honey is stealing and stealing is bad' – which was a really simple way to put it.

How long have you been vegan?
Since 2012.

What has benefited you the most from being vegan?
Exercise and training is a big part of my life, so the thing I've noticed the most is energy levels.

What does veganism mean to you?
It's looking after myself in a way that doesn't harm others.

TRAINING

What sort of training do you do?
Weight training and cardio.

How often do you (need to) train?
It depends on my schedule. Right now I do weight training 6 times per week for an hour and 1-2 cardio sessions usually 30 minutes in duration. My favourite training though was while I was living in Japan - I was able to train 9 times per week doing weights. I wasn't doing any cardio so I didn't feel very fit, but I gained 2kg of muscle in 3 months and was in the best shape of my life, which I really enjoyed.

Do you offer your fitness or training services to others?
Definitely. I work as a Gym Instructor in Brisbane where I help people with their training in the gym. I'm also a group exercise instructor, which is what I enjoy the most. I like to take classes where I combine resistance training and cardio together like an indoor boot camp. But I'm at heart a minimalist, so I like to use as little equipment as

possible. I'm working on a website at the moment which is focused on putting aside the illusion that vegans are either weak or skinny. It's an 8-week training program complete with a vegan eating plan, containing whole food recipes designed for fitness and muscle gain combined with strength and conditioning programs. The goal is to help people get a fit, athletic body on a vegan diet.

What sports do you play?
None at the moment. I used to play rugby but because of my work, I can't afford to be injured anymore. I exercise almost every day for my job so even to sprain an ankle can be a big hassle.

"I think veganism started off really well as a nutritious diet, but nowadays the same mistakes are being made by processing things, adding sugars, and thinking they're still healthy because they're made from plant foods."

STRENGTHS, WEAKNESSES & OUTSIDE INFLUENCES

What do you think is the biggest misconception about vegans and how do you address this?
That they have to be outspoken. For me veganism has been a personal journey, I don't look at someone eating meat and think that they have to change their ways. Everyone is on their own path and doing their best with their own level of awareness. If someone is interested in trying a vegan diet, I will help them as much as I can. If someone had approached me the day before I switched to a vegan diet and said, 'You shouldn't be eating meat, meat is murder!' I probably wouldn't have made the switch. I don't think anyone likes to be told what to do.

What are your strengths as a vegan athlete?
I don't really have a particular strength, my personality is that I'm terribly inconsistent and am always looking for variety. Having said that, I've been doing resistance training in the gym for 10 years now - I wouldn't say it's my strength because it's something I do for fun, but it's certainly what I've been most consistent at.

What is your biggest challenge?
Vegan-only restaurants. They're not that common where I'm living so when I find a place with a large variety of vegan options, I never know what to choose. I end up ordering too much and leaving with a stomachache and an empty wallet.

Are the non-vegans in your industry supportive or not?
Definitely supportive.

Are your family and friends supportive of your vegan lifestyle?
Yeah of course, my brother loves to cook and he always modifies my dish so it's vegan. Whenever my mum sees a new organic vegan food or shop/cafe she always rings me to tell me about it or will buy me something as a surprise.

What is the most common question/comment that people ask/say when they find out that you are a vegan and how do you respond?
They ask me 'So what exactly do you eat?' I have so much fun with this question, my last response was that I sneak into bird sanctuaries and steal their seeds because that's all vegans really eat. It usually gets a laugh or a weird look and then I just run through what I would normally eat in a day.

Who or what motivates you?

It's all intrinsic now, I switched my diet after watching "Forks Over Knives" and reading the health statistics, but now I'm motivated by how good I feel and the energy I have each day.

FOOD & SUPPLEMENTS

What do you eat for Breakfast?

Smoothie and a coffee. Usually with a banana, macadamia milk and rice protein at the core, and then a mix of greens, powders and berries depending on what I have in the cupboard. This is usually before training.

What do you eat for Lunch?

Tofu and vegetables with pasta sauce and a bowl of steamed vegetables.

What do you eat for Dinner?

This is always different, a mix of vegetables and maybe tofu or tempeh depending what I've had during the day.

What do you eat for Snacks - healthy & not-so healthy?

My diet has always had the fundamental of being for my health so although I do eat some processed foods occasionally, I don't include them in my everyday diet. My snacks are tomatoes and carrots, which I just eat whole. I love cucumber and also a bowl of blueberries. Macadamias and mixed nuts are also another favourite. Every now and again, I'll eat something sweet like a slice of mint cake and am reminded why I don't eat them.

What is your favourite source of Protein?

Tofu, tempeh, rice protein powder or nuts.

What is your favourite source of Calcium?

No idea - it's never been something I've had to worry about.

What is your favourite source of Iron?

I don't think about it anymore. I had tests done 3 months after switching my diet and my Iron levels were a lot higher than when I ate meat.

What foods give you the most energy?

My morning smoothie and my organic coffee.

Do you take any supplements?

Only protein at the moment but I've taken Vitamin B in the past as well.

ADVICE

What is your top tip for gaining muscle?

Eat plenty of plant-based protein, don't waste time with processed foods or snacks and do whatever training you enjoy the most.

What is your top tip for losing weight?

Avoid the processed crap. I think veganism started off really well as a nutritious diet, but nowadays the same mistakes are being made by processing things, adding sugars, and thinking they're still healthy because they're made from plant foods. Coconut ice cream is not going to do you any favours in this department! Also, one quote that has really stuck with me was 'When hungry, eat. When tired, sleep' by the Dalai Lama. I change it slightly to 'When hungry, eat. When not hungry, don't eat.' It sounds so basic but many people eat out of habit rather than listening to their body.

What is your top tip for maintaining weight?
Eat and train.

What is your top tip for improving metabolism?
Weight training. I think it's a very individualistic thing, but for my body type, eating more combined with weight training always leaves me leaner than if I eat less and do cardio. Regular resistance training allows your body to be in a constant state of muscle repair so your metabolism is always increased.

What is your top tip for toning up?
Eat and train.

How do you promote veganism in your daily life?
Be it. When I see people who inspire me, I ask 'What do they do to be like that?'

How would you suggest people get involved with what you do?
At the moment, I have a YouTube channel, which I use for personal vlogs called Other Ways of Life. When my other website is up and running I'll announce it on in my videos.

"A vegan misconception is that they have to be outspoken. For me veganism has been a personal journey, I don't look at someone eating meat and think that they have to change their ways. Everyone is on their own path and doing their best with their own level of awareness. If someone is interested in trying a vegan diet, I will help them as much as I can. If someone had approached me the day before I switched to a vegan diet and said, 'You shouldn't be eating meat, meat is murder!' I probably wouldn't have made the switch. I don't think anyone likes to be told what to do."

"Do all the good you can, by all the means you can, in all the ways you can, in all the places you can, at all the times you can, to all the people you can, as long as ever you can."
- John Wesley

Your Vibe Attracts Your Tribe

ROB BIGWOOD
VEGAN PROFESSIONAL ARM WRESTLER

New York City, New York, USA
vegan since: 2009

blog.rbigwood.com
rbigwood.com
SM: *FaceBook, Tumblr, Twitter*

Rob Bigwood is a New York City based Interactive Art Director and a top-ranked Professional Arm Wrestler (PAC). Rob has won over 40 state tournaments, as well as the PAC's World Championship in 2006 (left handed). He has also been featured in VegNews magazine's "The Hot List," Maxim magazine's "He-Man Vegans", John Joseph's book "Meat is for Pussies", the Vegan Society Magazine, and been interviewed on countless other sites for breaking the vegan stereotype.

WHY VEGAN?

How and why did you decide to become vegan?
It all started back in 2002 at a State Fair when a group of piglets caught my attention. It was adorable watching them interact with each other, and it was no different than watching puppies. I got ill thinking that I had eaten a bacon and egg sandwich for breakfast that morning. I've always been an animal lover and when I actually made the connection, it made me sick. I researched and discovered how disgusting and inhuman the factory farming industry is.

How long have you been vegan?
I have been a vegetarian for years but vegan since 2009.

What has benefited you the most from being vegan?
The biggest benefit is that I know I'm thriving on a cruelty-free diet and that no animals have to endure any pain or suffering for my personal benefit. I use to weigh around 290lbs (131kg) and felt extremely lethargic. Now I'm 225lbs (102kg) and feel like a new person. I've never felt healthier in my entire life and it has been one of the best decisions I ever made.

What does veganism mean to you?
I made an ethical decision to give up all animal products and was willing to face any consequences. It is more important to stand up for what I believe in than to worry about being an amazing arm wrestler. Veganism is a lifestyle that more people should get behind.

"Most people are intrigued when they find out I'm vegan. We were always raised to believe that the only way to get protein is meat. I educate them about my diet and where I get my protein."

TRAINING

What sort of training do you do?
Torque exercises that simulate arm wrestling, heavy weights and cable training.
Forearms, biceps and back are the most important body parts to train for this sport.

How often do you (need to) train?
For a tournament, I'm in the gym 4-5 days a week. I also arm wrestle with a group of guys every few weeks.

Do you offer your fitness or training services to others?
Sure, if they have any interest in my sport.

What sports do you play?
Professional Arm Wrestler.

STRENGTHS, WEAKNESSES & OUTSIDE INFLUENCES

What do you think is the biggest misconception about vegans and how do you address this?
I blitz any misconceptions by beating over-sized meatheads on the arm wrestling table.

What are your strengths as a vegan athlete?
Muscle endurance and tendon strength.

What is your biggest challenge?
Drinking too much beer, liquor and wine.

Are the non-vegans in your industry supportive or not?
Surprisingly yes, but this might be because I'm successful.

Are your family and friends supportive of your vegan lifestyle?
Absolutely! My dad loves the food and my mom makes sure I have everything needed for when I go home to New Jersey.

What is the most common question/comment that people ask/say when they find out that you are a vegan?
"Where do you get your protein?".

Who or what motivates you?
I motivate and push myself. I have always been the type of person to never settle for anything less than the best.

"I made an ethical decision to give up all animal products and was willing to face any consequences. It is more important to stand up for what I believe in than to worry about being an amazing arm wrestler. Veganism is a lifestyle that more people should get behind."

FOOD & SUPPLEMENTS

What do you eat for Breakfast?
I usually mix oatmeal and almonds, sunflower seeds, flaxseeds, and raisins. If I'm feeling lazy, I'll eat organic cereal with almond milk and a banana.

What do you eat for Lunch?

A variety of salads.

What do you eat for Dinner?
I love Indian, Thai, Mexican and Japanese food and a few of my favorite places in NYC are Gobo, Blossom, Terri, Soy and Sake, and Candle 79.

What do you eat for Snacks - healthy & not-so healthy?
Vegan ice cream and New York's Dun-Well Donuts.

What is your favourite source of Protein?
Sunwarrior and Vega protein shakes, Builder protein bars, almond milk, legumes, nuts, tofu, tempeh, seitan, and mock meat.

What is your favourite source of Calcium?
Tofu, almond milk, and dark green leafy vegetables eg bok choy, broccoli, collards, kale, spinach.

What is your favourite source of Iron?
Dark green leafy vegetables and beans eg lentils, soybeans, spinach, quinoa, chickpeas.

What foods give you the most energy?
Fruits, vegetables, nuts and freshly squeezed juices. I also have more energy when I eat fewer calories.

Do you take any supplements?
Only when I train for a competition, I take protein shakes and a multivitamin. I also take flaxseed oil and glucosamine for my elbows.

ADVICE

What is your top tip for gaining muscle?
Eat more protein and calories. Also, do between 8-12 repetitions of each set at the gym.

What is your top tip for losing weight?
Eat fewer calories and add more cardio to your workouts.

What is your top tip for improving metabolism?
Spend more time exercising.

What is your top tip for toning up?
I'm the wrong guy to ask - but check out Robert Cheeke or Jimi Sitko.

How do you promote veganism in your daily life?
I have a blog where I post related topics. Most people are intrigued when they find out I'm vegan. We were always raised to believe that the only way to get protein is meat. I educate them about my diet and where I get my protein.

"Veganism for me started back in 2002 at a State Fair when a group of piglets caught my attention. It was adorable watching them interact with each other, and it was no different than watching puppies. I got ill thinking that I had eaten a bacon and egg sandwich for breakfast that morning. I've always been an animal lover and when I actually made the connection, it made me sick. I researched and discovered how disgusting and inhuman the factory farming industry is."

ROB DOLECKI
VEGAN FREESTYLE BMX RIDER

Philadelphia, Pennsylvania, USA
Vegan since: 1997

doleckivisuals.com
SM: *FaceBook, Instagram, Twitter*

Rob Dolecki will hop fences, risk arrest, and sleep in moving vans to get a good photo, but he can't stomach coffee or pistachios. He travels around the world riding bikes and shooting BMX photos, occasionally stopping to rest at his home in Philadelphia, which he shares with his girlfriend and two cats. In addition to being a photographer for DIGBMX.com, he also freelances and has a few independent projects in the works, such as a three-part print photo 'zine series under the name Maintain.

WHY VEGAN?

How and why did you decide to become vegan?
I stopped eating meat and eggs in 1996, which transitioned into weaning myself off of dairy over the following year. Veganism was just the obvious next step for myself after the personal progression of my outlook on living in a positive way - from health, ethical, spiritual and environmental aspects.

How long have you been vegan?
Since 1997.

What has benefited you the most from being vegan?
A body that functions as efficiently as I could possibly want.

What does veganism mean to you?
It's the most important way for me to show respect daily for everything that also lives on Earth.

TRAINING

What sort of training do you do?
I wouldn't necessarily call it "training," but I ride my BMX bike about 2-6 days a week. That can involve trying to cruise a skate park, my neighborhood, or trails (BMX dirt jumps) like a maniac for anywhere from an hour to most of the day. I also pedal around with an excessively large camera back weighing over 40 lbs a few days a week. Thanks to the encouragement from my lady Nicole, I may actually make yoga a more common practice too. I've done a few classes, and man, that will stretch your body and stress muscles in ways I never thought possible. It's also enlightened me to the fact that I am absurdly not limber in certain stretches.

How often do you (need to) train?
Whenever I have the urge to ride my bike, or the need to shoot BMX street photos. Both are usually at least a few times a week, on average.

Do you offer your fitness or training services to others?
If someone wanted to be an assistant and carry my camera bag around, I would gladly "train" him or her.

What sports do you play?
Freestyle BMX takes up most of my free time. Occasionally, I'll push around on a skateboard, shoot some hoops, or attempt to body board.

STRENGTHS, WEAKNESSES & OUTSIDE INFLUENCES

What do you think is the biggest misconception about vegans, and how do you address this?
That veganism is unhealthy. It can be, if all you ate were French fries and bagels. But, based on everything I've ever been exposed to, the evidence is more common than ever these days that a whole foods plant-based diet is the most beneficial diet; the proof is in the chia seed pudding.

What are your strengths as a vegan athlete?
Lots, but probably the two main things from an athletic standpoint are most likely common goals of any athlete: strength and stamina.

What is your biggest challenge?
Finding a delicious meal in certain food deserts around the world, especially when there is a language barrier.

Are the non-vegans in your industry supportive or not?
I'd say so. Outside of the occasional light-hearted jokes, I usually encounter nothing but respect and tolerance for how I choose to eat. Sometimes there is a lack of understanding why, but I wasn't any different when I was in my early twenties and younger.

Are your family and friends supportive of your vegan lifestyle?
Even though no one in my family besides Nicole is vegan, everyone is very respectful of my eating choices, even if turkey is the main dish being served at Thanksgiving dinner.

What is the most common question/comment that people ask/say when they find out that you are a vegan, and how do you respond?
Usually, they say how they could never do it. I thought the same thing over 17 years ago.

Who or what motivates you?
Trying to enjoy every day that I can.

FOOD & SUPPLEMENTS

What do you eat for Breakfast?
At home - Any combination of fruit, green juice, green smoothie, and steel-cut oatmeal, occasionally homemade whole grain waffles or pancakes with a variety of healthy and delicious toppings.

On the road - Whatever I can get my hands on.

What do you eat for Lunch?
At home - Any combination of a veggie sandwich on Ezekiel bread (avocado, hummus, etc), homemade soup, salad, fruit, etc.

On the road - Whatever I can get my hands on.

What do you eat for Dinner?

At home - Any combination of salad, lightly cooked greens, squash, beans, tofu scramble, veggie and bean/rice pasta casserole, bean tacos, polenta, stir-fries, etc. Occasionally eating out at Ethio (Ethiopian), Vegan Tree, New Harmony, The Nile, Soy Café, Essene buffet, Govinda's, Vgë, Mi Lah, and Su Tao - all restaurants in the Philadelphia area.

On the road - Whatever I can get my hands on.

What do you eat for Snacks - healthy & not-so healthy?

At home - Fruit, banana and chocolate shake, apple crisp, avocado mousse, air-popped popcorn, rice cakes with almond butter and apple butter, homemade trail mix, coconut date rolls, homemade sugar-free, gluten-free cookies, etc.

On the road - Larabars, fruit, hummus and veggies, and on those occasions when I'm unprepared and stuck at a gas station in the middle of nowhere, occasionally I'll eat some kind of junky chips for a snack.

What is your favorite source of Protein?
Any type of beans.

What is your favorite source of Calcium?
Dark leafy greens.

What is your favorite source of Iron?
Lentils and dark leafy greens.

What foods give you the most energy?
Smoothies, green juices, bowl of steel-cut oatmeal with walnuts, blueberries, flax seeds and soy or almond milk.

Do you take any supplements?
Multi-vitamin, zinc, vitamins C and D, and green powder a few times or more a week; B12, glucosamine, DHA & EPA a few times a week.

ADVICE

What is your top tip for gaining muscle?
Exercise, and eat lots of beans, unprocessed fats, and greens.

What is your top tip for losing weight?
Exercise, and minimize the excessive oil, fried foods, sugar and white foods.

What is your top tip for Maintaining weight, Improving metabolism & Toning up?
Exercise, and eat a whole foods, plant-based diet. Recurring theme for all.

How do you promote veganism in your daily life?
I'm not one for preaching about something that works for me on a personal level. I just do what I do, and someone is interested, they may realize that if I can do it, they can too.

How would you suggest people get involved with what you do?
Get a bike and just start cruising around.

"Being vegan is the most important way for me to show respect daily for everything that also lives on Earth."

ROB TILLING
VEGAN CYCLIST

United Kingdom
Vegan since: 1993

E: rob.tilling@phonecoop.coop

Rob Tilling has been vegan for over 20 years and will not be going back to animal exploitation. He is a determined environmentalist who avoids motor vehicle use and aeroplanes as well. Many aspects of Rob's life are geared towards a "green" result. He loves to cook quality, vegan, and whole food meals but still enjoys a bit of cake or chocolate from time to time.

WHY VEGAN?

How and why did you decide to become vegan?
I became aware of animal rights issues gradually as I grew up, and by the time I was a teenager I understood that I would become a vegetarian. It just seemed like an obvious thing to do. As a teenager, I came across veganism and only spent around a year as a vegetarian before giving up milk and eggs. I found milk consumption distasteful throughout childhood and I do not believe that I can digest it properly so the giving up of dairy was very easily achieved.

How long have you been vegan?
Over 20 years.

What has benefited you the most from being vegan?
My weight has become stable and I am no longer overweight. As a child, I was always carrying extra pounds.

What does veganism mean to you?
Veganism is now second nature to me. I have spent my adult life as a vegan and it makes up a large part of my identity. Veganism impacts upon many areas of life; social; political; work; lifestyle, etc and it cannot be unwoven easily from my life without questioning every part of my behaviour and motivation. It has become part of me and I generally do not even think of it, having been following a vegan lifestyle for such a long time.

TRAINING

What sort of training do you do?
I am a cyclist. I cycle around 1000miles (1609km) per month. More in the summer and a bit less in the winter. I cycle for utility, work and leisure as well as in organised rides and for "personal development."

How often do you (need to) train?
I will do at least one 50-80 mile (80-128km) ride every weekend, but this can easily be doubled in the summer. I will sometimes ride on an evening, after work, 3-4 times in the summer months and even on dark, cold winter nights I attempt at least one or two rides through the week.

Do you offer your fitness or training services to others?
No, I am willing to try and push beginner cyclists along where possible but they are not cycling at my level. I have taken new road cyclists out on occasion and introduced them to rides, which are a little longer than they are used to!

What sports do you play?
I have never considered myself to be a true sportsman. I cycle and attempt to run and climb at a very basic level. I enjoy walking, in particular up hills and fells - or even mountains.

STRENGTHS, WEAKNESSES & OUTSIDE INFLUENCES

What do you think is the biggest misconception about vegans and how do you address this?
Perhaps the notion that we are torturing ourselves by depriving ourselves of the joy of eating flesh and dairy. All I can do to address this is to look happy with the delightful meals I prepare for myself on a daily basis, come across as a lover of food and be knowledgeable about the very wide range of foods available to vegans.

What are your strengths as a vegan athlete?
Not having to feel the urge to stuff in "crap" when visiting cafes. I carry decent food and enjoy it whilst others fork in heaps of lard and cream.

What is your biggest challenge?
Cycling Lands End to John O'Groats (the length of Britain) - I haven't done this yet.

Are the non-vegans in your industry supportive or not?
Occasionally, but generally I feel that cyclists have a negative attitude to veganism.

Are your family and friends supportive of your vegan lifestyle?
Yes, they have had to get used to it. If they want to have me visit or visit me then vegan food needs to be on the menu.

What is the most common question/comment that people ask/say when they find out that you are a vegan and how do you respond?
Perhaps "Oh, that must be difficult" to which I reply that it isn't hard to prepare delicious vegan meals at home when my cupboards are over-flowing with quality vegan whole foods. I point out that vegans typically have a far greater culinary and dietary repertoire than most "conventional omnivores."

Who or what motivates you?
I am self-motivated. If I were the only vegan in the world, I'd still not start eating animal products. Die hard.

FOOD & SUPPLEMENTS

What do you eat for Breakfast?
Porridge with sultanas and banana, or muesli followed by toast and yeast extract. Some fruit usually too. Strong tea if I'm riding or chamomile tea otherwise. If I've ridden a lot the day before I usually eat some corn cakes with peanut butter and jam as well.

What do you eat for Lunch?
Mostly just fresh fruit - a lot of apples and oranges in particular and rarely bananas.

What do you eat for Dinner?
Curries and rice or chapatti, stews with dumplings, soups, roasts, pizza, sushi, pasta

dishes and plenty more. Usually I look to see which vegetables need eating up and add beans, pulses or tofu to it. I'll serve it with whatever starchy food goes best with it.

What do you eat for Snacks - healthy & not-so healthy?
A lot of dried figs and dates. I don't get much of a kick from eating junk food and almost never eat crisps or drink fizzy drinks. I have chocolate and biscuits from time to time. If it's cake then I'd like a fruit cake best of all - these "treats" are rare though.

What is your favourite source of Protein?
Chick peas or "braised" tofu - it comes in a tin.

What is your favourite source of Calcium?
Figs - by far.

What is your favourite source of Iron?
Beetroot and green leafy stuff.

What foods give you the most energy?
Dates.

Do you take any supplements?
Veg 1 from The Vegan Society UK - for B12 and vitamin D in Winter. It contains other nutrients too.

ADVICE

What is your top tip for gaining muscle?
Eat some protein every day and vary the source.

What is your top tip for losing weight?
Cut back on the big portions of starchy food.

What is your top tip for maintaining weight?
Exercise regularly. Eat organic whole foods. Do not eat junk foods including hydrogenated fats.

What is your top tip for improving metabolism?
Cycle regularly and quickly.

What is your top tip for toning up?
Cycle regularly.

How do you promote veganism in your daily life?
By being active and staying fit and healthy. By staying happy and continually challenging the misconceptions about veganism by getting on with life and not dwelling on the petty nature of some people who feel threatened by our lifestyle.

How would you suggest people get involved with what you do?
Get a decent (light) bike. Get some quality instruction on how to cycle safely. Ride whenever and wherever possible. Stop eating animal products and junk foods today.

"Veganism impacts upon many areas of life: social, political, work, lifestyle etc and it cannot be unwoven easily from my life without questioning every part of my behaviour and motivation."

RODOLFO PALMA
VEGAN SWIMMER & TRIATHLETE

Eugene, Oregon, USA
Vegan since: 1995

veganfitness.net
SM: FaceBook

Rodolfo was born in Chile, and was a child during the Pinochet dictatorship until he moved to upstate New York. It was as a youth in New York that he found a love for swimming, which he pursued throughout most of his life. One spring afternoon after his senior year of high school, Rodolfo went straight from eating meat to being 100% vegan. Rodolfo played water polo briefly for the University of Michigan, but took a hiatus from sports. After college Rodolfo found sports again. He soon joined Ann Arbor Masters and started competing again. In 2001 Rodolfo and his wife Melissa moved to Chile. There, Rodolfo swam for the Universidad de Chile swim team and missed Olympic cut by just a few seconds. Upon moving back to the USA, Rodolfo began coaching Ann Arbor Masters. He coached for nearly a decade. In 2008, Rodolfo tried his first triathlon, and he was hooked. In 2011, he tried his first purely open water swim and was also hooked. Now, Rodolfo competes regularly in swim meets, triathlons, open water races, and the occasional road running race.

WHY VEGAN?

How and why did you decide to become vegan?
I went vegan for Animal Rights reasons. This happened slightly on a whim. I was a meat-eater and had even dated a vegetarian but found it silly. A friend and I went to eat at a Middle Eastern restaurant and he suggested that we read the book, "Diet for a New America" by John Robbins. He said it was about veganism. I realized that inadvertently, my meal had already been vegan, so I decided to stick to veganism for the rest of the day as I read the book. I finished the book quickly, and had already been vegan for a few days without really noticing it being difficult. I just kept going, day by day as a vegan. That was in 1995.

How long have you been vegan?
I've been vegan for over 20 years, or just over half of my life.

What has benefited you the most from being vegan?
I am happiest living in step with my ethics. I can look at myself in the mirror - happy with my (food) choices daily.

What does veganism mean to you?
It means a simple step towards living ethically. I do not think that my going vegan will change the world, but it certainly allows me to feel good about who I am. Begin vegan is now a part of my identity.

TRAINING

What sort of training do you do?
I swim approximately 4 times a week (3000miles+/4828km+ per session), cycle about 3 times a week (10miles/16km per session), and run about twice a week (5miles/8km per session). Occasionally, I play soccer, water polo, weight lifting or other sports for cross training.

How often do you (need to) train?
When work and life allows, I train twice a day six days a week, with one day off for recovery. Unfortunately, that happens only once or twice a year. I need to train at least once a week.

Do you offer your fitness or training services to others?
I am a Masters swim coach, but my current full-time work has made my part-time work of coaching more marginal in my life. Now I do personal training for former clients and swimmers.

What sports do you play?
As a competitive swimmer, I swim the 200 Individual Medley (IM), 200 Breaststroke, 200 Butterfly, 100 Butterfly, 400 IM, 200 Freestyle and 100 Backstroke. I swim those events at least twice a year, but often in 5 meets a year. I also do open water swims, specifically a yearly 5km (3mile) Open Water Swimming (OWS). I also do approximately 5 sprint distance triathlons a year. Last, I do at least one foot-race per year, usually a 10k (6mile) run in the spring and a 5k run in the fall.

STRENGTHS, WEAKNESSES & OUTSIDE INFLUENCES

What do you think is the biggest misconception about vegans and how do you address this?
Folks don't perceive vegans as doing sports. I make sure that people know I'm vegan with my race kit, and in my conversations.

What are your strengths as a vegan athlete?
I find it easier to avoid the garbage diet that most athletes fall into because I'm already avoiding a lot of mass produced fitness foods.

What is your biggest challenge?
When I do find an easy vegan fitness food, like vegan sports bars, I tend to over-rely on them rather than on the vast amount of healthier whole foods out there.

Are the non-vegans in your industry supportive or not?
Mostly.

Are your family and friends supportive of your vegan lifestyle?
My wife and kids are supportive of our collective veganism, but my parents and in-laws and others are not particularly helpful. They do not interfere with my veganism, but they rarely help or know how to help.

What is the most common question/comment that people ask/say when they find out that you are a vegan and how do you respond?
The most common question is, "Where do you get your protein?" I respond that if you eat enough calories, it's impossible to not get enough protein. I show them my kids, and myself, as examples.

Who or what motivates you?
I am motivated because I love swimming and the feeling of racing.

FOOD & SUPPLEMENTS

What do you eat for Breakfast?
Tofurky sandwich with Veganaise, avocado, tomato, lettuce, and salt.

What do you eat for Lunch?
Salad with spinach, tofu, garbanzo beans, sprouts, lemon juice, salt, tomatoes, hearts of palm, and Artichokes. Prepared tofu "mock chicken" sandwich from local organic grocery store. Vegan ice cream sandwich.

What do you eat for Dinner?
Vegan pizza and a vegan donut.

What do you eat for Snacks - healthy & not-so healthy?
Vegan snack bar and/or 95% chocolate and organic peanut butter.

What is your favourite source of Protein?
Tofu and seitan.

What is your favourite source of Calcium?
Soymilk.

What is your favourite source of Iron?
Fortified grains and greens.

What foods give you the most energy?
All foods give me energy equally. However, high sugar foods like vegan ice cream tend to give me energy, but sap it afterwards. I tend to avoid high sugar, processed foods before races. I do eat fresh bananas and I find I like eating them before races.

Do you take any supplements?
Not regularly. Occasionally, I'll take an Emergen-C pack before I get a cold, or eat my kid's multi-vitamin when our kids have them.

ADVICE

What is your top tip for gaining muscle?
Lift high resistance weights, and eat plenty and often - especially high calorie-dense foods.

What is your top tip for losing weight?
Track your foods using a food log and track your calories. What you eat matters more to weight loss than exercise.

What is your top tip for maintaining weight?
Exercise often and adjust your food intake according to your changing metabolism.

What is your top tip for improving metabolism?
High-intensity interval training (HIIT) of any kind to increase metabolism, but most of all, gaining muscle mass. That means doing weight lifting somewhat regularly, but never cutting calories so much that your body starts to slow its metabolism.

What is your top tip for toning up?
Weight lifting is ideal for toning, while not over-eating.

How do you promote veganism in your daily life?
I wear my veganism on my sleeve. Everyone at work knows I'm vegan, and most of my competitors know I'm vegan. Having healthy vegan kids also helps. Doing well and living healthily are what I do now. However, in the past, what I did most was Animal Rights activism. I still prefer that, but I cannot do it often these days.

How would you suggest people get involved with what you do?
Support your local vegan athletes!

RUTH HEIDRICH
VEGAN TRIATHLETE

Honolulu, Hawaii, USA
Vegan since: 1982

ruthheidrich.com
SM: *FaceBook*

Ruth Heidrich is a six-time Ironman Triathlete and a lifelong runner who is named one of the Ten Fittest Women in North America. She is holder of a World Fitness Record at the famed Cooper Clinic, and has run over 67 marathons including Boston, New York, and Moscow. She co-hosts the Healing & You radio show, and is author a variety of books including "A Race for Life", "CHEF", and "Senior Fitness, Lifelong Running."

WHY VEGAN?

After a diagnosis of breast cancer, I enrolled in a clinical research study to determine the effect of a low-fat vegan diet on my cancer. She co-hosts the Healing & You radio show, and is author a variety of books including "A Race for Life", "CHEF", and "Senior Fitness, Lifelong Running."

How and why did you decide to become vegan?
After only a few days on the diet and seeing all the other advantages, I realized that this was the diet I should have been on all along.

How long have you been vegan?
It's now been over 30 years, since 1982.

What has benefited you the most from being vegan?
Where to begin? The vegan diet reversed my cancer, got my high cholesterol down to normal, reversed my arthritis and got me off the drug prescribed for that, got me un-constipated for the first time in my life, and gave me the strength and energy to do the Ironman Triathlon.

What does veganism mean to you?
It is much more than a diet. It's a philosophy of life that embodies abundant health for not just me but for the animals and the planet. It embraces compassion, awareness, sensitivity, and a joie de vivre.

TRAINING

What sort of training do you do?
Running, cycling, swimming, and weight-lifting. Having struggled to reach an Ironman fitness level, I decided I would never let training go.

How often do you (need to) train?
I train 2-3 hours daily with at least an hour on the bike and an hour running with alternating days of swimming and weights.

Do you offer your fitness or training services to others?
On my website, there is an "Ask Dr. Ruth" box where I answer questions people have on both nutrition and training.

What sports do you play?
Besides running, cycling, and swimming, I enjoy table tennis and hiking.

STRENGTHS, WEAKNESSES & OUTSIDE INFLUENCES

What do you think is the biggest misconception about vegans and how do you address this?
That vegans are weak, scrawny, and couldn't be very healthy from lack of protein. Addressing this is a challenge due to the pervasiveness of misinformation from advertising of products touting protein from animal products. I try to educate people through my four books: ""A Race for Life" - how I went from being a cancer patient to a six-time Ironman Triathlete; "CHEF" - my cooking and raw eBook covering all I think people need to know about nutrition; "Senior Fitness" - covers both the diet and exercise components leading to the top ten killers of people and how to reverse them; and "Lifelong Running" which demolishes myths that surround running and how it is suitable for most every person, anytime, anywhere.

What are your strengths as a vegan athlete?
Some people call me "disciplined" in my training but I call it "having fun."

What is your biggest challenge?
Aging! Although I can slow down some of the indicators of aging such as muscle and bone loss, I haven't yet figured out how to stop them completely.

Are the non-vegans in your industry supportive or not?
I think we're in such a minority that the answer has to be "no."

Are your family and friends supportive of your vegan lifestyle?
Although I generally get respect for having won over 1,000 gold medals in the years after going vegan, most of my family and friends don't seem to be able to see themselves doing this.

What is the most common question/comment that people ask/say when they find out that you are a vegan and how do you respond?
It is, "Where do you get your protein?" Even after all these years of trying to get the message out that ALL plants have protein, it's still the most common question I hear. Then, of course, the second-most common question, "Where do you get your calcium if you don't drink milk?" I tell them that leafy greens have abundant protein AND calcium!

Who or what motivates you?
A passion and a mission! I enjoy keeping on top of the latest research on nutrition and aging.

"The vegan diet reversed my cancer, got my high cholesterol down to normal, reversed my arthritis and got me off the drug prescribed for that, got me un-constipated for the first time in my life, and gave me the strength and energy to do the Ironman Triathlon."

FOOD & SUPPLEMENTS

What do you eat for Breakfast?
A large bed of leafy greens with mango and banana.

What do you eat for Lunch?
A carrot or two and an apple.

What do you eat for Dinner?
Another large bed of leafy greens with a tomato, bell pepper, broccoli, dressed with salsa, curry, and mustard.

What do you eat for Dessert?
A large bowl of blueberries, 9-10 dried plums, and a handful of walnuts. I also add about an inch of finely sliced fresh ginger to all my meals for a nice, tangy zing.

What is your favourite source of Protein, Calcium & Iron?
Leafy greens.

What foods give you the most energy?
All plant foods are high in carbohydrates, which are converted to glucose to glycogen - the fuel for our muscles. For the brain, glucose is the only fuel that passes through the blood-brain barrier.

Do you take any supplements?
Only B12.

ADVICE

What is your top tip for gaining muscle?
Find a sport you love and do it often, preferably daily.

What is your top tip for losing weight?
In my eBook, "CHEF", I suggest "a green fast" for rapid, healthy, short-term weight loss.

What is your top tip for maintaining weight?
In general, our appetites tell us how much we need to eat to match our caloric expenditure as long as we are eating a healthy, whole-food diet.

What is your top tip for improving metabolism?
Definitely exercise. Our bodies are meant to move - we die if we don't.

What is your top tip for toning up?
Again, exercise.

How do you promote veganism in your daily life?
By taking whatever opportunities arise to show how veganism helps solve whatever problem is under discussion whether it's our health, our treatment of our fellow Earth inhabitants (animals), or any of the environmental problems coming up in the news of the day.

How would you suggest people get involved with what you do?
First, get educated. The more knowledge we have in what we see as the problems, the better able we are to make a difference in people's lives. This includes areas such as the sky-rocketing rates of obesity, health-care (disease-care) costs threatening to bankrupt us, or the tendency for our medical system to turn to pharmaceuticals – "a pill for every ill" kind of mentality which now arguably is the third most frequently cited cause of death. With a little more help, we can do better!

SABINA SKALA
VEGAN STRENGTH & CONDITIONING COACH

London, England, UK
Vegan since: 2011

cjscombat.com
SM: *FaceBook, Twitter*

Sabina Skala hails from Poland, is a certified and highly experienced Strength and Conditioning Coach, and Sports Massage Therapist currently based in London, UK. She has trained under numerous world top coaches, has presented at national exhibitions and workshops in the United Kingdom and worldwide that explore the potential of strength training for athletic development.

As a former athlete herself - having competed in kayaking for five years - Sabina has a great understanding of the demands a professional sport places on a contestant. Working out of CJS Combat in London, Sabina's stable of clients includes athletes from various disciplines ranging from endurance sports like cycling to professional Mixed Martial Arts (MMA) athletes and other top combat sports professionals. She is one of the founders of Fighters Development Program, which supports talented upcoming fighters in their training and career development.

WHY VEGAN?

Initially it was not a conscious life time decision. It was a wager for fun, which was supposed to last one month, instead it completely changed my view on nutrition.

How and why did you decide to become vegan?
It was by accident. One of my clients is a strict vegan. I was born and bred Polish and grew up eating meat. One day we had a bet. He said I would not last a week on a strict vegan diet, I said make it a month. It was 4 years ago and I haven't looked back since.

How long have you been vegan?
Over 4 years.

What has benefited you the most from being vegan?
I am much more aware of what I eat, and have become much more creative with cooking. I had to spend some time researching and learning new recipes at the beginning, as I felt a bit lost and limited with what I could eat. After the first month, I had it all in place. My energy levels are great, my training is going very well and I haven't noticed any problems with strength and recovery etc.

What does veganism mean to you?
The reasons why I became vegan are mostly performance and health related. I guess what it means to me is to be conscious of how the quality and amount of food affects the athletic performance and health. It also transferred to the other parts of my life. I started seeking information about topics I was never interested in before like factory farming, GMO's, testing cosmetics on animals etc. I guess I am more aware about how important it is to keep healthy nutrition, and that unhealthy and stressed animals cannot provide us with healthy products whether it is meat, milk or eggs etc.

TRAINING

What sort of training do you do?

My training has changed during recent months. I used to do gymnastics training, however shoulder injury makes me unable me to continue. At the moment I strength train 4 times a week, dance once a week, run 4 times and swim once a week. At the moment, in my strength phase, the training will look like: I concentrate on deadlifts, back squats, weighted chin-ups, strict presses, power cleans etc. Supplemental work will include: 1 arm pushups, ab wheel roll outs, various mobility drills and rehab work.

How often do you (need to) train?

I train 6 days a week, mostly twice a day. The training intensity varies accordingly - after high intensity, heavy days, I will have a day of more recovery based activities, like mobility, easy runs, swims or dance technique.

Do you offer your fitness or training services to others?

I work with combat athletes e.g. Mixed Martial Arts (MMA) and Brazilian Jiu-jitsu (BJJ), I also have some endurance athletes in my books (triathletes and cyclist), plus regular private clients.

What sports do you play?

My sports background is kayaking, which I have retired from. For the last few years I have been preparing for fitness competitions, so the core of my training was gymnastics and strength work in the gym. However, shoulder injury doesn't allow me do continue with gymnastics or any ballistic work. At the moment, I am looking into doing Blenheim triathlon, which is going to change my training to more endurance based.

"I strongly believe people should have information of how food and other goods are produced, and make their own mind whether they want to support that industry and whether consuming animal products is actually healthy and good for them."

STRENGTHS, WEAKNESSES & OUTSIDE INFLUENCES

What are your strengths as a vegan athlete?

Recovery after training - since turning vegan my recovery is much better.

What is your biggest challenge?

I find the vegan diet pretty easy to follow when I am at home and able to cook for myself. The biggest challenge so far is finding restaurants that cater for vegans when I travel. It is surprisingly hard to find a place that serves good, clean vegan food.

Are the non-vegans in your industry supportive or not?

Everyone is very supportive. Some of my family and friends in Poland always try to tempt me with some grilled kielbasa (sausage) but I hope they are about give up with that soon.

Are your family and friends supportive of your vegan lifestyle?

Yes, other than making fun of me during BBQs etc, they keep asking for some vegan recipes and have included quite a few vegan dishes in their diets as well. Also, nearly all of my friends have either given up dairy or at least replaced cow's milk with coconut milk or coconut cream.

What is the most common question/comment that people ask/say when they find out that you are a vegan and how do you respond?

"What do you eat?" I say, "Loads of yummy food."

Who or what motivates you?

I am motivated by how I feel. I have never felt better and I love the way my nutrition looks like at the moment. I also look up to Mike Mahler a lot. He is by far the strongest man that I know who is on vegan diet. He is also a very supportive of animal rights, which I totally identify with.

FOOD & SUPPLEMENTS

What do you eat for Breakfast?

Smoothie with pea protein, cinnamon, ginger, nutmeg, coconut oil or nut butter, frozen blueberries, frozen spinach, juiced cucumber and celery, with water or coconut milk.

What do you eat for Lunch?

I don't have a meal for lunch. It would be just coffee with coconut milk, or I juice carrots, apple, beetroot and ginger and have it as a energy drink.

What do you eat for Dinner?

Examples would be a homemade veggie burger on a portobello mushroom (instead of a bun), with salad (lettuce, cucumber, avocado, tomatoes etc) or peas with homemade pesto.

What do you eat for Snacks - healthy & not-so healthy?

I don't really snack, but I made some really nice ice cream a couple of days ago for my guests.

What is your favorite source of Protein?

I use plant-based protein powders (pea, hemp or rice), also I add nuts and seeds to my meals.

What is your favorite source of Calcium?

Kale, either added to smoothies or to salads.

What is your favorite source of Iron?

Lentils, cooked spinach and dried prunes.

What foods give you the most energy?

I feel very energetic after drinking my smoothies or juices - fresh ginger seems to be doing the trick.

Do you take any supplements?

Yes, Exclzyme, Myomin, Vitamin C, pea or hemp protein powder, Mike Mahler's Magnesium oil.

"The reasons why I became vegan are mostly performance and health related. I guess what it means to me is to be conscious of how the quality and amount of food affects the athletic performance and health. It also transferred to the other parts of my life. I started seeking information about topics I was never interested in before like factory farming, GMO's, testing cosmetics on animals etc. I guess I am more aware about how important it is to keep healthy nutrition, and that unhealthy and stressed animals cannot provide us with healthy products whether it is meat, milk or eggs etc."

ADVICE

What is your top tip for gaining muscle?
This can be tricky and depends on the individual. Some athletes are genetically gifted to put on muscle mass quickly, for some it is a struggle. It will depend on the person, but it requires increasing calorie intake and specific hypertrophy and strength/hypertrophy targeted training, also minimum of 8 hours of sleep and minimum stress. Assuming you are a well-conditioned athlete, I would limit the long slow cardio (for me long and slow starts from 20 mins+) to minimum (1 session a week as a recovery ie easy swim or jog) and add short sprint intervals.

What is your top tip for losing weight?
Weight loss starts in the kitchen. 4 hours break between meals, limit the meals to 3 times a day, remember to portion control, and instead of counting calories, focus on eating fresh, local, organic produce. Eat loads of green leafy veggies. In the morning, just after waking up drink warm water with lemon and a pinch of cayenne pepper.

What is your top tip for maintaining weight?
It depends, if you have lost weight and want to maintain it, you have to watch how you react to certain foods. Consuming some refined carbohydrates can cause temporary water retention and weight gain, so just be aware how different foods affect you. For anyone who has gained weight and wants to maintain it - monitor the training and sleep, make sure you get enough calories a day. If eating a lot becomes problematic, try to get more calorie-dense foods in your diet eg. nuts, dried fruit, nut butter etc.

What is your top tip for improving metabolism?
Take a minimum of 4 hrs breaks between meals, if able add heavy weight training to your regimen and 1-2 session of sprinting (hill and chosen distance - I do 5 x 400m sprints once a week and 1 session of 10 lots of hill sprints)

How do you promote veganism in your daily life?
I just try to lead by example. In my line of work, health, physical performance and appearance are very important, and I hope so far I have been a good ambassador for vegan nutrition. I also post recipes, some informative videos related to vegan lifestyle, animal rights etc online. I get involved in different projects that promote vegan nutrition i.e books etc.

How would you suggest people get involved with what you do?
The most important thing is to be aware of how unhealthy food can be - and I am not only talking about meat and dairy (thought these are especially toxic), but also about non-organic fruit and vegetables. Also search for information about how animals are treated - in the meat and dairy industry, beauty and fashion. I believe that if all of us had the knowledge of what happens in fur factories, factory farms etc, we all would either refuse to support that industry or at least think twice before buying fur etc.

I strongly believe people should have information of how food and other goods are produced, and make their own mind whether they want to support that industry and whether consuming animal products is actually healthy and good for them. If people want to get involved, search for information and share it – it's the best way.

"Initially going vegan was not a conscious life time decision. It was a wager for fun, which was supposed to last one month, instead it completely changed my view on nutrition. One of my clients is a strict vegan. I was born and bred Polish and grew up eating meat. One day we had a bet. He said I would not last a week on a strict vegan diet, I said make it a month. It was 4 years ago and I haven't looked back since."

SAMUEL HARTMAN
VEGAN FITNESS FANATIC & ROAD CYCLIST

Midwest, USA
Vegan since: 2006

thenailthatsticksup.com
SM: *FaceBook, Instagram, Twitter*

Samuel Hartman is a vegan athlete, activist, and writer living in the midwest of the US. He has written for VegNews and other publications, always trying to take a positive look at ways in which we can better ourselves through eating and living. When he's not doing vegan outreach, Sam enjoys playing music, having lengthy philosophical discussions, and cooking delicious meals for his friends.

WHY VEGAN?

How and why did you decide to become vegan?
I became vegan after becoming interested in vegetarianism back in 2005. I had several vegetarian and vegan friends, who were never pushy, and at the same time, I was reading a lot about the health effects of red meat. I decided to try vegetarianism, more as a challenge than anything, and ended up sticking with it. I went vegan six months later, buying stuff like crazy to veganize my entire life (I now caution people not to move so quickly) and haven't looked back since.

How long have you been vegan?
Since January 1, 2006.

What has benefited you the most from being vegan?
Awareness, or "consciousness-raising" to borrow a phrase from Richard Dawkins. Of course, I discovered the horrors of factory farms, and the environmental toll of animal agriculture, but I never thought that I could be so passionate about a cause. I found that passion with veganism because of how easy it is to remove animal exploitation from our lives. I am proud to be living healthy and contributing to a more sustainable society, but overall I want to be known as a positive person and inspire others to act positively - be that veganism or any other cause.

What does veganism mean to you?
Veganism means the intention of eliminating the exploitation, or the use, of animals, worldwide, now, and forever. This is a never-ending goal, but one that with every meal and act we can move towards.

TRAINING

What sort of training do you do?
Around the time I went vegetarian I got really interested in running and quickly became addicted. As many runners know, it's easy to get caught up in your sport, the love of fitness, and not pay attention to your body. I did this, and succumbed to injury a

year or two later. During this time, I learned more about weightlifting for strengthening purposes and also cycling as a way to get cardio without the stress on the joints. In cycling, I found a new love: road racing, and raced at an amateur level for three years in Louisville, Kentucky. The fitness, camaraderie, and culture of the sport are unmatched; it's why the Tour de France is so glamorous and amazing.

How often do you (need to) train?
For road cycling, it's pretty much a year-round pursuit with only a couple months off in September and October. From November to February, you build your endurance, and then intensity starts to rise, peaking around June or July, which is the height of the road season in the U.S. This year I've decided to focus more on weights, running, and try some new sports (rock climbing!) so I have a much more flexible training schedule. I typically work out five to seven times a week.

Do you offer your fitness or training services to others?
I don't, but if anyone wants to come to my gym or go on a ride with me, they are welcome to! Unless you have a strict pace you need to follow (be it intervals or a weightlifting circuit), it's almost always more fun to have a friend to workout with. Some of my best rides and workouts have been my friends and I just goofing around, trying to see who could go faster or longer.

What sports do you play?
I enjoy running and road cycling a lot, but I've also done a fair amount of mountain biking and what could be considered power lifting. I also enjoy yoga and rock climbing.

STRENGTHS, WEAKNESSES & OUTSIDE INFLUENCES

What do you think is the biggest misconception about vegans and how do you address this?
I would assume the protein issue is still out there, but it's fading fast with more and more people becoming interested in vegetarianism and veganism. It is so ridiculously easy to get enough protein. If people think vegans are 'weak' they're typically just stating an insecurity they have about their cultural and habitual food choices: they're nothing intrinsic about animal foods that makes us strong, at least in the 21st century.

What are your strengths as a vegan athlete?
Even when I do eat "junk food" it's typically cleaner than what my omnivorous counterparts are having. The big plus I see is that by not eating meat and dairy I'm fueling myself for training and for a healthy lifestyle years down the road. If you're looking for protein in meat and eating lots of it, that's not a recipe for living to 100+. It doesn't correlate directly with veganism, but not drinking alcohol (I'm straight-edge) provides some benefits in the recovery and relaxation department.

What is your biggest challenge?
There have been times when I was skeptical of not taking in enough calories, but like any serious athlete, you have to make time for planning and cooking your meals. In the middle of the season I would typically eat 3,000-3,500 calories a day, but that wasn't difficult if I made each meal a solid one with veggies, protein, grains, and so forth.

Are the non-vegans in your industry supportive or not?
There aren't any vegan cyclists where I live, but there many online (veganfitness. net) and around the world. In general, cycling is a sport dominated by culture and habit - and that mostly comes from Europe where animal foods are widely eaten. That

being said, American teams like Garmin-Cervelo have changed up their teams' diets to include gluten-free stuff, and they have one of the sole vegan riders, Dave Zabriskie, on their team. I would say running or triathlons have it a little easier: there are quite a few vegans in those sports. Weightlifting has it the worst, of course, as it's dominated by protein-obsession, which means meat-obsession. However, veganbodybuilding.com is doing its best to counteract that!

Are your family and friends supportive of your vegan lifestyle?

Absolutely, and that's always been a pretty awesome part of it all. My Mom ended up going vegan a few years ago and others try their best to be veg after seeing how easy it is to eat and cook vegan meals. I try to exude positivity and compassion and show people that eating vegan makes you happy and positive. Not only because of all the health, environmental and ethical benefits, but because it allows you to see that change is possible. Most of my friends are pretty stoked on that aspect of me, and know that veganism extremely important to me.

What is the most common question/comment that people ask/say when they find out that you are a vegan and how do you respond?

It's often not a question, but something along the lines of: "Oh, that's cool...I could never do that" or "I don't eat much meat...but I could never give up my cheese." Most people are interested but intimidated, specifically with regard to dairy because of how addictive it is. I try to tell them I went through all that, that I used to love meat and dairy, and that I was able to overcome all that and feel awesome because of it. There is lot of talking points out there, and it really just depends on the person I'm speaking to. If they love dogs or cats, that's a great "in" right there.

Who or what motivates you?

Any time I'm doing activism with a group and someone comes up to us with an open mind, it's such a good feeling. It can take a long time to change your beliefs and your habits, but I've seen a lot of people do it, and that really drives me to continue being active. I've met so many people who were vegetarian or vegan and had no idea there were others out there who shared their beliefs. What motivates me is allowing my compassion to foster community in my city and spread across the world. If I can get people to realize that they are capable of profound change, then their actions will resonate with others, and the "love" will spread outwards.

FOOD & SUPPLEMENTS

What do you eat for Breakfast?

I used to be pretty obsessed with cereal for breakfast but I've tried to add in more protein, so lately it's been black beans, onions, spinach, and perhaps some "chicken-less" strips by any of the various brands. I also really enjoy a good tofu scramble with nutritional yeast.

What do you eat for Lunch?

My midday meals are so scattered that it's usually just a lot of snacking until dinner. I love kale salads or any bean dish; homemade hummus is awesome of course. One thing I will never grow tired of is Tofurky sausages; so high in protein and so versatile in cooking. I eat a lot of "soy meat" or "wheat meat" but it's the taste and texture I want, not some carry-over of killing from my meat-eating days.

What do you eat for Dinner?

Dinner is usually my biggest meal of the day and while this is backwards to a lot of dietary advice, it works for me. I include all the macronutrients, though the carbohydrate ratio changes depending on what kind of training is going on, and I use spices and sauces liberally. Stir-fries are my go to meal: a good protein source along with onions, broccoli, carrots, mushrooms, and some greens like Swiss chard. If I need carbohydrates, I'll go with brown rice or quinoa. There's a lot you can do with squash, which is in season right now in the Midwest – I love sweet potatoes and spaghetti squash. I try to eat local when I can, though a cold frozen plain makes that difficult here. In general, my food options are pretty diverse, but always vegan and always tasty.

What do you eat for Snacks - healthy & not-so healthy?

Carrots and hummus are the ultimate healthy snack, I think. Nuts and seeds are great, and I usually rotate some sort of nut butter depending on my mood: peanut, almond, cashew. I really love the vegetarian jerky products, though those with the other soy meats can put you in the soy-overload category. When the U.S. finally gets its act together and starts making a lot of hemp products I think that will be my go-to food - hemp is so healthy and nutrient dense it's definitely worth eating a lot of.

As for "vegan junk food," I have no bounds, I love it all! Right now, I make Sundays my "cheat day" in which I eat anything and everything from vegan candy bars (Go Max Go!) to coconut ice cream and Tofutti Cuties. Anything by Sweet and Sarah or Liz Lovely is incredible and of course, I make my own brownies, cakes, cookies, etc. I cannot get enough of this stuff, which is why, for the moment; I restrict it to one day. The practicalities of a diet like this are mixed and I'd be happy to have a discussion with anyone about it. However, for me, it works.

What is your favourite source of Protein?

I think the best source is beans, at least the most natural. I love black beans and garbanzo beans like no other. The tastiest source is those Tofurky sausages – 27g of protein per sausage!

What is your favourite source of Calcium?

Calcium often appears in fortified soymilk or tofu now, but it's also in the leafy greens and nuts I eat. I've had some nasty spills on the bike and zero broken bones, so I think they're strong and healthy with the amount of calcium I take in on a normal vegan diet.

What is your favourite source of Iron?

I use a cast-iron pan for just about every stir-fry, mostly because of how easy it is to re-use and clean, but this does impart small amounts of iron into every meal. However, I get iron through nuts, soy products, beans, and some fortified stuff like cereal, too. My iron count at the blood bank has always been spot on.

What foods give you the most energy?

To really perform well I've found the best thing I can do is to eat a high-carbohydrate meal the night before. As far as direct food to energy connections, there are too many variables to really say. Mental preparation plays a huge part for sport, and if that gets messed up, it doesn't matter how much energy, caffeine, sugar, or glucose you have in you. During races and around events I prefer easy sources of food like Clif bars or gels.

Do you take any supplements?

Over the years, I've tried all kinds of stuff, but two I really like are a solid multivitamin (Now brand, for instance) and a good probiotic for digestion and gas. Vegans eat a lot of gassy stuff and the probiotic, in my opinion, really helps with any stomach issues. For sport performance, I've tried everything from green tea to maca to CLA. Who knows if it works – the diet is the most critical component at the end of the day.

ADVICE

What is your top tip for gaining muscle?
Lift heavy, rest a lot, and lift again. Seriously, don't spend two hours in the gym with 50 different lifts. Squats, deadlifts, and bench presses are (almost) all you need.

What is your top tip for losing weight?
Cut the carbs. I know, I know, but I've seen it work for me and so many others. Excess carbohydrates get turned into fat, which - unless you are training 15 hours (or so) a week, and mostly cardio - will just stay there. A "slow carb" diet of protein and veggies for six days and chaos on the seventh has worked for me.

What is your top tip for maintaining weight?
This one's easy. Eat when you're hungry, and exercise a few times a week to keep your body active. If you eat the right foods you'll live quite a long time.

What is your top tip for improving metabolism?
Supposedly garlic, green tea, and a host of other supplements help with this, and you are welcome to try them, but I would recommend adding some weight routines into your work-out if you haven't already done so. Most people focus on cardio so much; but everything will improve if you do some lifting. If you run for an hour, make it 45 minutes and do 15 minutes of work with free weights or a bar (squats, bench press) etc. Bigger muscles = more calories burnt, and your sport will improve because of it. Eat some protein in the morning, for breakfast, and don't sit down all day. I've tried to convert a lot of my workspaces into standing desks for this very reason. It seems weird at first, but now I love it. Oh, and caffeine. Who can argue with a cup of coffee in the morning? Some, I'm sure. However, I love it, and there are health benefits too.

What is your top tip for toning up?
Again, this is a carbohydrates thing; all of us have a 'six pack' buried under there somewhere, but burning calories only does so much. Especially for men, our fat likes to sit around our midsection, and I believe the best way to get at that is to stop fueling it with excess carbohydrates. Strength training will help, but up the protein and fat (with good stuff like olive oil!) and lower the carbs for a better effect.

(Note: this should not be considered professional dietary advice - I'm just a vegan dude with my own experiences.)

How do you promote veganism in your daily life?
Every time I eat a vegan meal, or question the societal norm of animal exploitation I promote veganism. The number one thing that I, or anyone can do, is live a good life. Strive to be positive, re-think negative actions, and act with compassion, not anger or violence. If people see vegans living well, then they will be interested in that, and seek out information.

How would you suggest people get involved with what you do?
Find a local vegan or vegetarian advocacy group in your area, and if there isn't one, start it! There are compassionate people everywhere, and the Internet is of course a huge resource for this. Again, just living by example we can affect change, so don't be afraid to live the way you want, and when people ask questions, tell them honestly why you're doing what you do. If you hear about injustice to animals, speak up, but with kindness, not anger. Most people are simply unaware of the horrors that animals go through daily, whether for food, clothing, or entertainment. If we make them aware and offer alternatives, without forcing it, those with an open mind will seek to change.

SANDRA LAWSON
VEGAN WEIGHT LIFTER

Atlanta, Georgia, USA
Vegan since: 2009

sandralawson.org
SM: *Twitter*

Sandra Lawson is a Rabbinical student, a sociologist, a weight lifter, bike commuter, a new lover of trail running, and a vegan. She is passionate about fitness and Judaism and calls them the two loves of her life. She is the first African-American student accepted at the Reconstructionist Rabbinical College Rabbinical Program, and the first black queer student accepted at any rabbinical school. She really wants to make the world a better place and make the world a better place for Jews of color, queer Jews and all Jews.

WHY VEGAN?

How and why did you decide to become vegan?
So first of all, I am 45 years old and I started lifting weights when I was 18, and have been lifting consistently since I was 21. In my 20s I became a power-lifter, and was able to pack on a ton of muscle and gain a lot of strength - often out-lifting a lot of men that I knew.

In my mid-20s, I became a vegetarian and a Personal Trainer, and in my 30s, some friends persuaded me to enter my first bodybuilding competition. None of us knew anything about being a vegetarian and competing as bodybuilders. There was some information out there but not a lot, and all of my friends and fellow bodybuilders were all omnivores and so I acquiesced and started eating fish. I cannot even begin to tell you how much fish (mostly Tuna) and how many egg whites I ate for that first competition.

Well, needless to say I got very bored with that diet and could not eat it any more of it. As my love of the sport of bodybuilding grew, so did my meat consumption and I threw out my vegetarian diet completely. I stopped bodybuilding to go to graduate school but continued to lift and eat meat. I continued my weightlifting regimen and working as a personal trainer and over the course of a few years my healthy diet deteriorated and I gained 40 pounds (18kg). I knew I needed a change and I felt like crap. I wanted to go back to being a vegetarian but for some reason I didn't.

Then one day in February 2009, I saw Rip Esselstyn on "The Today Show" and that changed my life. On the show, Esselstyn talked about being vegan and eating a strong plant-based diet and offered a 28-day challenge to try the vegan diet. I didn't have any serious plans to be a vegan, I just wanted to follow his plan for 30 days and get back on track to at least be vegetarian. From February to May or June, I dropped 30 pounds (13kg) and eventually lost over 50 pounds (22kg) and I became a committed vegan. Although I became a vegan for vanity reasons, and health, I have since stayed a vegan for ethical, environmental and religious reasons.

How long have you been vegan?
Over 6 years.

What has benefited you the most from being vegan?
My health, my energy, and I also feel more compassionate.

What does veganism mean to you?
Veganism is my life.

TRAINING

What sort of training do you do?
I lift weights, cycle and run on trails.

How often do you (need to) train?
I lift weights about 4 to 5 times a week, and run on the trails several times a week.
Cycling is more like bike commuting.

Do you offer your fitness or training services to others?
Yes.

What sports do you play?
Not currently playing any sports.

STRENGTHS, WEAKNESSES & OUTSIDE INFLUENCES

What do you think is the biggest misconception about vegans and how do you address this?
I think the biggest misconceptions are that vegans are weak and we don't get enough protein. I try to educate people about how muscle is created and that all food contains protein, and by eating a variety of food loaded with nutrients, I am getting what my body needs - including enough protein.

What are your strengths as a vegan athlete?
My strength is my strength. I am proving that one does not need to eat animals or animal by-products to be strong and athletic.

What is your biggest challenge?
Can't think of one.

Are the non-vegans in your industry supportive or not?
Yes.

Are your family and friends supportive of your vegan lifestyle?
Yes.

What is the most common question/comment that people ask/say when they find out that you are a vegan and how do you respond?
The biggest question I get is, "How do you get your protein?" My answer depends on how the person asked the question. If they are sincere, I will be sincere in my answer.

Who or what motivates you?
Me.

FOOD & SUPPLEMENTS

What do you eat for Breakfast?
Fruit.

What do you eat for Lunch?
Mostly fruit but maybe a salad.

What do you eat for Dinner?
Mostly salad or it could be something else.

What do you eat for Snacks - healthy & not-so healthy?
Love vegan pizza.

What is your favourite source of Protein, Calcium & Iron?
Spinach, kale, broccoli and beans.

What foods give you the most energy?
Dates and bananas.

Do you take any supplements?
Nope.

"One day in 2009, I saw Rip Esselstyn on "The Today Show" and that changed my life. On the show, Esselstyn talked about being vegan and eating a strong plant-based diet and offered a 28-day challenge to try the vegan diet. I didn't have any serious plans to be a vegan, I just wanted to follow his plan for 30 days and get back on track to at least be vegetarian. From February to May or June, I dropped 30 pounds and eventually lost over 50 pounds and I became a committed vegan. Although I became a vegan for vanity reasons, and health, I have since stayed a vegan for ethical, environmental and religious reasons."

ADVICE

What is your top tip for gaining muscle?
Lift weights.

What is your top tip for Losing weight & Maintaining weight?
Eat plants - lots of them - and exercise.

What is your top tip for improving metabolism?
Eat plants and exercise.

What is your top tip for toning up?
Exercise.

How do you promote veganism in your daily life?
Not sure if I am promoting veganism. People who know me, they know that I am a vegan. I think I provide a good example of how to be fit and without eating animals.

How would you suggest people get involved with what you do?
They can contact me through my website, or on Twitter.

SCOTT SPITZ
VEGAN MARATHON RUNNER

Indianapolis, Indiana, USA
Vegan since: 1992

runvegan.wordpress.com
whitepinedistancetraining.com
SM: *FaceBook, Instagram*

Up until 2013, Scott Spitz was a long distance competitive runner. His marathon personal record is 2:25:55, and he was chasing a US Olympic Marathon Trials qualifier (2:19), when he was suddenly sidelined by a rare form of stomach cancer (PMP). He underwent intensive surgery, was kept alive by machines for days, before spending months recovering. Scott slowly built back up to running and cycling during his chemo regimen then underwent the same surgery in August 2014. He hopes to be training again without the effects of chemotherapy, and chasing down a marathon PR. He's been a ethical vegan for over 20 years.

WHY VEGAN?

How and why did you decide to become vegan?
I was involved in a musical subculture (straight-edge) where drug-free living, veganism and care for the earth were foundational ethical principles, so being exposed to those issues through pamphlets, books and music, I made the decision that eating animals was unnecessarily cruel. When I made the visceral connection between what was on my plate and how it got there, I simply stopped eating it without ever looking back.

How long have you been vegan?
Over 20 years.

What has benefited you the most from being vegan?
Initially it was the satisfaction that I was not involved in the cruel confinement and production of animals for food. Knowing that I had successfully removed myself from that process gave me a sense of calm and compassion that I carry to this day. Beyond that, paying attention to food and what I put into my body has expanded my knowledge of food choices and experiences, enriching my life more than I could have imagined.

What does veganism mean to you?
Above all else, it is my attempt to change the world for the better - by doing a small part to let animals (human and non-human) live their existence free from confinement and undue suffering.

"I'm always inspired by the reality of the lives of animals, the unimaginable suffering they experience at the hands of our drive for convenience and disassociated lifestyles. The use of animals is beyond cruel, it's sadistic, and that knowledge always keeps me focused, motivated and driven."

TRAINING

What sort of training do you do?

Now that I've been off chemotherapy since my last surgery, I've been able to run with only minimal side effects and overall damage from surgery. I'm currently fluctuating between 80 and 90 miles (128-144km) a week of running, consisting of 2 high-intensity workouts and a long run. I'm training myself to run a benefit ultra-run, and so my long runs are creeping up towards 30 miles (48km). I include various body weight exercises and light yoga to supplement my run specific training.

How often do you (need to) train?

I run every day of the week, only taking breaks if my body sends me distinct warning signs or life obstacles make it a necessity. I could get away with running less, but I enjoy the daily effort and routine. I'm still pushing towards a half-marathon race goal, along with preparing myself to complete my benefit ultra-run, which will push my body and mind to a place I've never been previously.

Do you offer your fitness or training services to others?

I have been coaching runners for the past year at White Pine Distance Training.

What sports do you play?

Running is my passion, but I also really enjoy bike commuting and hiking in the woods when the opportunity is available.

"The best part about running is all you need is the ability to put one foot in front of the other. Do that over and over again, and suddenly you're a runner! Do it to your abilities, your motivations and your needs – and that's it.

It's not too different with veganism. Just put your fork somewhere else on your plate, that isn't into an animal products or by-products, and you will already be on your way to a new life and new perspective – and the non-human animals will benefit as well!"

STRENGTHS, WEAKNESSES & OUTSIDE INFLUENCES

What do you think is the biggest misconception about vegans and how do you address this?

At one point, I would say it was that we are inherently weak due to our non-protein based diets, but I think the mass of vegan athletes in all sports has pretty much killed that idea. Now, it seems there is a perception of vegans as hyper-pacifists who are drawn to new-age ideas and extreme fringe cultures. Although stereotypes exist for a reason (because there is some truth to them), I'm certainly not of that category of vegan, and I combat this by spreading specific messages that aren't necessarily related to veganism. I promote science, reject new-age ideas, and let it be known that I'm not a tree-hugging hippy when the opportunities arise.

Veganism, in no way, has to be associated with an identity. It's simply about doing what is necessary to not bring harm onto animals. One can own a gun, be a CEO, and reject new-age religion while still doing so.

What are your strengths as a vegan athlete?

My strengths would be my ability to run through the voice in my head that tells me to take a break, ease up, and slow down. I have a drive to get better and better and I constantly find ways to push myself as the efforts get harder and harder. Sometimes that involves a number of motivations, whether that is inspiring others, seeking my goals, or keeping in mind the plight of animals.

What is your biggest challenge?
Right now, it's getting past cancer and getting back to my life of consistent training. Before cancer, it was managing my daily life responsibilities, but still getting in all the training and doing all the tiny things that would push me closer and closer to my goals.

Are the non-vegans in your industry supportive or not?
They are really. To be honest, it's hard to discredit my dietary choices when I'm succeeding as an athlete. If I was getting worse and worse as a runner, then maybe people could point to my diet and say, "See, it's not working." But, that was never the case. I was continuing to win races throughout my running career, and even now, I'm thriving through this cancer experience and shocking the doctors with my recovery and abilities, so it's still hard for anyone to not support my decisions. The proof is in the vegan pudding, right?

Are your family and friends supportive of your vegan lifestyle?
Families are always more difficult to persuade, but they are very supportive. My parents have come to adopt some of my dietary choices in small ways and my Mom enjoys making vegan options for me. As far as friends go, I surround myself with people I admire and appreciate, so I have a lot of vegan friends or people who aren't so judgmental about non-normative lifestyles, so yes, they are quite supportive as well.

What is the most common question/comment that people ask/say when they find out that you are a vegan and how do you respond?
Usually it's, "How long have you been vegan?" They are always quite surprised when I give them the number of years and they usually don't ask much more. Because I "fly the flag", so to speak, I get a lot of specific questions about nutrition (for themselves, not me) and I do my best to give them reliable answers and ways to incorporate veganism into their lives.

Who or what motivates you?
My community of friends - those I've met and those I haven't - who are in my feedback loop of effort, compassion and inspiration. We promote our lives, our politics and our physical efforts to let each other know that we aren't alone, that we can always do more and that our lives are better for it in the end.

Fundamentally, I'm always inspired by the reality of the lives of animals, the unimaginable suffering they experience at the hands of our drive for convenience and disassociated lifestyles. The use of animals is beyond cruel, it's sadistic, and that knowledge always keeps me focused, motivated and driven.

FOOD & SUPPLEMENTS

What do you eat for Breakfast?
More than anything, oatmeal that I create with oats, bananas, raisins, cocoa, cinnamon, ginger, almonds, flaxseeds and any number of other ingredients I have at the time.

What do you eat for Lunch?
Depending on my needs - how much I've been running, how hungry I am, etc. - it could be a more substantial snack of sorts, a kale salad, or something similar. Sometimes I "graze" a lot, so lunch isn't a big, solid meal for me.

What do you eat for Dinner?
Among many things I create, stir-fry is my go-to. It's quick, easy and nutritious. I'll use

frozen stir-fry veggies, nutritional yeast, almonds, ginger, turmeric, etc. and then add either rice or couscous as a base.

What do you eat for Snacks - healthy & not-so healthy?
Not-so healthy are the cookies I enjoy making - oatmeal or coffee chocolate chip. The healthy snacks might be smoothies, energy bars or kale salad, and plenty of fruit - oh, and peanut butter on a spoon. I'm known to dip into peanut butter all the time.

What is your favourite source of Protein?
Definitely peanut butter (or any nut butters). I don't eat many fake meats often, especially with current digestive issues. I do enjoy tofu and tempeh, but get protein through nut butters, grains and beans primarily.

What is your favourite source of Calcium?
I put a lot of spinach and kale in my foods, so I get a decent amount there, but also through fortified foods such as soy milk, tofu, etc.

What is your favourite source of Iron?
Again, a lot of green leafy veggies, beans, etc.

What foods give you the most energy?
I've never been able to pinpoint anything that gives me a significant boost of energy, aside from coffee. I eat primarily whole foods and often have a lot of energy, so I attribute everything to my diverse diet as a whole. All the veggies and beans and nuts and fruits and grains are constantly supplying me with necessary energy.

Do you take any supplements?
I do. I take B-12 once or twice a week, but that's it. On the other hand, most of our foods are fortified and, to me, that is no different than supplementation, just in different amounts.

"Although stereotypes exist for a reason (because there is some truth to them), I'm certainly not of that category of a hyper-pacifist vegan. I spread specific messages that aren't necessarily related to veganism. I promote science, reject new-age ideas, and let it be known that I'm not a tree-hugging hippy when the opportunities arise.

Veganism, in no way, has to be associated with an identity. It's simply about doing what is necessary to not bring harm onto animals. One can own a gun, be a CEO, and reject new-age religion while still doing so."

ADVICE

What is your top tip for gaining muscle?
I wouldn't be much help in this category. I'm always focusing on endurance and speed rather than muscle building. For me, the muscle building comes with repetition in running and the inherent body weight strain put on all my necessary muscles. The only specific attempts I've made for muscle building have been through injury, when I needed to start a body resistance routine to correct muscular imbalances in my legs and when I engaged in core workouts to help that part of my body.

What is your top tip for losing weight?
I've been able to keep a consistent weight through my general activity, but also

through eating a primarily whole foods diet. I've found that I can eat a lot of food, but the calorie counts aren't excessive due to a lack of additions of sugars, fats and other unnecessary ingredients. Paying attention to eating good foods will go much further in weight loss than going to the gym every day.

What is your top tip for maintaining weight?

Physical activity isn't the best for losing weight when you have already adjusted your diet in both portions and calories, but it can certainly help in maintaining weight. It helps burn those added calories you may intake from time to time without knowing it. I personally don't calorie count, never have, but don't worry about it because I know whatever calorie surplus I have in a day or two will be equalized with physical activity in my life.

What is your top tip for improving metabolism?

I don't have a professional knowledge to be able to answer this question properly. I'll leave that one up to the experts.

What is your top tip for toning up?

Toning for runners is just about running consistently. The more you run, the more unnecessary weight will be shed and your "tone" will show through. It's that simple.

How do you promote veganism in your daily life?

By living vegan first and foremost, but also by sharing stories, thoughts and articles I think are effective in persuading others. I won't flood people with veganism, but rather consider what people will be receptive to the most and push that, but always keeping an ethical perspective on everything. To me, ethical veganism is the most important and long lasting of all the motivations to adopt the vegan lifestyle. I also push it through my blog by making it front and center in everything I display on the page. Beyond all that, I continue to try and perform at a high level, despite my current obstacles, and just be a person that others enjoy and respect.

How would you suggest people get involved with what you do?

The best part about running is all you need is the ability to put one foot in front of the other. Do that over and over again, and suddenly you're a runner! Do it to your abilities, your motivations and your needs - and that's it.

It's not too different with veganism. Just put your fork somewhere else on your plate, that isn't into an animal products or by-products, and you will already be on your way to a new life and new perspective - and the non-human animals will benefit as well!

Don't Get Sidetracked By Those Not on the Same Path as You

Seba Johnson
VEGAN OLYMPIC SKI RACER

West Coast, USA
Vegan since: 1973

sebajohnson.com
SM: *FaceBook, Twitter*

Seba Johnson was born in the United States Virgin Islands. Her mother is a native of New Hampshire, and her father is a native of Burundi, Africa. At the age of 5, Seba was standing on a ski slope in St. Moritz, Switzerland, and instantly became in awe of the graceful skiers gliding down the slopes, and 9 years later, she was at the start gate of the Winter Olympic Games, as the Youngest Alpine Ski Racer in Olympic History at age 14. Seba is now a member of the Screen Actors Guild pursuing a career in acting and Public Speaking as she writes her book. As an ethical vegan since birth, her commitment to speaking up for animals and to never wear, eat, nor use animal products paved the way for the compassion she has for all living beings.

WHY VEGAN?

How and why did you decide to become vegan?
I was raised vegan since birth. My mother became vegan in her early 20's and promised herself to raise her kids vegan if she were to ever have children. I remember watching undercover investigation videos and reading the pamphlets that were mailed to the house when we were kids - I felt deeply for the animals at an early age. I remember how the other parents of my childhood friends would either get upset or interested when their kids would come home after sleepovers at my house - I felt it was my duty to show my friends what was happening to animals.

How long have you been vegan?
I was born a vegan and have been for my entire life – over 4 decades.

What has benefited you the most from being vegan?
The benefit for me is the knowledge that I am saving so many lives and not taking one to sustain my own. I am living proof that it can be done. Children can successfully be fed plant-based foods and grow into healthy strong vegan adults! And maybe it's my father's Tutsi Burundi, African genes, but I like to attribute the fact that I look younger than my actual age because of my organic vegan lifestyle.

What does veganism mean to you?
Veganism is the ultimate form of compassion. As I've quoted at the 2013 Animal Rights Conference (where I received the first ever Outstanding Vegan Athlete Award) "I believe that we will express sincere respect towards each person's gender, ethnicity, ability or disability, and will survive only when we turn to a vegan lifestyle - the human evolution of compassion that starts in the heart, not the stomach." I never considered my being vegan was for health reasons - it was always for the love and respect I had for animals. And because of that love and respect I have for non-human animals, my compassion flows over to all living beings, of all types.

TRAINING

What sort of training (did) you do?

During my Olympic training, I was blessed with a complimentary membership to a gym overlooking Lake Tahoe in Sierra Nevada while I was in High School. It was either the gorgeous view or my love for skiing that encouraged me to weight train every day after school. On weekends, I would ski eight hours a day and then back to the gym I would go. During the week, I also worked out with my high school ski team - lifting weights and stretching - then taking the ski lift chair to the mountaintop where I would train Slalom and Giant Slalom. The main muscle groups I worked were: legs, stomach, back, and arms – all of which were important for staying strong on courses with speeds up to 90 miles an hour.

In between ski seasons, I would do dry-land training and ski training on glaciers during summer ski camps in Mount Hood, Oregon; Portillo in Chile, or Hintertux in Austria with the best international ski coaches.

How often do you (need to) train?

I trained all year round. Four years after I became the youngest Alpine Ski Racer in Olympic History in 1988, I qualified for the 1992 Winter Olympic Games in Albertville, France, competing in the Giant Slalom and Slalom ski events. As an animal rights advocate I protested the following Winter Olympic Games in 1994 held in Lillehammer, Norway and decided not to participate due to the fact that Norway lifted their moratorium and resumed their practice of commercial hunting for minke whale.

Do you offer your fitness or training services to others?

Before I moved to LA almost 5 years ago, I taught inner city youth from Boston how to ski. For most of the kids, it was their first time out of the city. Once I find a vegan venue and money to afford it I would love to get my Yoga Teacher Certification so I can continue to help people.

What sports do you play?

Since I retired from ski racing, I used to ski every year just for fun, until 2008 when I broke my pelvis in 3 places and had to learn how to walk again. I skied for the first time since in 2012, to commemorate the accident that almost took my life four years prior. These days I enjoy Yoga at least 3 times a week (though I shoot for more), Zumba, spinning classes, or an hour of cardio with 400 crunches and weights. I also love swimming and hiking.

STRENGTHS, WEAKNESSES & OUTSIDE INFLUENCES

What do you think is the biggest misconception about vegans and how do you address this?

The misconception is that we are deficient in necessary nutrients. I explain that every nutrient my body has ever needed can be found in a plant source.

What are your strengths as a vegan athlete?

As an athlete: I honestly don't think I reached my highest potential, I was 10 years younger than the winners of the ski races I was competing in. So perhaps my strength as a vegan athlete was the fact that I made history twice; as the youngest ever and the first black female in Olympic alpine ski racing history. I retired before my prime due to the racism I found difficult to endure.

As a vegan: We do not become clogged with dairy products or bogged down by heavy meat and dead foods. We strive to have healthy bodies and minds, and not make ourselves walking graveyards for dead animals and their products.

What is your biggest challenge?

As an athlete, my biggest challenge was finding sponsors who would support my ethical vegan needs. Thankfully, I was able to have a great relationship with my clothing sponsor who graciously accommodated my every need of having ski suits and apparel that did not contain wool, leather, fur, silk, nor down. I was once disqualified from a World Cup ski race because I refused to wear a ski suit (of another clothing company) that had a patch of leather sewn into it - they would not understand that for moral and ethical reasons I just couldn't wear it.

Are the non-vegans in your industry supportive or not?

In the sport of ski racing, it wasn't necessarily that the non-vegans weren't supportive, it was the people who opposed seeing a black person in what they called "a white man's sport." At the tender age of 14, my experience was a startling eye opening to the various forms of jealousy and the reality of prejudice that exists in the world. But what I chose to embrace for the years that I competed as a two time Olympian, was the support and words of encouragement I received from various celebrities and devoted fans here in the USA and overseas. Children would write to me from grade schools asking what my favorite color was, and it was these experiences that led me to take tours of elementary and high schools between the ski seasons. I gave inspirational talks, based on my experiences, for those who wanted to attain their own special dream that seemed impossible.

Are your family and friends supportive of your vegan lifestyle?

My mother, yes naturally, since it was her idea to raise me vegan. But it was certainly hard going to family holiday dinner parties at my Grandmother's house with all of my uncles, aunts, and cousins - most of whom would chastise my mother for raising her kids vegan, in front of my sister and I. Even though my mother would bring vegan dishes to share, eventually we were no longer invited. We have never been quiet about our stance on preventing the suffering of animals and even though we didn't realize it then, we were planting the seeds of change in their minds.

What is the most common question/comment that people ask/say when they find out that you are a vegan and how do you respond?

The first question is always, "How long have you been vegan?" and I respond, "Since birth." Then there is always a confused look of shock and disbelief!

Who or what motivates you?

I am encouraged by compassionate souls and the love I see in the eyes of those I've committed my life to stand up for.

"I was raised vegan since birth. My mother became vegan in her early 20's and promised herself to raise her kids vegan if she were to ever have children. I remember watching undercover investigation videos and reading the pamphlets that were mailed to the house when we were kids – I felt deeply for the animals at an early age."

FOOD & SUPPLEMENTS

What did you eat when competing?

At the Olympic village the chefs were very understanding and did their best to provide a non-dairy, strict vegetarian diet for me. I insisted on berries, which became abundantly available when other Olympians saw me flourishing off them. Organic soy products gave me energy and I avoided anything with honey. Pure maple syrup and raw organic almond slivers on oatmeal found my Olympic morning meals satisfying and energetic.

What is your favourite source of Protein?

Almonds, quinoa, and tempeh.

What is your favourite source of Calcium?

Kale - I love kale.

What is your favourite source of Iron?

Lentils and spinach.

What foods give you the most energy?

Raw dishes for certain - and anything with kale. Freshly juiced ALL greens, or organic carrot, beets, parsley, and ginger root juices. Organic kale, frozen blueberries, frozen banana, maca powder, ginger root, cacao powder, cinnamon, and almond milk smoothies.

Do you take any supplements?

When I feel my body craves it I buy vegan formula B12 and vegan calcium tablets derived from sea kelp.

ADVICE

What is your top tip for losing weight?

Trying to figure out this one ever since my accident in 2008...

What is your top tip for maintaining weight?

If there is a vegan supplement or protein shake company that would like to sponsor me in my weight loss endeavor, please let me know!

What is your top tip for improving metabolism?

Green tea has helped me in the past.

How do you promote veganism in your daily life?

Via social networking and in every opportunity where someone is willing to listen. I visit schools and youth camps to speak about veganism and respecting animals, as well as speaking at various veg festivals and animal rights conferences. Via any national or international radio, television, magazine, or newspaper interview I would be sure to make mention of my ethical vegan upbringing and the myriad of benefits living vegan has - by simply eating compassionately and not contributing to the suffering of animals.

How would you suggest people get involved with what you do?

There's so much a person can do to help animals. Volunteer at any of the animal rights organizations, your local animal shelters, and speak up if you see an animal being harmed. Or simply GO VEGAN today - don't wait. Your life and countless others will be better off for it. I am available for speaking engagements, public appearances, mentoring and acting projects. Please contact me via my website.

SEBASTIAN GRUBB
VEGAN DANCER & CHOREOGRAPHER

San Francisco, California, USA
Vegan since: 2003

sebastiangrubb.com
SM: *FaceBook, Twitter*

Sebastian Grubb is a certified Personal Fitness Trainer and certified Health Coach, emphasizing "whole moves and whole foods" as the basis for a healthy life. Based in San Francisco, he runs Sebastian's Functional Fitness, where his clients use simple equipment and their own body weight to increase strength, endurance, and agility in every session. A vegan since 2003 and trainer since 2006, Sebastian was crowned the 2014 Champion of the "Battle of the Best Trainers" in San Francisco. He is also a professional contemporary dancer and choreographer, touring nationally and internationally.

WHY VEGAN?

How and why did you decide to become vegan?
I'm a logic-based person, so when I finally heard the full argument for veganism from the perspectives of environmental impact, disease prevention, animal compassion, politics, and health in general, I could only say Yes. Taken together, the reasons for following a vegan diet are just so compelling. Much more compelling than the reasoning behind any other way of eating, which usually focuses on just one aspect of food, such as weight loss. With a whole food, vegan diet based around nutrient-dense plants, you get fat loss, environmental protection, a longer lifespan, responsibility to animals, lower risk of cancer and heart disease, and other benefits. There are a lot of details to go into, but that's the big picture.

How long have you been vegan?
Since 2003.

What has benefited you the most from being vegan?
Since going vegan I have far fewer conflicts between my food choices and moral values.

What does veganism mean to you?
It's a confluence of ethical values we can use to lead better lives. It's not the only way, but it's a good one.

TRAINING

What sort of training do you do?
I do bodyweight-based functional fitness training, including strength circuits, sprint training, endurance running and cycling, and dancing. I'm a professional contemporary dancer, so I have to adjust my non-dance training based on how intense my rehearsals are.

How often do you (need to) train?
6-7 days per week, 1-4 hours each time. The total number of hours depends on the intensity.

Do you offer your fitness or training services to others?
I run Sebastian's Functional Fitness and see about 30 clients a week. Most are fitness-focused, but some are clients focused on nutrition or weight loss.

What sports do you play?
Dance is currently the sport of choice.

STRENGTHS, WEAKNESSES & OUTSIDE INFLUENCES

What do you think is the biggest misconception about vegans and how do you address this?
Aside from the ubiquitous protein question, a number of people have told me that I'm the first fit, healthy vegan they've met. A few of these folks were then motivated to become vegan themselves. This is why I believe vegans have a responsibility to be as healthy as possible.

What are your strengths as a vegan athlete?
I have a lot of leg power for jumping and sprinting. I also have a high strength-to-bodyweight ratio, so I excel at bodyweight-based activities. In the dance world I'm known for my uncommon strength and also cardiovascular endurance.

I'm the 2014 Champion of the "Battle of the Best Trainers" in San Francisco. This was a fitness competition for trainers based on bodyweight exercises and I won by a significant margin.

What is your biggest challenge?
Balancing my own training program. I find it much easier to balance the program for other people and then overdo my own training and get injured.

Are the non-vegans in your industry supportive or not?
They don't criticize how I eat anymore, which I like to think is because of what I can do with my body. But I don't really know.

Are your family and friends supportive of your vegan lifestyle?
In general, yes. My parents have really supported me, and eventually have come to follow a more plant-based eating pattern.

What is the most common question/comment that people ask/say when they find out that you are a vegan and how do you respond?
They want to know where I get my protein. I tell them that all whole foods contain protein, and that legumes are a particularly dense plant source.

Who or what motivates you?
I'm motivated by my sense of responsibility of being a good role model. I also strive for excellence in general and that means a big commitment to hard work.

"Taken together, the reasons for following a vegan diet are just so compelling. Much more compelling than the reasoning behind any other way of eating, which usually focuses on just one aspect of food, such as weight loss. With a whole food, vegan diet based around nutrient-dense plants, you get fat loss, environmental protection, a longer lifespan, responsibility to animals, lower risk of cancer and heart disease, and other benefits."

FOOD & SUPPLEMENTS

What do you eat for Breakfast?
Oatmeal with nuts and berries; sprouted whole grain bread with nut butter and berries or banana; and/or Larabar when running out the door.

What do you eat for Lunch?
Huge salad with whole grains, beans, nuts or seeds. Several vegetable sandwiches on whole grain bread, with beans or tofu on the side.

What do you eat for Dinner?
Steamed veggies with whole grains, beans, nuts or seeds; veggie soup with corn tortillas etc.

What do you eat for Snacks - healthy & not-so healthy?
Apples, citrus fruits, Larabars, dates, trail mix, corn thins and hummus, whole grain bread with nut butter.

What is your favourite source of Protein?
Black beans and split red lentils.

What is your favourite source of Calcium?
Dark green vegetables (check out collard greens, for instance.)

What is your favourite source of Iron?
Dark green vegetables.

What foods give you the most energy?
Dates. Fast-digesting and high in sugar. I eat them often right before or during long workouts.

Do you take any supplements?
B-12, D3, Omega-3s. All vegans must supplement B-12! Do more research on this one if you are not currently taking it - many vegans are deficient, which increases risk of heart disease and nerve damage, among other things. 42% of Americans are deficient in Vitamin D. And I take an algae-derived supplement for omega-3s, aside from what I get from ground flaxseed, hemp seeds, chia seeds, and walnuts.

ADVICE

What is your top tip for gaining muscle?
Do intense strength-training 3-4 days per week and eat a lot (of healthy) food!

What is your top tip for Losing weight & Improving Metabolism?
Do circuit training and cardio training that emphasize high intensity intervals. Base your diet around vegetables, fruits, and beans. Eliminate processed foods, flour-based foods, and alcohol.

What is your top tip for maintaining weight?
Do a mix of the above. If you want to lose a little, eat more vegetables and no processed foods. If you want to gain a little, eat more nuts and seeds.

What is your top tip for toning up?
Same as Losing Weight and Improving Metabolism above. One thing to discuss is what "toning" even means. Most people say this when they want to lose some body fat so they have more defined/visible muscles. Sometimes they also want slightly larger muscles. This means they need to follow an extremely healthy diet and do circuit strength training

and interval cardio training (total 6-7 days per week). Just to set the record straight: having "toned" muscles literally means muscles with increased "tone", ie increased "tonus", meaning more tension when at rest. The more you exercise and do strenuous activities, the more "tone" your muscles will have, regardless of whether or not they are covered in a fat layer, but this isn't what most people mean when they use the word.

How do you promote veganism in your daily life?
I lead by example, discuss healthy habits with people, and am ready to answer questions in a compassionate way. I also write and publish articles on health topics via my website.

How would you suggest people get involved with what you do?
Check out my website and come train with me if you are ever in San Francisco! I also frequently post awesome findings from recent scientific studies. You can catch all this by finding me on FaceBook and Twitter.

"Do not let what you cannot do interfere with what you can do."
- John Wooden

Vegans don't only care about animals, so let's start to act like it - especially online.

Let's learn more about each other and the world around us.

SIMONE COLLINS
VEGAN FIGURE COMPETITOR

Melbourne, Victoria, Australia
Vegan since: 2009

simicollins.com
SM: *FaceBook, Instagram*

Simone Collins is an active figure competitor with the International Federation of Body Builders (IFBB) and is passionate about health and fitness. She initially went vegan for ethical reasons but also learned about the health and ecological benefits of a plant-based diet. Simone is currently studying Certificate III and IV in Fitness to become a certified personal trainer.

WHY VEGAN?

How and why did you decide to become vegan?
I went vegetarian at 13 years of age due to ethical reasons. Even as a child I never wanted to eat meat - I was always an animal lover, and I despised the fact that I was eating them. When I turned 13 my parents allowed me to make a choice, and I chose never to eat meat again. I went vegan for the same reasons. I came to realise through campaigns run by Animal Liberation Victoria, that the dairy and egg industries are just as guilty for enslaving, exploiting and mistreating animals as the meat industry. I vowed to go vegan and never use or consume any animal products. I also make sure any cosmetics or household products I use are cruelty-free and not tested on animals.

How long have you been vegan?
I went vegetarian in 1999 and vegan in 2009.

What has benefited you the most from being vegan?
I have never felt healthier or more energised since going vegan. I have been able to get in the best shape of my life, build muscle, and compared to other figure competitors, I am able to keep more variety in my diet and do less cardio when preparing for a show. I also feel peace of mind, and more at-ease with the world, knowing that I am doing my best to lead a positive, compassionate, healthy and more sustainable lifestyle.

What does veganism mean to you?
To me, veganism is not a "diet." It means to live respectfully and compassionately, to understand all sentient beings are equal in their right to live in freedom and happiness, without suffering - human and non-human alike.

TRAINING

What sort of training do you do?
I used to do mainly old-school bodybuilding-style training with weights, but recently have started CrossFit and I LOVE it! So now I do a bit of both.

How often do you (need to) train?
5-6 days a week, for about an hour.

Do you offer your fitness or training services to others?
This is something I will be offering face-to-face and online when I have completed my certificates.

What sports do you play?
I compete in bodybuilding and figure competitions, and have just started competing in CrossFit as well. I also do the occasional fun run or obstacle course.

STRENGTHS, WEAKNESSES & OUTSIDE INFLUENCES

What do you think is the biggest misconception about vegans and how do you address this?
The obvious - that we need to eat meat! Especially in sports like mine, where building muscle and getting lean is primarily associated with the consumption of large amounts of animal protein. I address this by explaining that vegan sources of protein are better for you - they are free from saturated fat and cholesterol, they are non-carcinogenic (unlike meat and dairy) more easily absorbed by the body, and are alkalising rather than acid-forming. I also use my results in the gym to prove my point that building muscle and strength is just as achievable as a vegan, but far more beneficial to health, the animals and the environment.

What are your strengths as a vegan athlete?
Applying my training and diet to build strength and muscle. My upper-body is my strong point, and for power lifting the bench press is my best lift.

What is your biggest challenge?
Genetically my upper body builds a lot more easily than my abs or legs, so I have a hard time increasing muscle mass in these areas. Squats are a challenge for me and are my weakest lift. There's also a lot of fun to be had in a challenge so I use it as motivation to improve.

Are the non-vegans in your industry supportive or not?
Generally they are. I think a lot of people who have seen my transformation during my training changed their views on veganism, and a few have even joined me. Most people who don't know already are often surprised when I tell them I'm vegan, and are instantly and genuinely interested in what I eat. The people who aren't supportive are usually those who don't know me and haven't seen how far I have come in just a few years as a vegan athlete.

Are your family and friends supportive of your vegan lifestyle?
I was the first in my family to become vegan, however both my sisters are now vegan. My parents are not vegan, but have always been supportive of me.

FOOD & SUPPLEMENTS

What do you eat for Breakfast?
Oats, berries, flax oil, cinnamon and a vegan protein powder mixed in with water.

What do you eat for Lunch & Dinner?
Tofu, tempeh or seitan, vegetables, brown rice or lentils, and raw salad topped with salsa, natural sea salt and nutritional yeast.

What do you eat for Snacks - healthy & not-so healthy?
Healthy - Vegan protein shakes, nuts, rice cakes, nut butter, seeds, wraps, superfood balls, vegan snack bars.

Not-So Healthy - Chocolate, vegan ice-cream, vegetable chips, chocolate soy milk, vegan cakes, brownies, muffins, cup cakes and anything sweet (I have a big sweet tooth) but generally I try to keep these kind of foods to a minimum.

What is your favourite source of Protein?
Tofu, tempeh, seitan and protein shakes.

What is your favourite source of Calcium & Iron?
Green leafy vegetables.

What foods give you the most energy?
I love nuts. They really keep my energy up between meals.

Do you take any supplements?
Not all the time, but sometimes I cycle creatine, or use BCAA's during my workouts. I often get Vitamin D deficient, so when my levels are low I take an organic vegan D3 capsule made from fungi.

ADVICE

What is your top tip for gaining muscle?
Eat a lot, especially plenty of vegan protein, and lift heavy.

What is your top tip for losing weight?
Cut back on junk food and incorporate a bit of cardio training.

What is your top tip for maintaining weight?
Keep a mostly clean diet, train with weights and minimal cardio.

What is your top tip for improving metabolism?
Eat regular meals and be aware of your caloric needs - make sure you are eating enough to support your training.

What is your top tip for toning up?
Keep a healthy diet and lift weights regularly, maybe 2-4 times a week. If you can't get to a gym, try some plyometric or bodyweight exercises.

How do you promote veganism in your daily life?
I try to send out a positive and inspiring message about veganism though my passion for training - by building up my strength and muscle, getting involved in the health and fitness scene, and competing in bodybuilding. I hope to show people that you don't need animal protein to succeed in your sport. That being vegan is not a disadvantage. That you can achieve anything as a vegan. I hope that I can motivate and inspire others to also lead a compassionate, healthy vegan lifestyle.

How would you suggest people get involved with what you do?
I cannot wait to be able to take on clients, to be able to help others on their vegan fitness journeys, and to offer training, diet plans and online coaching for a plant-based lifestyle. I recommend following my blog, Facebook and Instagram. I also recommend doing an online search to find out more about vegan fitness, muscle, strength, health and activism.

"Even as a child I never wanted to eat meat – I was always an animal lover, and I despised the fact that I was eating them. When I turned 13 my parents allowed me to make a choice, and I chose never to eat meat again. I went vegan for the same reasons."

SPENCER PUMPELLY
VEGAN PROFESSIONAL RACING DRIVER

Atlanta, Georgia, USA
Vegan since: 2010

spencerpumpelly.com
SM: *Twitter*

Spencer Pumpelly is professional racing driver and a two-time class winner in the Rolex 24 at Daytona, having won the GT class in 2006 and 2011. He has won races in the Tudor United Sportscar Challenge, American Le Mans Series, Grand Am Rolex, Continental Challenge, and Pirelli World Challenge and holds class victories in six major sportscar endurance races. Spencer currently lives in Atlanta, Georgia with his wife Lindsay, son Ryder, and daughter Parker. When not racing he enjoys running, ice-hockey, jiu-jitsu, and flying helicopters.

WHY VEGAN?

How and why did you decide to become vegan?
In 2003, my father began having heart issues. I knew that I would be at risk if I didn't make some changes so I tried to go vegetarian for a little bit just to see if I could. It was easier than I thought so I continued and have not (intentionally) eaten meat since. While vegetarian, I began searching the web for more vegetarian information, and became aware of all the cruelty that went into the production of animal products. I had always considered veganism to be extreme and assumed that it would be impossible for me given that I'm on the road over 180 days in the typical year.

As time went on, I became more and more aware of both the health risks and cruelty involved with eating things like eggs, cheese, and dairy. I can't pinpoint exactly what pushed me to finally go vegan, but when I did I found that while difficult, it was possible to be on the road and find vegan food. I can't see myself ever going back.

How long have you been vegan?
Vegan since 2010, vegetarian since 2003.

What has benefited you the most from being vegan?
I have seen all sorts of benefits. For one I am about 20lbs (9kg). lighter than I was as a vegetarian. When we race, the cars are weighed without the drivers in them so while the cars cannot be lighter than the minimum weight, the car and driver combination can be 20lbs (9kg). doesn't sound like much, but in our sport we have to optimize everything when lap times are measured in hundredths of seconds. I also have much better endurance in the car so I can attack at the end of a long race. Outside of the car I have seen improved focus and my cholesterol went from very high to well into the normal range.

"Racing is unlike other sports where you can practice every day. It's cost prohibitive and you need to be near a racetrack – which isn't the case for me in downtown Atlanta. The only thing I can really do to prepare is show up to the track in great shape."

What does veganism mean to you?

Veganism is justice. While life isn't fair, societies for centuries have sought and valued the concept of justice and have gone to great lengths and struggles to try and create an ever more just world. There is no way anyone who seeks to be part of a just society can endorse the extreme suffering and torment of the innocent. We have a choice every time we eat or shop to make things better or worse. Unfortunately, many otherwise caring and compassionate people have let societal norms lead them to avert their consciousness and support things they would not if they knew they had a choice. Veganism is about becoming aware, and then acting when rationalizations seem much easier.

TRAINING

What sort of training do you do?

It is hard to describe to someone who hasn't raced just how physically demanding it is, but in order to keep a car at its absolute limits - with the heat and G-forces all while making thousands of critical decisions in a very stressful environment - you have to be in great shape. The type of cars I race take more cardio fitness to drive than muscular strength, so running makes up the majority of my training. I like running because I can do it almost anywhere, and by entering 5Ks, 10Ks, and half marathons I can quantify my training and fitness bases on my results. I set a (post high school) 5K personal best last summer at a 19:21 which isn't bad for a 40 year old.

How often do you (need to) train?

Racing is unlike other sports where you can practice every day. It's cost prohibitive and you need to be near a racetrack - which isn't the case for me in downtown Atlanta. The only thing I can really do to prepare is show up to the track in great shape. I typically run three to six miles, three days a week. Twice a week I mix in a different sport of equal intensity and the other two days I rest and recover. In season, I reduce the number of runs per week and taper off before each event, but my time in the race car makes up for the reduced workouts.

Do you offer your fitness or training services to others?

I do private coaching for aspiring drivers but we don't often get to work on fitness.

What sports do you play?

I supplement my running by playing ice-hockey and training in Brazilian jiu-jitsu once a week. Both activities are somewhat new to me, but by mixing them into my weekly workout schedule I get some strength and interval workouts that I can't get from running alone. For me the key is enjoying the workout whatever it is. You'll find me on the ice, mat, or trail but never in a gym.

STRENGTHS, WEAKNESSES & OUTSIDE INFLUENCES

What do you think is the biggest misconception about vegans and how do you address this?

I am finding fewer people with true misconceptions as veganism becomes more popular. A few people still think of it as a hippie-inspired counterculture trend, much like I did a few years ago. I feel now when it comes up in conversation I get good questions from people who are truly interested.

What are your strengths as a vegan athlete?

Since becoming vegan I have improved my overall fitness, first by personal best 5K and 10K times, run my first half marathon, and dropped 20lbs (9kg). I also feel more motivated to train so it's easier to stay in shape. This translates to better performance on the track. My first year as a vegan I won 5 of the 15 races I entered and finished on the podium in 10 of them.

What is your biggest challenge?
Finding healthy food on the road is by far my biggest challenge. It's easy to find vegan food, but when you're on the road sometimes what you eat isn't the healthiest. I often have to choose between things like potato chips or nothing at all. Planning ahead when I can helps, and at the track our team has caterers who do a decent job of providing healthy options.

Are the non-vegans in your industry supportive or not?
Some like to kid me about it. I have a buddy who texts me a picture of his food every time he eats a steak. But, for the most part everyone is supportive and respectful.

Are your family and friends supportive of your vegan lifestyle?
Yes, very much so. My wife Lindsay is also vegan, as are my mother and her husband. Our children are being raised vegan and are welcome to eat meat when they can buy it with their own money - that might be a while.

What is the most common question/comment that people ask/say when they find out that you are a vegan and how do you respond?
"Where do you get your protein?" I get it less and less, but I still get it. I went to a screening of "Forks Over Knives" here in Atlanta and got to hear Rip Esselstyn tell the audience how he responds and I use his response sometimes. When asked he says, "Protein? Never really thought about it, how much do you think I need?" Brilliant!

Who or what motivates you?
I love my job and I want to keep racing well into my 50's. The problem with racing is that for every driver making a living racing cars, there are hundreds of equally motivated drivers on the sidelines who would kill to take your seat. My love for what I do pushes me to be the best so I can continue to have the privilege. I am also a small part of a big team. We have over 30 people on our team working hard at what they do, giving their all - year round. They inspire me to work as hard as they do so their work isn't wasted on a driver that can't push because he's tired.

I am also motivated to stay healthy by my family. I want to be around to see my great grand kids which means giving myself the best odds at beating disease. If that isn't enough, all I have to do is think of the suffering on factory farms and that's motivation in itself.

FOOD & SUPPLEMENTS

What do you eat for Breakfast?
Vegan Vega shake with soymilk, with a banana, and decaf coffee. Cereal with almond milk. On a cheat day a (faux) sausage, egg and cheese biscuit from either Sevenanda or La Dolce Vegan here in Atlanta.

What do you eat for Lunch?
Salad with tahini-based dressing. Whole grain wraps with fake meats, Field Roast frankfurters are my favorite.

What do you eat for Dinner?
Pastas, Mexican, Asian, or we eat out at places like Cafe Sunflower or Soul Vegetarian. Pre-race meal is whole grain pasta with veggies.

What do you eat for Snacks - healthy & not-so healthy?

Almonds, sliced veggies, popcorn, and fruits. For not healthy stuff I love the Earth Balance sour cream and onion chips and I have a Sweet Tart addiction I should probably find a 12-step program for.

Do you take any supplements?

I supplement with B-12. My B-12 levels were off the charts last time I had blood work done, but I know I don't get enough on the road so I supplement it in season.

ADVICE

How do you promote veganism in your daily life?

I have to be very careful. I try to only directly talk about it to those who ask. It's very easy to get preachy and turn people off. I promote veganism by first being 99% vegan - there are still no FIA approved racing shoes that are leather free - but I am working on it. I try to find good hand me downs from other drivers. That's the only thing that keeps me from 100%. I tweet about animal cruelty often and support places like Farm Sanctuary. Everyone knows I'm vegan without me having to shout about it.

Here in Atlanta, I have also started a project called Vegan Identifier. We find restaurants with at least one vegan option and get them to sign on to our network. They display our logo in their storefront and train their servers on how to get you that option when you ask for vegan food. It's a way to make being vegan easier and we are getting a lot of good feedback.

How would you suggest people get involved with what you do?

Follow me on Twitter and catch our races on Fox, Fox Sports 1, or imsa.com. A full schedule of my races can be found on my website.

"Veganism is justice. While life isn't fair, societies for centuries have sought and valued the concept of justice and have gone to great lengths and struggles to try and create an ever more just world. There is no way anyone who seeks to be part of a just society can endorse the extreme suffering and torment of the innocent. We have a choice every time we eat or shop to make things better or worse. Unfortunately, many otherwise caring and compassionate people have let societal norms lead them to avert their consciousness and support things they would not if they knew they had a choice. Veganism is about becoming aware, and then acting when rationalizations seem much easier."

STEPHANIE BELLIA
VEGAN PERSONAL TRAINER

Brisbane, Queensland, Australia
Vegan since: 2013

movenimprove.com.au
SM: *FaceBook, Instagram*

Stephanie is a 40-year old vegan personal trainer who has been running her own personal training business Move 'n' Improve for the past 13 years. Fitness has been a huge passion for her since the age of 17 when she was drawn to buying her very first Fitness & Bodybuilding Magazine. She discovered Cory Everson, 8-times Miss Olympia who became her idol, inspiration, model and drive. Something had clicked there, and from that moment on she knew what her purpose in this lifetime would be: helping, supporting and encouraging others on their very own health and fitness journey. Originally from France, Move 'n' Improve personal training was created when Australia became Stephanie's new home. She believes in a holistic approach to health and fitness, placing a strong emphasis on eating a plant-based diet, combined with exercise, along with a positive, focused mind.

WHY VEGAN?

How and why did you decide to become vegan?
From the age of 17, I developed two huge passions: one being fitness and the other animals. I knew in my heart that they were going to be the driving factor of all I would undertake in this lifetime. After doing extensive research on the health benefits of living a meat-free lifestyle, as well as looking deeper into what happens to the animals before they end up on our plates, I instantly decided that being vegetarian was the only way. What I didn't realise during my 20 years of being vegetarian, is that I was still contributing to tremendous animal cruelty by still consuming dairy and eggs. It is only just over two years ago that I became vegan, thanks to an incredible animal activist and owner of a farm animal rescue sanctuary who simply exposed me to the truth. My only wish is that it would have been done sooner. Soon after becoming vegan, I started experiencing almost immediate health benefits which only re-enforced my convictions that it was the right path for me, the earth and all living creatures.

How long have you been vegan?
I have been vegan for over two years.

What has benefited you the most from being vegan?
Having been a fitness fanatic my whole life, I noticed an immediate difference in the way I was feeling with a surge of new found energy. The headaches I was having on a weekly basis just disappeared. I started sleeping better. My pre-menstrual symptoms were significantly reduced, which of course made a huge difference to my life. The best part was that I felt physically, mentally and spiritually more balanced. I started feeling more in tune and in harmony with my environment.

What does veganism mean to you?
Veganism means compassion. It means I deeply care for the earth, the animals and my health. It means nobody gets hurt.

TRAINING

What sort of training do you do?
I do weight-lifting mostly using free-weights and kettle bells. I use the TRX suspension training system. Calisthenics, running and mountain-biking.

How often do you train?
I train 6 days a week - alternating my routine to suit my body's needs and maximise results.

Do you offer your fitness or training services to others?
Yes I do. I have been a certified Personal Trainer for 13 years. I have been fortunate to be living the dream everyday having turned my passion into my occupation.

What sports do you play?
I don't play any sports outside of my weekly training routine.

STRENGTH, WEAKNESSES & OUTSIDE INFLUENCES

What do you think is the biggest misconception about vegans and how do you address this?
The biggest misconception is that vegans can't get enough protein and are vitamin deficient. The way I address this is leading by example. I am my own walking advertising to the cause, so to speak. I try to inspire and educate people by practicing what I preach, and showing others that we can be vegan and have a fit, strong, athletic body. There is nothing I love more than the look of surprise on people's faces when I tell them that I am vegan. This is usually when they run out of valid arguments.

What are your strengths as a vegan athlete?
I have a lot more energy than I used to, which allows me to more easily address the high physical demands that running a personal training business involves. Very importantly, it still leaves me with plenty more readily available energy to attend to my own training outside of work. I feel stronger and healthier than I have ever been. I am able to keep raising the bar and set new goals and new challenges on a regular base because I know that both my mind and body will take me there. There is an inner trust that I am giving my body the best chances to perform.

What is your biggest challenge?
Consuming enough calories to sustain muscle mass, and sitting down long enough to allow my body to recover.

Are the non-vegans in your industry supportive of your vegan lifestyle?
They mostly seem to think I come from another planet. But this mentality will only change once trainers start thinking outside the box, and not just believe what we were taught in the nutrition classroom. Fortunately, more professionals are bringing a more open mind to the industry and are willing to listen and learn of different ways, especially when backed up with undeniable facts and evidence. Again, here my job is to lead by example.

Are your family and friends supportive of your vegan lifestyle?
My family lives on the other side of the planet, so I actually haven't been around them since I've gone vegan. But, they have always been very supportive of my vegetarian lifestyle with two of my sisters following in my footsteps. I am fortunate to have a family who has always supported my choices. As for my closest friends, they have also been behind me 100% and have even been open to new, healthier ways. Some I have lost along the way, but the real ones stayed close. Becoming vegan has made me reach out to the vegan community via Social Media, and I have made some wonderful new supportive friends, which is essential as a minority.

What is the most common question/comment that people ask/say when they find out you are vegan and how do you respond?
It's usually, "But where do you get your protein from?" Shortly followed by, "I love my meat - I just couldn't do it." I usually follow this with a rather extensive list of all the plant-based protein sources, which I usually carry around with me in the form of a flyer being a personal trainer. If that's not enough, I can always do a little flexing of my muscles for the most skeptical ones.

Who or what motivates you?
Although health and fitness is a huge part of my life and I have some people I look up to for inspiration and motivation, I have to say that my biggest motivation is the animals. The thought of billions of animals being tortured and slaughtered on a daily basis is my driving force. My mission is to open people's eyes to a better way of life, a healthier way of life, but most importantly a cruelty free way of life.

FOOD & SUPPLEMENTS

What do you eat for Breakfast?
A green smoothie, and a bowl of oats with a blend of pumpkin seeds, sunflower seeds, sultanas and raw almonds with rice milk.

What do you eat for Lunch?
A large salad with lots of greens, heaps of vegies, mixed beans, seeds, sprouts, tofu and a homemade dressing.

What do you eat for Dinner?
Usually cooked food. Stir-fries with lots of greens and vegies, tofu, chick-peas, kidney beans, lentils. With some form of grains such as quinoa, brown rice or gluten-free buckwheat pasta. Roasted sweet potatoes and pumpkin are my favourites.

What do you eat for Snacks - healthy & not-so healthy?
Green smoothies, bananas, dates, gluten-free bread with organic peanut butter and coconut spread.

What is your favourite source of Protein?
Tofu, it is very versatile.

What is your favourite source of Calcium & Iron?
Greens.

What food gives you most energy?
Green smoothies, bananas and dates.

Do you take supplements?
Only B12 and Iron.

ADVICE

What is your top tip for gaining muscle?
Eat enough food! Make sure you eat enough calories. Lift heavy and be consistent with your training while allowing recovery time for muscle repair and growth.

What is your top tip for losing weight?
Only eat clean, fresh foods and stay away from processed foods, sugar and alcohol. Find a balance between cardiovascular activities and weight training. Implement circuit training and interval training for optimum fat burning.

What is your top tip for maintaining weight?
Be consistent. Organisation and preparation is the key to staying on track with proper nutrition. Allow yourself a special treat occasionally.

What is your top tip for improving metabolism?
Eat 5-6 meals a day, no calories restricting. Drink plenty of water.

What is your top tip for toning up?
Eat clean and train dirty!

How do you promote veganism in your daily life?
I promote it daily through my business Move 'n' Improve Personal Training and online.

How would you suggest people get involved with what you do?
See my website or my FaceBook page.

"What I didn't realise during my 20 years of being vegetarian, is that I was still contributing to tremendous animal cruelty by still consuming dairy and eggs. It is only just over two years ago that I became vegan, thanks to an incredible animal activist and owner of a farm animal rescue sanctuary who simply exposed me to the truth. My only wish is that it would have been done sooner."

Permanent Change leads to Permanent Results

STEPH DAVIS
VEGAN PROFESSIONAL CLIMBER

Moab, Utah, USA
Vegan since: 2002

highinfatuation.com
climb2fly.com
SM: FaceBook, Instagram, Twitter

Steph Davis is a professional climber who lives in Moab, Utah, USA. She started climbing when a freshman at the University of Maryland in 1991. Climbing is her anchor and passion. It's as much a part of her as eating or walking. For Steph, living half-tamed feels right. She love high places, and seeing the world from above. Steph started skydiving and base-jumping seven years ago and has learned that climbing really is a metaphor for life in many ways.

WHY VEGAN?

How and why did you decide to become vegan?
I started eating vegan in 2002. I was experimenting with different eating systems to improve my climbing performance. I tried four different diets for four months each. When I was finished, I did the master cleanse. When I started to eat food again after the cleansing fast, I found that the only things I wanted to eat were whole-food, non-meat items, and I decided to just go with it. I quickly discovered that I was climbing and feeling better than before, and that's why I stayed vegan.

How long have you been vegan?
Over 12 years.

What has benefited you the most from being vegan?
Athletic performance and overall health.

What does veganism mean to you?
To me, it means being healthy, eating mindfully, respecting the environment and causing less harm to other living creatures.

TRAINING

What sort of training do you do?
I climb and train for climbing 5 days a week. I base-jump (carrying my gear to the top of the cliff or mountain) 4 days a week. I trail run 2-4 times a week.

How often do you (need to) train?
See above.

Do you offer your fitness or training services to others?
I own a company called Moab Base Adventures, which offers climbing clinics, climbing coaching, base-jumping guiding and base jumping instruction.

What sports do you play?
Climbing, base-jumping, wing suit flying, trail running and Nordic skiing.

STRENGTHS, WEAKNESSES & OUTSIDE INFLUENCES

What do you think is the biggest misconception about vegans and how do you address this?
I feel it's changed a lot over the years, but climbers used to think that you needed animal protein for climbing performance. I've also heard people say that males and endurance athletes "need" animal protein, despite what we see from ultra-runners like Scott Jurek.

What are your strengths as a vegan athlete?
Beyond just being vegan, I'm very interested in nutrition - eating whole foods, nothing processed, and no refined sugar.

What is your biggest challenge?
I don't like to rely on refined wheat products to fill me up, and it can be harder when traveling to find good food, depending on the part of the country or world I'm in.

Are the non-vegans in your industry supportive or not?
Yes.

Are your family and friends supportive of your vegan lifestyle?
Yes.

What is the most common question/comment that people ask/say when they find out that you are a vegan and how do you respond?
"How do you get protein?" I explain that people can actually process much less protein than the common perception, and that eating excess protein is actually just a waste.

Who or what motivates you?
At this point in my life, my main motivation for being vegan is to remove my consumer dollars from the factory farming system, and in that way cast my vote for halting animal abuse.

FOOD & SUPPLEMENTS

What do you eat for Breakfast?
Homemade granola and soy or brown rice milk, or just fruit if I'm not very hungry. Also ginger tea.

What do you eat for Lunch?
Usually I don't eat an official lunch, rather I eat throughout the day as I feel hungry.

What do you eat for Dinner?
In the summer, salad with nuts and sauteed tofu. In the winter, brown rice or quinoa with tofu and veggie stir-fry. Sometimes brown rice pasta with grilled vegetables.

What do you eat for Snacks - healthy & not-so healthy?
Homemade hummus with red peppers and cucumbers is a real favorite, nuts, fruit and dried fruit, Clif Mojo bars and shot Blocks.

What is your favourite source of Protein?
Tofu, lentils, garbanzo beans, black beans, almonds, and walnuts.

What is your favourite source of Calcium?
Kale, chard and spinach.

What is your favourite source of Iron?
Spinach.

What foods give you the most energy?
Hummus and vegetables.

Do you take any supplements?
I take B vitamins, creatine and sometimes Iron.

"At this point in my life, my main motivation for being vegan is to remove my consumer dollars from the factory farming system, and in that way cast my vote for halting animal abuse."

ADVICE

What is your top tip for Gaining muscle, Losing weight, Maintaining weight, Improving metabolism, and Toning up?
For all of the above, lots of exercise, being mindful of including protein sources in meals and eating lots of whole grains and vegetables.

How do you promote veganism in your daily life?
I love cooking, so I always cook for people and bake for people, and I share recipes on my blog.

How would you suggest people get involved with what you do?
Go to a climbing gym, or go to a drop zone and make a tandem skydive!

The Environmental Impacts of a Mainstream Diet

The link between animal food products and climate change involves many inter-related factors, such as:

- Livestock's inherent inefficiency as a food source
- The massive scale of the industry, including tens of billions of animals slaughtered annually
- Land clearing and degradation
- Greenhouse gases, including carbon dioxide, methane and nitrous oxide
- Other warming agents, such as black carbon

(Source: 'Protecting Global Climate with Vegan Challenge' & 'Omissions of Emissions: A Critical Climate Change Issue' both by Paul Mahony)

Suzanna McGee
VEGAN TENNIS PLAYER

Venice Beach, California, USA
Vegan since: 2013

tennisfitnesslove.com
SM: *FaceBook, Google+, Instagram, Pinterest, YouTube*

Suzanna McGee is a former Ms. Natural Olympia drug-free bodybuilding champion, now competitive tennis player, expert athletic trainer, speaker and author of "The Athlete's Simple Guide to a Plant-Based Lifestyle" and "Tennis Fitness for the Love of it". She is certified by the National Academy of Sports Medicine as a performance enhancement specialist and corrective exercise specialist. She has over twenty years of experience in athletic training. With great success, Suzanna has become a plant-based athlete, raw vegan, and has earned a certificate in plant-based nutrition at eCornell University. Besides her love of sports, learning, and teaching, Suzanna has two master's degrees in computer science, and speaks six languages. This Czech native resides with her vegan chocolate Labrador in Venice Beach, California, USA.

WHY VEGAN?

How and why did you decide to become vegan?
I used to be a drug-free bodybuilder (and former Ms. Natural Olympia champion) and I used to eat so many animal products because I believed I need them to grow, just like many bodybuilders 15-20 years ago used to believe. Then I started to play competitive tennis and slowly transitioned to a lighter diet, with very little meat, but still a lot of dairy. I was almost vegetarian. Then a few years ago, many of my still young friends and family member started to pass away from cancers and heart disease, and I felt this is not how it is supposed to be. We should be able to live until at least 100 years old, so I started to do more research and learn so many amazing things about the plant-based diet and the dangers of animal products. I became plant-based. As I was promoting the health message of eating plants to my students and friends, I was looking more into how the animals are treated and I was horrified. The animals don't deserve to live and suffer for us like this. I became vegan.

How long have you been vegan?
I have been vegan for the past two 2 years after being semi-vegetarian for maybe 6 years. The last year, I've become a raw vegan.

What has benefited you the most from being vegan?
Besides the feeling that I am doing something really great for the fellow animals, who I love so much, I also feel great health benefits and performance advantage in my tennis and strength training. I have a lot of unlimited energy, I recover really fast, and I plainly enjoy all the plants I eat. There is no better feeling than eating all the crunchy, juicy, plants and knowing that I have saved another animal life.

What does veganism mean to you?

Compassion for every living being. I love animals and nature so much, and it doesn't make any sense to treat animals so viciously and destroy our environment and nature at the same time, while we are making ourselves sick, fat, and slowly dying. I have supported many different animal organizations all my life and being vegan makes absolute sense to me. I just don't understand why I hadn't transitioned to this state much earlier. Even my dog, chocolate labrador Zuzi, is a vegan dog and she is thriving. We both are great examples for many other animal lovers out there.

TRAINING

What sort of training do you do?

After being a cross-country skier in my teens, then downhill skier in my 20s, drug-free bodybuilder in my 30s, I became a tennis player in my 40s. I love all sports. Now I mostly focus on tennis and to be a great player, I need to work on my strength, agility, endurance, and flexibility.

How often do you (need to) train?

I train almost every day. I take a day off maybe every other week, if I feel like I am getting rundown. Being on a raw vegan diet gives me so much energy, that I feel I need much fewer off-days. I walk or jog every morning with my dog, for about one hour – I've been doing that every day, for the past six years. I play tennis about 5-6 hours a week, do strength training for about another 5-6 hours per week. Stretching or yoga and myofascial release, I do every day a little bit.

Do you offer your fitness or training services to others?

Yes, I am a performance coach and an injury prevention specialist. I love to focus on tennis players, because I have realized how tennis players need good fitness training, and they are not even aware of it until they get a lot of imbalances and then many injuries. Even though tennis players are my main focus, I do also train seniors and enjoy that very much because it feels like I give them another 20 years of youth when they feel strong, balanced, and fit. I train a few juniors as well, and many non-tennis players, too. With my experience of at least 20 years of training athletes, and participating in many different sports through all my life, I can offer good training to almost anybody.

What sports do you play?

Tennis is my main sport now. Strength training and building the body in the gym is a part of my focus on being balanced, fit, healthy, and strong. Yoga is good for my flexibility and my mind. I do love many other sports, like swimming, roller-dancing, skiing, running, etc. but I only have time for the above mentioned.

STRENGTHS, WEAKNESSES & OUTSIDE INFLUENCES

What do you think is the biggest misconception about vegans and how do you address this?

I think there are two major misconceptions that I am observing. The first one is physical. People think that vegans are weak, scrawny, sickly people who just melt away and die after a while. This is so far from the truth. The other one is that people often think that vegans are aggressive, pushy, and rude by promoting their message of not hurting the animals and eating plants. They don't realize that the majority of advertisements all around us are from the meat eaters and meat industries. They don't see that as pushy or aggressive.

Addressing the physical misconception is easy - I just flex my muscles while telling them that I am raw vegan. I also mention many other super strong and fit vegan athletes. Then I explain that the scrawny people possibly don't eat enough calories and that such people are among all groups, vegans or non-vegans. A little education goes always long way. Regarding the second misconception, that one is a bit harder, because if I get too much into it, then I confirm to them that I am "pushy and aggressive." I often choose a mellow and more educational approach. I explain about the indoctrination of animal products, the TV ads, the health issues caused by the animal foods, and when they start getting more interested, I can win them over.

What are your strengths as a vegan athlete?
I have amazing amounts of energy and mental clarity. I recover really fast, I feel quick on the tennis court and strong in the gym.

What is your biggest challenge?
My personal challenge may be that I love nuts. I am a nut addict, I could almost say. While this doesn't sound so bad, I really can eat a pound (450g) or more every day, which definitely is too much. Being raw vegan, not all nuts are raw. I always buy peanut butter for my dog, and then I am "stealing" spoons from her jar. It is really challenging to control myself. Otherwise, I don't have challenges like some other people may have, that they crave some non-vegans food. I love my lifestyle and I am not tempted ever to eat non-vegan foods.

Are the non-vegans in your industry supportive or not?
I find that people do not understand well what being vegan means. They don't understand how healthy and delicious it is to eat all the plants. After I explain, they are more open. But, in the gym - among the weight lifters, bodybuilders, and fitness competitors - it is much harder. The majority believes that animal products are extremely important to grow muscles, and it is hard to get through to them. I understand that, because I used to be like that too.

If somebody is open-minded, I very gladly explain to him or her all the benefits. In the beginning of my vegan journey, I had so many naysayers and negative people discouraging me, but now when I can show the great results, it is much easier. I've always turned the negativity into fueling me and helping me to achieve what they thought was impossible. I have also published a book for athletes and how to transition to the plant-based lifestyle - that gives me more credibility too and people leave me alone now.

Are your family and friends supportive of your vegan lifestyle?
They are now, but in the beginning they were a bit against it, they thought I was crazy and that I couldn't do it, it's not healthy and many other reasons. I always educate myself well before I do something, so every negative comment just kept me going and made me learn more.

What is the most common question/comment that people ask/say when they find out that you are a vegan and how do you respond?
The first question is the famous one, "How do you get your protein?" I often reply with a question "How do you get yours and how much do you get?" They are often very surprised because they don't have a clue. Then I explain to them how much we actually need - it's not as much as they believe - and how the plant-based diet supplies the perfect amounts of protein. The next question is, "What do you eat?" I patiently explain all the great foods I eat. I don't eat any processed foods - everything is mostly fruits,

vegetables, nuts, seeds, legumes, and meals out of those. When I start describing some delicious meals, they are truly impressed and feel like they want to try some of them.

Who or what motivates you?

I am a quite self-motivated and driven person. However, sometimes I need to keep the fire going. So for my training, I look at the athletes who are persistent, disciplined, hardworking and never complain. Their drive drives me. Especially the vegan athletes who have to go through similar negativity from people, and they keep going, thriving, achieving, and motivating others. In my personal life, all the people, who tell me that I am a great inspiration for them with my training, social presence, and my writings, motivate me. Each time I hear a "thank you", I am determined to help another few. This is the best feeling. Because I am an author and a promoter of this great vegan and plant-based lifestyle, I feel like I need to be in great shape to show that I practice what I preach. That motivates me.

FOOD & SUPPLEMENTS

What do you eat for Breakfast?

I have figured out that the best breakfast for me is a freshly squeezed juice. I drink about 40-48oz (1-1.5L) of it, and it gives me amazing energy for my training (which I do after the breakfast) while my stomach and digestive tract is nicely light and empty. Sometimes I have a smoothie instead of a juice, but I think I feel more energy with the juice.

What do you eat for Lunch?

If I don't need to hurry to my next client, I make myself a huge bowl of salad, with different greens, veggies, some fruits, nuts, avocado, sprouted lentils, etc. It is a huge bowl, maybe 4 pounds (1.8kg) of salad. I take all the time to chew slowly and enjoy this moment of peace. If I am in a hurry to get somewhere, I make a nutritious smoothie and have the salad for dinner.

What do you eat for Dinner?

Either a salad that I didn't have for lunch. Or if I had the salad, I am often still pretty full, so I make something light, maybe squeeze another juice, or just a few pieces of fruit, or some nuts and dehydrated homemade snacks.

What do you eat for Snacks - healthy & not-so healthy?

Fruits are the best snack for me. Then I also love to snack on nuts, but as I mentioned before, I try to avoid this because when I have one nut, I am able to eat the whole pound. I have no self-control when it comes to nuts!

What is your favourite source of Protein?

Sprouted lentils or other legumes. Spirulina and hemp that I add into my smoothies. Peas and dried peas as a snack. Occasionally, I add a plant-based protein powder.

What is your favourite source of Calcium?

All the leafy green vegetables that I add into my smoothies or salads; raisins that are my favorite snack; oranges that I add to salads or make a smoothie from. All the nuts that I try not to over consume are great too.

What is your favourite source of Iron?

Sprouted lentils, green leafy vegetables, sprouted quinoa, and nuts.

What foods give you the most energy?
It's my morning freshly-squeezed juice from carrots and apples, with ginger and turmeric (anti-inflammatory).

Do you take any supplements?
Not daily, but sporadically I take vitamin B12. I also take probiotics sometimes, and if I have huge meals, I may take extra digestive enzymes when I feel like my digestion is a bit weaker e.g. when I am too tired.

ADVICE

What is your top tip for gaining muscle?
Work hard in the gym and eat enough calories - I cannot stress this enough! Often vegan athletes don't eat enough because of the volumes of foods they need to eat to get the calories in. I don't have this problem, because I love to eat.

What is your top tip for losing weight?
Create a deficit about 500 calories a day and don't rush the weight loss. Be patient, train hard, eat a bit less than normally, and don't starve yourself. You need energy for all your training.

What is your top tip for maintaining weight?
With some experience, you will find your caloric needs to maintain your weight. Keep weighing yourself daily so you know where your weight is heading, and preferably keep a food log as well, so you can reevaluate when something goes differently than you've planned.

What is your top tip for improving metabolism?
Train hard - gain a lot of muscles.

What is your top tip for toning up?
Toning up is losing body fat so you would look leaner. It means that you need to cut your calories slightly and train hard. As your body fat gets lower, you will look more "toned."

How do you promote veganism in your daily life?
I educate people, very gently. I tell them how great my meals taste, how much energy I have, and how greatly I recover. All these things are easy for people to accept and they are tempted to try. Then I go deeper into how the animal products are unhealthy and how the poor animals are mistreated. This is often a very sensitive subject, so I have to show some tactfulness when I get into it, so I won't scare people away. On Social Media, I publish healthy, motivating messages and try to encourage people to add more plants in their diets. From my experience, if they add a bit more, then even more, eventually they may become completely plant-based because they feel so great. From plant-based to veganism is just a little step. It is often a very natural progression.

How would you suggest people get involved with what you do?
I am very active on FaceBook and Instagram, where I post motivational photos of training and raw vegan foods. People can connect with me there or through my website. My book "The Athlete's Simple Guide to a Plant-Based Lifestyle", is available on Amazon and I think it could help anybody, athlete or non-athlete, to get more involved with this great lifestyle.

"I love animals and nature so much, and it doesn't make any sense to treat animals so viciously and destroy our environment and nature at the same time, while we are making ourselves sick, fat, and slowly dying."

TIA BLANCO
VEGAN SURFER

San Clemente, California, USA
Vegan since: 2013

tiablanco.tumblr.com
SM: *FaceBook, Instagram, Twitter*

Tia Blanco is an 18-year-old vegan surfer who loves animals and yoga. She is a member of the USA surf team, who surfs with power and style, and took 3rd overall in the 2014 World Juniors. Tia became one of the most talked about amateurs in women's surfing when she was 17, winning both the NSSA Southwest Women's under 18s and Surfing Prime America Women's under 18s seasons. In 2015, she has won The Ron Jon's Pro, Women's Gold in ISA World Surfing Games, NCampion in the SSA Western Conference, and Winner of the Surfing America Championships. Also an outspoken vegan athlete, Tia has become an ambassador for PETA2 and is frequently featured in vegan, vegetarian and health media as a role model and athlete.

WHY VEGAN?

How and why did you decide to become vegan?
I am vegan for the animals, for my health, and for the environment.

How long have you been vegan?
I have been vegetarian my whole life and vegan since 2013.

What has benefited you the most from being vegan?
There have been so many positive benefits: my surfing performance, saving animals, spreading the word, and being enlightened to a cruelty-free way of living.

What does veganism mean to you?
Veganism means love.

"When I see that veganism is trending it inspires me to keep the ball rolling. Every time I look at the hashtag #vegan on Instagram it goes up 1,000,000... Crazy."

TRAINING

What sort of training do you do?
I surf, practice yoga, run, and practice surf training.

How often do you (need to) train?
I like to stay active every day!

Do you offer your fitness or training services to others?
Haha no. I can teach someone to surf, but not as a fitness trainer.

What sports do you play?
Surfing.

STRENGTHS, WEAKNESSES & OUTSIDE INFLUENCES

What do you think is the biggest misconception about vegans and how do you address this?
Protein! I get that question almost every single time my diet is brought up. I try to explain to people that it is the quality of the protein, not the quantity.

What are your strengths as a vegan athlete?
I feel lighter and always energized.

What is your biggest challenge?
Traveling with the vegan diet, but I always make it work.

Are the non-vegans in your industry supportive or not?
No, most of them don't think I get enough protein. I try to explain to them I get more than enough. Too much protein produces toxic ketones, increase your chances three times of getting cancer, promotes kidney failure, and is hard on your liver making it very hard to process. Animal protein is also very acidic to the body. Even though protein is essential, it is important to eat the cleanest and healthiest protein and that is plant-based protein. Pound for pound, kale and spinach have more protein than a piece of steak. How do you think the strong vegan animals like gorillas get their protein? GREENS.

Are your family and friends supportive of your vegan lifestyle?
My immediate family is vegan, so yes.

What is the most common question/comment that people ask/say when they find out that you are a vegan and how do you respond?
And again the protein misconception...

Who or what motivates you?
When I see that veganism is trending it inspires me to keep the ball rolling. Every time I look at the hashtag #vegan on Instagram it goes up 1,000,000... Crazy. When I saw Ariana Grande's Twitter post about veganism it made me want to re-post. To inspire and be inspired.

FOOD & SUPPLEMENTS

What do you eat for Breakfast?
Green smoothie with any kind of leafy greens like kale, any kind of frozen fruit like berries, with chia seeds, bananas, spirulina, mint, chlorella and water.

What do you eat for Lunch?
Stuffed bell peppers with quinoa.

What do you eat for Dinner?
Lentil soup.

What do you eat for Snacks - healthy & not-so healthy?
I snack on fruit throughout the day.

What is your favourite source of Protein?
Quinoa.

What is your favourite source of Calcium?
Almond milk.

What is your favourite source of Iron?
Leafy greens and beets.

What foods give you the most energy?
BANANAS.

Do you take any supplements?
No.

ADVICE

What is your top tip for gaining muscle?
PiYo.

What is your top tip for losing weight?
High carb, low-fat, vegan.

What is your top tip for maintaining weight?
Eat until you're full, and no more.

What is your top tip for improving metabolism?
Eat throughout the day and never deprive your body.

What is your top tip for toning up?
Running and yoga.

How do you promote veganism in your daily life?
I try to promote veganism by setting and sharing a positive example. I try my best to eat clean, stay active, and be happy.

How would you suggest people get involved with what you do?
I would suggest following me on my two Instagram channels - you can catch up on my daily food diary and activities there.

"Too much protein produces toxic ketones, increase your chances three times of getting cancer, promotes kidney failure, and is hard on your liver making it very hard to process. Animal protein is also very acidic to the body. Even though protein is essential, it is important to eat the cleanest and healthiest protein and that is plant-based protein. Pound for pound, kale and spinach have more protein than a piece of steak. How do you think the strong vegan animals like gorillas get their protein? GREENS."

TIFFANY BURICH
VEGAN FITNESS MODEL & TRAINER

Miami, Florida, USA
Vegan since: 2008

noexcusestrainer@gmail.com
SM: *FaceBook, Instagram, Twitter*

Tiffany Burich has over 10 years experience in the fitness and nutrition industry. She is a vegan figure competitor, vegan athlete, fitness model, an American Council on Exercise (ACE) certified personal trainer, has a B.S. in Exercise Science and a B.S. in Biology/Pre-Med.

WHY VEGAN?

How and why did you decide to become vegan?
I saw an article about a "downer cow" and was immediately mortified and surprised that a human being could do something like this. I immediately cut out red meat and pork, and then continued to do research on factory farming and the meat industry. I was a biology/pre-med student at the time but had already been "cruelty-free" as far as purchasing products: cleaners, make up, etc.

How long have you been vegan?
I've been vegan since 2008. I really wanted to stick with it so the year before that I cut out a different group of meat every two months, ending with giving up dairy and all animal by-products.

What has benefited you the most from being vegan?
A lot! Long term: I haven't been sick in 5 years, my endurance and recovery time in the gym is better, and I recently rehabilitated myself from a torn meniscus (when the doctors were saying surgery) through vegan supplements and my own Exercise Science knowledge. Short term: I tried eating chicken again about two months after I cut it out of my diet (as an experiment) and I immediately felt what I can only describe as "toxic". Physically, I felt sick but more importantly, my mood was definitely changed. I just "feel better" all around as a vegan.

What does veganism mean to you?
Veganism means many different things to me (positive & negative). People can advocate veganism because 1. They have experienced the benefits 2. They want to stop suffering and cruelty to animals and 3. They want to save humans from disease. I am motivated by all three! The negative (for me) is just staying hopeful and not letting the images I've seen affect me by haunting me to the point of emotional imbalance. I am driven by the sadness of what I can't currently fix, but I'm able to control it to deliver the whole message in an effective and educational way.

"Be consistent with meals and food choices, drink at least 3L of water a day, stick to your workout plan, allow rest days and cheat meals."

TRAINING

What sort of training do you do?
A mixture of steady state cardio, High-intensity interval training (HIIT), traditional weight training, CrossFit, metabolic training, and running.

How often do you (need to) train?
5-6 days a week, sometimes two workouts a day - depending on what my goals are.

Do you offer your fitness or training services to others?
Yes, I have been a trainer for ten years and offer personal training, online training, nutritional coaching, online competition prep coach, and CrossFit coaching.

What sports do you play?
I am a figure competitor in bodybuilding, weight lifting, running (marathons), CrossFit and tennis.

STRENGTHS, WEAKNESSES & OUTSIDE INFLUENCES

What do you think is the biggest misconception about vegans and how do you address this?
That our diets are boring, we don't get enough protein, and are weak or feeble. I compete in endurance competitions and bodybuilding, I get people coming up to me all the time in the gym to compliment my physique or training style, and they are always shocked when I say I'm vegan – I love it!

What are your strengths as a vegan athlete?
My endurance and my recovery time. I can do an hour on the stairs and then beat anyone's time in heavy lifting or CrossFit workouts right after. I'm also very competitive but I am working hard for those who do not have a voice or choice.

What is your biggest challenge?
To not over train and to take rest days. I also have to defend myself sometimes and try not to show my annoyance - talking about veganism is the ONLY time I can control my emotions actually. I know people are turned off and look at the extreme activists as just being "crazy" or "hippies." While I feel just as passionate about veganism as they do, I have a knack for approaching people in a less extreme manner - plus I get asked about my physique a lot so that helps.

Are the non-vegans in your industry supportive or not?
Everyone has an opinion about veganism, regardless of what they do for a living. Fortunately forming the Plant Built Vegan Muscle Team in 2013 has made a huge impression in the bodybuilding industry. Our group of 15 completely dominated the competition, multiple placings in every category, and even earned a few pro-cards!

Are your family and friends supportive of your vegan lifestyle?
No one in my family gives me a hard time, they can see I'm healthy and mostly just ask questions.

What is the most common question/comment that people ask/say when they find out that you are a vegan and how do you respond?
"What do you eat?" "I could never give up (blank)", "How do you get enough protein?" "Do you eat eggs? Fish?" Haha! I never really understood the miscommunication on the fish question. I respond with a short answer and try VERY hard not to be irritated.

Who or what motivates you?

The images of suffering and abused animals TATTOOED in my brain is what motivates me! I definitely have some vegan athletes who I've looked up to and recently had the pleasure of meeting. Obviously everyone from my Plant Built team; but to name a few: Robert Cheeke - who turned me onto vegan bodybuilding and I was totally star-struck when I met him. Mindy Collette - who I also followed and is now one of my best friends, we clicked immediately. Dani Taylor - who did my nutrition for my first competition and her fiancé Giacomo Marchese - who put this team together. Stephanie Rice, Sara Russert, Yolanda Presswood and Jaclyn Gough for their encouraging texts and messages on a daily basis; and Big Bald Mike from Bonebreaker Barbell - he's been my rock and shoulder for sure.

"It can be hard to stay hopeful and not let the images I've seen affect me by haunting me to the point of emotional imbalance. I am driven by the sadness of what I can't currently fix, but I'm able to control it to deliver the whole message in an effective and educational way."

FOOD & SUPPLEMENTS

What do you eat for Breakfast?
Orgain organic plant-based protein powder, oats, unsweetened vanilla almond milk, Warrior Force elite green protein, and fruit.

What do you eat for Lunch?
Kale, veggies, beans, and Beyond Meat chikin strips.

What do you eat for Dinner?
Tempeh or Beyond Meat, lentils, veggies, and rice.

What do you eat for Snacks - healthy & not-so healthy?
I snack two or three times a day on my "famous" Seitan choco-coconut protein muffins, nuts & fruit.

What is your favourite source of Protein?
Beyond Meat, tempeh, kale, lentils, Warrior Force supplements, and ORGAIN organic plant-based protein.

What is your favourite source of Calcium?
Almond milk (unsweetened vanilla), spinach, and broccoli.

What is your favourite source of Iron?
Beans (pinto, black, garbanzo), spinach, and kale.

What foods give you the most energy?
Bananas, coconut water, and nuts.

Do you take any supplements?
Branched-chain amino acid (BCAA)s & Glutamine.

ADVICE

What is your top tip for gaining muscle?
Supersets, lifting heavy and eating carbohydrates. Don't be afraid of carbs, you just

gotta eat the right ones at the right time.

What is your top tip for losing weight?
Eating small meals all day, lifting heavy and doing cardio.

What is your top tip for maintaining weight?
Be consistent with meals and food choices, drink at least 3L of water a day, stick to your workout plan, allow rest days and cheat meals.

What is your top tip for improving metabolism?
Lift heavy - the more muscle mass you have, the more fat you are burning when you're not even in the gym - you will not get bulky! Eat small meals and snacks every three hours.

What is your top tip for toning up?
Alternate high repetition and light-weight days with low repetition and heavy weight days.

How do you promote veganism in your daily life?
I bring up veganism on Social Media by sharing stuff. Also every time I get a compliment on my physique or working out routine – or when anyone brings up the subject of food - I use it as an opportunity to educate others.

How would you suggest people get involved with what you do?
Contact me via email or through my website, follow me on Social Media and check out other athletes at the PlantBuild team website.

"Compassion is the foundation of everything positive, everything good. If you can carry the power of compassion to the marketplace and the dinner table, you can make your life really count."
- Rue McClanahan

Invest in you, your health and your life.

TUMERIA LANGLOIS
VEGAN PERSONAL TRAINER

Maynard, Massachusetts, USA
Vegan since: 2002

fit-2-a-t.com
SM: *FaceBook, Google+*

Tumeria Langlois became interested in fitness and nutrition at the age of 14, when following major surgery, she gained 65 pounds (30kg). Through diet and exercise, Tumeria was able to lose the weight within 1 year. In addition to weight loss, exercise improved her body image, self-esteem, general health, endurance and love of life. It helped her maintain a positive attitude and gave her a feeling of accomplishment. Upon graduation from high school, Tumeria enrolled in the Exercise Specialist/ Physical Education major at the University of New Hampshire, graduated Cum Laude and obtained her Bachelor of Science degree. For over 27 years she has dedicated her life to helping others make fitness a part of their lives.

WHY VEGAN?

How and why did you decide to become vegan?
I became vegan for spiritual reasons. I always loved animals and even had a very close relationship with a baby cow when I was a child. As I began my spiritual search I realized that I was connected to all living things. I started eating less and less animal products. It just didn't feel right any more. I recognized that all animals were sentient and deserved the right to live their lives.

How long have you been vegan?
Over 13 years.

What has benefited you the most from being vegan?
My soul feels free; my body feels clean and healthy.

What does veganism mean to you?
It is a lifestyle and a commitment to living a life of compassion for all living beings - human and non-human alike.

TRAINING

What sort of training do you do?
I lift weights and do cardiovascular training.

How often do you (need to) train?
I train 5 to 6 days per week, with a 3 on, 1 off lifting schedule. Day one is chest and back, day two is legs, day three is shoulders and arms.

Do you offer your fitness or training services to others?
Yes, I am a certified personal trainer and I hold a degree in exercise science. In the past year I have opened up my own personal training studio in Maynard, Massachusetts.

What sports do you play?

None. I am into fitness and health rather than competitive sports.

STRENGTHS, WEAKNESSES & OUTSIDE INFLUENCES

What do you think is the biggest misconception about vegans and how do you address this?

That we are radical and feel superior to everyone else. In fact it is just the opposite. We are vegan because we don't feel superior to any other life form. We respect all of life. I firmly believe in teaching by example. I also believe in educating the people I come in contact with if they are open. I let them ask the questions rather than impose myself on them. They have to be open and receptive.

What are your strengths as a vegan athlete?

I find that I recover more quickly from my workouts, even at the age of 54. Having a good amount of muscle mass shows that even a vegan girl can put on muscle and not be protein deficient.

What is your biggest challenge?

I never look at life as a challenge. I look at life as an opportunity to grow and evolve.

Are the non-vegans in your industry supportive or not?

Yes, The people who work at my gym are very supportive. They have reduced their meat consumption as well. I remind them to eat healthier.

Are your family and friends supportive of your vegan lifestyle?

Yes. Most of my friends are vegan but those who are not are very accepting and supportive.

What is the most common question/comment that people ask/say when they find out that you are a vegan and how do you respond?

"Where do you get your protein?" Seriously, I get asked that a lot! I tell them beans, nuts, seeds legumes, dark green leafy greens.

Who or what motivates you?

I have always motivated myself. As part of my spiritual evolution, I have learned to look within myself for my strength and motivation.

Do research. Educate yourself. Make connections with farm animals. Go to a farm sanctuary and meet animals. Pet them; play with them – it won't take long to realize they are all unique individuals. Do some soul searching. Every person is on their own path. My path is unique to me. Everyone must find their own in their own time in their own way.

FOOD & SUPPLEMENTS

What do you eat for Breakfast?

Oatmeal with walnuts and a banana. I add some ground flaxseeds, cinnamon and date sugar to sweeten it some.

What do you eat for Lunch?

Vegetable soup with beans and red rice mixed in, a handful of nuts (cashews or pistachios), and fruit like pineapple.

What do you eat for Dinner?
I always cook some sort of grain - red rice, brown rice, barley, millet or quinoa.
Then add any and all kinds of veggies into a big pot - carrots, sweet potato, broccoli,
mushrooms, tofu, zucchini, summer squash, kale, spinach, Swiss chard - you name it.

What do you eat for Snacks - healthy & not-so healthy?
Usually fruit: cherries, pears, apples and bananas. Once a week a sweet indulgence is
allowed like a vegan whoopie pie.

What is your favourite source of Protein?
Tofu, beans and nuts.

What is your favourite source of Calcium?
Dark green leafy vegetables, beans, and almond milk.

What is your favourite source of Iron?
Spinach and beans.

What foods give you the most energy?
Whole grains and fruit.

Do you take any supplements?
B12, Vitamin D2 in the Winter, DHA Omega 3's from algae.

ADVICE

What is your top tip for gaining muscle?
Strength train and be consistent. Don't be afraid to push yourself.

What is your top tip for losing weight?
A combination of strength training, cardio, exercise and diet - eliminate processed
foods, refined sugars and eat a whole foods, plant-based diet.

What is your top tip for maintaining weight?
Find your balance. Monitor your weight and note fluctuations. I have a weight range
of 5 pounds (2.3kg) that I keep within. If my weight sneaks up to the higher end of the
range, I cut back a little. If it goes to the lower end of the range I can indulge a little
more.

What is your top tip for improving metabolism?
Strength train is a must - muscle is metabolism.

What is your top tip for toning up?
Strength train. Women do not have to be afraid of it - you won't build bulky muscles.

How do you promote veganism in your daily life?
I live and teach by example.

How would you suggest people get involved with what you do?
Do research. Educate yourself. Make connections with farm animals. Go to a farm
sanctuary and meet animals. Pet them; play with them - it won't take long to realize
they are all unique individuals. Do some soul searching. Every person is on their own
path. My path is unique to me. Everyone must find their own in their own time in their
own way. You may become vegan for the animals, for the environment, for your health
or for spirituality like I did. I became vegan for my spiritual growth. That has now
changed. I am now vegan for ALL the reasons I have listed above.

Victor Rivera

VEGAN PERSONAL TRAINER

Los Angeles, California, USA
Vegan since: 2008

veganpowertraining.wordpress.com
SM: *FaceBook, Instagram, Twitter*

Victor Rivera moved to Los Angeles, CA in 2003 from Massachusetts, beginning his path to finding himself - and in the process, taking on the vegan lifestyle. Victor is a National Academy of Sports Medicine (NASM) certified personal trainer, as well as a student at University of California, Los Angeles (UCLA) where he is studying psychology. In his downtime, Victor eats lots of tasty vegan food with his wife and son, writes on his blog, takes care of their dogs, as well as visits shelters and animal sanctuaries.

WHY VEGAN?

How and why did you decide to become vegan?

My vegan journey began when I was reading "Fast Food Nation" and my wife, a long-time vegetarian, was reading "Skinny Bitch". After I finished reading both books, which explained the inhumane levels of animal cruelty, as well as many of the health, environmental and social issues that come from the meat and dairy industries, we both decided to go vegan.

How long have you been vegan?

Over seven years and counting!

What has benefited you the most from being vegan?

The biggest benefit I have received from going vegan is knowing that I am not contributing to the mistreatment of our fellow earthlings, as well as minimizing my carbon footprint. On the dietary level, the benefit for me has been better health - as I was able to lose about 60 pounds (27kg) and essentially get rid of my Irritable bowel syndrome (IBS) after going vegan.

What does veganism mean to you?

To me, veganism means awareness. Most of us were just given a plate full of meat without ever considering where it came from and how it ended up on our tables. So taking the time to understand the impact that our diets have on the animals, the planet, and our bodies is what being vegan is all about.

TRAINING

What sort of training do you do?

I tend to do full-body, functional training (as opposed to for instance, bodybuilding) with weights, kettle-bells, TRX, and body-weight. I also do what some call "Intuitive Training," meaning if my body isn't up for powering through a weight session, I'll go for a nice bike ride, jog, or do a little bit of yoga and stretching. Listening to my body comes first before a predetermined workout.

How often do you (need to) train?

I try my best to train with weights at least five times a week and do some light cardio the other two days. Your frequency of training depends on what your goals are, though. If you are just trying to be generally healthy, four days a week for half an hour at moderate intensity is good. If you're going for more advanced goals, training five to six days a week at a higher intensity is the way to go.

Do you offer your fitness or training services to others?

I am a personal trainer, certified through National Academy of Sports Medicine (NASM). I've been training clients since 2009 and love it. I'm also studying psychology at University of California, Los Angeles (UCLA), so I understand and help others with the mindset portion of diet and exercise.

What sports do you play?

I really enjoy playing baseball, basketball and football mostly. Basketball seems the easiest to play these days as I just need to grab my ball, head outside to my hoop and shoot around.

STRENGTHS, WEAKNESSES & OUTSIDE INFLUENCE

What are your strengths as a vegan athlete?

My strength as a vegan athlete is weight-training endurance. I seem to be able to keep going at the weights in terms of strength and form, while those around me need breaks or look super wobbly. My tip here is to focus on your breathing, as opposed to those thoughts that question why you're working so hard.

My biggest psychological strength is my ability to commit to something. If I'm going to do it, I'm going to go all the way. When I went vegan, it wasn't just something I was going flirt around with. I bought as many books as possible, visited all of the websites, and researched everything about it. When I decided to go back to school, I just put my head down, hit the books, and studied like crazy even on those many days where I just wanted to give up and watch TV.

What do you think is the biggest misconception about vegans and how do you address this?

Of course, the biggest misconception about vegans is that we can't contain muscle mass, we don't get enough protein and no way can we be athletes of any kind. I address this by basically saying, "Do I look like I don't get enough protein?" From there, I explain to those willing to listen how I get all of my amino acids, as well as all of the other nutrients people assume we are missing (B-12, Omegas, Calcium, etc.) I try to calmly educate those who question the capabilities as best as possible, while silently just wanting to bench press them.

What is your biggest challenge?

My biggest challenge physically is long-distance running. Between my stocky build, and how bored I get while jogging, I have always struggled with that type of training. I prefer to ride my bike or use the elliptical at the gym when I'm looking for some basic cardio.

I would say the biggest challenge I am working on personally is finding balance in my life. It's been hard for me to divide my time between my family, my schoolwork, my own training and my training business. I seem to be figuring it out, though, but still need some work. Wish me luck.

Are the non-vegans in your industry supportive or not?

The non-vegans in my industry seem be generally supportive. My fellow trainers know that at the end of the day, it's about facts and results. When they hear what I have to say and see me in action - as well as see the transformation that my clients go through - they're cool with it and actually usually like to learn more, as trainers tend to seek more information from each other.

Are your family and friends supportive of your vegan lifestyle?

My friends and family are very supportive of my vegan lifestyle, especially once they've eaten one of my wife's amazing meals. It's hard to deny how yummy vegan food is. I'm also fortunate to live in the Southern California area, where people seem to be more accepting of vegans. When I tell people in my old hometown in Massachusetts that I'm vegan, they usually say something like, "So you don't eat red meat?"

What is the most common question/comment that people ask/say when they find out that you are a vegan and how do you respond?

"Where do you get your protein?" Then I tell them that basically everything has protein in it, though some sources have more than others. I also explain that protein isn't some magical nutrient that you need in exorbitant amounts in order to be healthy. Protein is so overhyped now it's outrageous. Then, if they're really interested, I like to explain that the protein in meat isn't even efficiently absorbed, and the cost and benefit of meat as a source of nutrients is so risky. If I'm tired, I just flex, and ask them, "Do you think I'm not getting enough protein?"

Who or what motivates you?

My wife and son motivate me the most. There are plenty of days where I want to turn in a mediocre "performance," but when you have other people who depend on you, taking a day off is not an option. So being mentally present and driven benefits me personally, but also sets a good example for my son.

In the vegan community, I keep up with Eco-Vegan Gal, Robert Cheeke, Samantha Shorkey, and a host of others to keep me on the vegan and weight-lifting path.

FOOD & SUPPLEMENTS

What do you eat for Breakfast?

Oatmeal and fruit, or Nature's Path cereal with some soymilk.

What do you eat for Lunch?

A healthy burrito: brown rice, beans, avocados, tomatoes, onions, and lettuce in a whole-wheat wrap.

What do you eat for Dinner?

On a healthy day, I just love some basic brown rice noodles, tempeh or tofu with broccoli and carrots. When I want to treat myself, I LOVE vegan pizza!

What do you eat for Snacks - healthy & not-so healthy?

My favorite healthy snack is bananas. They're so satisfying as well as energy-packed. My not-so healthy favorite snack is a Clif Bar.

What is your favourite source of Protein?

Beans are my favorite healthy source of protein and Tofurky sausages on a junk food type of day.

What is your favourite source of Calcium?
Soymilk and tofu, as well as kale in my green drinks.

What is your favourite source of Iron?
Beans and lentils.

What foods give you the most energy?
Dense fruits like bananas and strawberries give me tons of energy, as well as peanut butter. Whenever I have a spoonful of peanut butter, I just feel so physically and mentally satisfied.

Do you take any supplements?
I like Vega's supplements and protein powders, as well as Orgain and Garden of Life protein powder when I'm on a budget. I take Deva B-12, Omega and a multi-vitamin pill, but try to get as much of my needs from whole foods as possible.

"Talk the talk, and walk the walk. Make yourself as a informed as possible so that you are up to date on which companies are still cruelty-free or vegan-owned; keep up with the latest health findings regarding animal products, meat recalls, the environment, etc., so that when non-vegans ask you questions, you are prepared."

ADVICE

What is your top tip for gaining muscle?
The best way to gain muscle is by adding more calories to your diet. To "Get Bigger," you're going to have to "Eat Bigger." The extra calories should be healthy though! And well distributed throughout the day (6-7 meals).

The training side of gaining muscle is to try to get as strong as possible, as well as increase your volume. This means 3-4 weeks of 4-6 reps, 3-4 weeks of 8-10 reps, and three weeks of 12-15 reps. Just think, more weight, more volume, more food.

What is your top tip for losing weight?
The best and safest way to lose weight is to really watch what you're eating, count your calories, and train for longer periods of time so that you're burning more calories. In order to watch what you're eating and calculate a weight loss goal (in a reasonable amount of time), I recommend the MyFitnessPal app. This way you are keeping track of what you eat, as well as eating a healthy amount of calories. Don't do extreme dieting (less than 100 calories a day) as this typically just leads to gaining all of the weight back plus more.

As for the training side, try to increase the length of your training sessions. If you generally lift weights and do some cardio and interval training for 45 minutes or less, try to increase your time at the gym (or wherever) to an hour. Do circuit-style cardio strength training and supersets when lifting weights so that you're not taking breaks and keep constantly burning calories. And try to be active during your general day by taking the stairs instead of the elevator, park far away at the mall, go for a short walk while you're making a phone call, etc. Your thought here is to have an active lifestyle.

What is your top tip for maintaining weight?
The best way to maintain your weight is a combination of the suggestions above. This means you are mixing up your weight training style so that your body is always being challenged via strength or endurance, and you are watching what you are eating either

through the MyFitnessPal app, your own food log, or just mentally monitoring your food. If you're gaining weight, you're eating too much and/or the wrong types of food. If you're losing weight, you're probably not eating enough.

What is your top tip for improving metabolism?

To improve metabolism, make sure you are eating smaller meals 5-6 times a day. Eating too large of a meal, as well as waiting too long between meals, slows your metabolism down.

To improve your metabolism through training, weights are the best, as well as interval training (sprints on a bike or elliptical for 30 seconds, followed by 30 seconds of a regular pace), and Tabata for a higher intensity training that will really boost your metabolism. While steady state cardio (i.e. a 30 minute jog) has its purposes, it doesn't tax your system in a way that speeds up your metabolic rate enough to get into fat-burning mode.

What is your top tip for toning up?

The best way to "tone up" is to do more of my style of training, which is a full-body, functional regimen, training each body part four times a week at least (every other day). This will keep your body more lean and athletic, as opposed to bodybuilding, which focuses on "Chest and Tricep" day, "Leg Day," "Back and Biceps," etc., once a week (or twice) per muscle group.

A functional style session looks like three sets of squat jumps, three sets of lunges, three sets of bench press, three sets of dumbbell shoulder press, and three sets of one minute of planks, completing a "Push Day." The next day would be Kettlebell swings, Back Extensions, dumbbell row, pull-ups, and medicine ball twists, completing a pull day. This way you are targeting all of your major muscle groups, but not overtraining them, so that you can train more frequently and get more of a toned look. The book "Men's Health Power Training" is a good place to start planning this type of routine.

How do you promote veganism in your daily life?

I promote veganism daily by putting posts up on my blog, or on Social Media. I wear Vegan Bodybuilding type shirts to the gym frequently, and answer questions whenever anyone reads my shirt and wants to know how it's possible. I sign petitions all of the time (i.e. Sea World Must Go Away), and tell people the truth when they say things like, "but I eat cage-free chicken..." I'm also involved in groups and just joined Bruins for Animals at UCLA.

How would you suggest people get involved with what you do?

I think the main way to get involved is to talk the talk, and walk the walk. Make yourself as a informed as possible so that you are up to date on which companies are still cruelty-free or vegan-owned; keep up with the latest health findings regarding animal products, meat recalls, the environment, etc., so that when non-vegans ask you questions, you are prepared.

Also, do whatever you're comfortable with. At first, I just wanted to stop eating meat, but wasn't quite asserting my beliefs out in the world. Once I became more confident and informed, I found my "vegan voice" and was able to comfortably post my findings on my sites, wear my vegan shirts in public with pride, and be as involved and part of the movement as possible.

WEIA REINBOUD
VEGAN HIGH JUMPER & JAVELIN THROWER

Utrecht, Netherlands, EU
Vegan since: 1982

at-a-lanta.nl/weia
SM: *FaceBook*

Weia Reinboud holds National Masters records in high jump, javelin throw, pole vault and heptathlon. Her first world record high jump was at the age of 50, followed by over sixteen other ones. She has participated in heptathlon, high jump, triple jump, hammer throw, javelin throw and pole vault. In August 2013, Weia restarted training for the multi-events, which lead to a world record heptathlon for women over 65 in 2015. Mid-2015 she already had four times jumped a world record in the high jump, one indoor and three outdoor. Besides this she twice improved the javelin national record. Now she concentrates on high jump and javelin for time reasons.

WHY VEGAN?

For ethical reasons.

How and why did you decide to become vegan?
Being vegetarian, I supposed there were no slaughter houses necessary for what I was eating: but spring 1982, I read an article about the killing of calves to keep the milk 'giving' going. The conclusion of that article was that some meat eating was okay, but I took the contrary conclusion, that no dairy products were okay. It took half a year to change my eating habits. At the time I did not know of veganism and there being others eating like that, we in a sense reinvented it.

How long have you been vegan?
Autumn 1982, so now more than 32 years.

What has benefited you the most from being vegan?
I just like to be vegan, to have a lifestyle that ethically fits me.

It's very difficult to say whether veganism and sports is a better combination than non-veganism and sports. It asks for difficult double-blind statistical studies. A long time ago, my mother was running an institute offering cooking courses etcetera. One was for vegetarians, and the instructor said she found those vegetarians so weak and pale, which could be her prejudice or just the situation for those needing cooking courses. My personal experience is completely different. I am giving high jump training and all my pupils are much younger, around forty years. We all do the same stuff and of course they have the strength of youth. But things like aching muscles seem to be the same, and when my recovery takes a bit longer age is the explanation.

What does veganism mean to you?

Veganism is one of those choices you make and never regret. When you see cows in a meadow with enormous udders you can say, "Sorry girls, I'm not the cause." Besides you have other advantages, you have a much smaller ecological footprint etcetera. I cannot see any disadvantage. You feel happy by living according your own choices and more important: these are ethical choices. The mainstream consumer searches for happiness in the act of consuming, but the ethical consumer consumes less and finds more happiness. This is the case for all ethical choices and veganism is the biggest of them.

TRAINING

What sports do you play?

My main disciplines are high jump and javelin throw. That means technical training, some running (sprints) and some strength training.

How often do you (need to) train?

Three times a week is the basics; some simple fitness stuff is added to that. In preparation of a record attempt in the heptathlon, training goes up to five times a week, with three trainings containing two long blocks, so in effect 8 blocks in total.

Do you offer your fitness or training services to others?

I am the high jump trainer at our athletics club.

STRENGTHS, WEAKNESSES & OUTSIDE INFLUENCES

What do you think is the biggest misconception about vegans and how do you address this?

The biggest misconception is that veganism is a diet that leads to dull meals. The best way to combat that is to serve an extremely nice vegan meal.

What is your biggest challenge?

Well, without research... There are three possibilities: as a vegan athlete, you are a better, equal or worse athlete compared to when you weren't vegan. I like to be modest about my accomplishments but it is the case that I am best of the world in my first discipline, the high jump, and one of the best of Europe in my second discipline, throwing the javelin (at this moment European champion in my age group). I do not know how much food adds to these successes, if any. But, it safely can be said that it is possible to play sport at the highest level as a vegan.

Are the non-vegans in your industry supportive or not?

In talking about sports and food it often is said that you need meat and milk and whatsoever. I can easily say that it's possible to do without, just a smile is enough. And because they know of my records they see they in fact have no point. I recently had a nice experience. The yearly meeting of all writers on the website of the National Athletic Federation was coming and after the meeting they are going to dine together – eating nasty things, not organic too. I said I wouldn't join, being vegan for over 33 years, and one of the vegetarians of the group immediately reacted with "Proud of you", he himself only being vegetarian. That's supportive!

Are your family and friends supportive of your vegan lifestyle?

They wouldn't be friends if not!

What is the most common question/comment that people ask/say when they find out that you are a vegan and how do you respond?

People can ask about protein. I personally very much like proteins. Nuts are one source, but I do not really like nuts, I hardly take them. Beans are another rich source and I especially eat beans in the right season: butter beans, fresh marrowfat peas etcetera. But, mostly I eat them as vegetables and like to have a 'real' protein product added. Here tofu is my favourite. I've know tofu since I was 15 or so, as it is a common ingredient in Indonesian cooking (where it's called tahu), which I love since my mother did a course in it. Tofu can be found in many prepared burgers or so, but I always prepare it myself. Indonesian-style or otherwise, a meal without tofu or sometimes tempeh can hardly be called a meal! Athletes need enough proteins and as I do not experience problems in recovery, tofu seems to be a sufficiently good source.

Who or what motivates you?

There is always enough internal and intrinsic motivation to have no need for other motivators.

"Veganism is one of those choices you make and never regret. When you see cows in a meadow with enormous udders you can say, "Sorry girls, I'm not the cause." Besides you have other advantages, you have a much smaller ecological footprint etcetera. I cannot see any disadvantage. You feel happy by living according your own choices and more important: these are ethical choices."

FOOD & SUPPLEMENTS

What do you eat for Breakfast?

First breakfast is fruit.

Second breakfast mostly a leftover of the day before, Italian pasta, Indonesian rice, and Dutch potatoes.

What do you eat for Lunch?

Bread. Mostly with Mediterranean stuff on it (olives, dried tomatoes etcetera.)

What do you eat for Dinner?

Salad quite a lot. Pasta, rice, potatoes, many vegetables, tofu, tempeh or sometimes beans. 100% organic by the way, for over 30 years.

What do you eat for Snacks - healthy & not-so healthy?

Potato chips (fried in olive oil, less salty than normal), and chocolate.

What is your favourite source of Protein?

Tofu in many kinds.

What is your favourite source of Calcium & Iron?

I never think about calcium or iron, it will be in the vegetables etcetera.

What foods give you the most energy?

All food!

Do you take any supplements?

Vitamin B12 of course.

"The mainstream consumer searches for happiness in the act of consuming, but the ethical consumer consumes less and finds more happiness. This is the case for all ethical choices and veganism is the biggest of them."

ADVICE

What is your top tip for gaining muscle?
High jumpers don't like too much muscles... However, as a typical high jumper, I simply am not muscled. Training with weights leads to better muscles, not more.

What is your top tip for losing weight?
Eat (a bit) less.

What is your top tip for maintaining weight?
Eat enough.

What is your top tip for Improving metabolism & Toning up?
Never felt a need for that.

How do you promote veganism in your daily life?
By just being there. I have written quite a lot (mostly in Dutch) about it, so have inspired others.

How would you suggest people get involved with what you do?
Feel free to contact me through my personal website.

Tips for a New Vegan from Leigh-Chantelle

Use your position of influence to promote positivity, inclusiveness and compassion in everything you do. Realise that you can educate more people with a soft tongue more than you will a sharp one. Be careful what you say to another online and in person. Remember that you may be the only vegan the person you are conversing with knows, so make it kind and respectful.

Remember to use your time wisely. Remember to have a break from activism. Remember to do the things you love and love the things you do. Remember to be kind. Compassion is always the answer.

YOLANDA PRESSWOOD
VEGAN FITNESS COACH

Riverside, California, USA
Vegan since: 2010

pwdfitness.com
elevatedfitness.net
SM: FaceBook, Instagram

Yolanda Presswood is a 39-year old stay at home/homeschooling mama with a teenage son and a preteen daughter. She's been married to the love of her life for over 19+ years. Yolanda has a 2 pups and 2 cats. She loves the beach, writes children's stories, and is obsessed with clouds and all things creation. Fitness has always been a part of her life in one way or another but it wasn't until Yolanda turned 35 that she started her full-force journey into living the life she had only been dreaming about.

As an International Sports Sciences Association (ISSA) certified fitness trainer, she is looking into her biggest ambition of opening her own gym. Yolanda wants people to know that some say you can't, some say you shouldn't, and some say you won't, but she's here to tell you that you CAN, you SHOULD, and you WILL - if you have the will! Motivate others, inspire from your heart, and live life alive and with compassion with every single breath that you take. Be authentic to who you are and live with intention. Don't let anyone steal your sparkle. Every single day is a gift!

WHY VEGAN?

How and why did you decide to become vegan?
I was a lacto-ovo vegetarian from the age of 16-19 and vegan for a short time at 19, then omnivore. I just didn't have the knowledge or anyone in my corner at the time. I always hated eating animals. It made me sick to look at blood and bite down on cartilage or see a vein in my chicken. After reading Dr. Michelle Schoffro's cookbook "The Ultimate pH Solution", my husband and I knew animal flesh and products had no place in our holistic healthy lifestyle. I like to say I returned to what I've always known is right. As we became further educated on the ins and outs of factory farming, it became more clear to us that it was not only for health, but for compassion for all life and that our consumption of animal flesh and products had a direct impact on not just our health but living beings and our planet.

How long have you been vegan?
Over 5 years.

What has benefited you the most from being vegan?
Hands down is that I've healed myself of hormone imbalance. I used to have severe Pre-menstrual Dysphoric Disorder (PMDD), insomnia, depression, rage, discontent, heavy periods with headaches and vertigo. I am happy to say I no longer deal with ANY of it - best thing ever!

What does veganism mean to you?

It means love, compassion, thought, and freedom. I'm liberated to peace in my own discovery of compassion. I can tell you that a side effect from living a compassionate life is the immense peace I hold in my heart, mind and soul. It was unexpected but definitely makes sense. It's not something I can explain fully. You must experience it for yourself to truly know.

TRAINING

What sort of training do you do?

I started out as a bodybuilder and have competed on stage. My first show was with the PlantBuilt alumni team in Austin, Texas at the Naturally Fit Super Show. My last show was the 7 Feathers Classic up in Oregon. In November 2014, I stumbled onto CrossFit after feeling stuck. I've always said I'm an athlete not just a physique competitor. When CrossFit found me it was a light bulb moment. I love everything from trail running to power lifting, Olympic lifting to gymnastics, plyometrics and power building. One thing that's new to me is swimming - crushing comfort zones there!

How often do you (need to) train?

I need to train daily as it's what allows me as a mother to have an energy outlet. I do CrossFit 5-6 days per week. A couple days a week I run my trails and do extra weight lifting or practice Olympic lifting skills.

Do you offer your fitness or training services to others?

I do. As an ISSA certified fitness trainer, I have a passion to motivate, inspire, and help others reach their personal fitness and health goals. I'm constantly learning through research of sports and nutrition sciences to better help each individual client. I also do bikini prep. Locally and worldwide coaching available.

What sports do you play?

I don't play any sports other than what's mentioned above but I'm always open to trying something new and fun.

STRENGTHS, WEAKNESSES & OUTSIDE INFLUENCES

What do you think is the biggest misconception about vegans and how do you address this?

I think the obvious misconception about vegans is that we're protein deficient and therefore weak. I address this by showing that you CAN build strong muscles with a compassionate lifestyle. Another funny one is that we secretly desire to eat meat like bacon. This is a tricky one and one I address with as much grace as I possibly can. This shows the lack of understanding for the vegan lifestyle, so it's always my aim to educate with kindness to hopefully help someone's eyes become opened just like mine were.

What are your strengths as a vegan athlete?

My strengths as a vegan athlete on a personal heart level are that I'm ambitious, I work hard, I push myself, I give myself grace, and I love every day no matter if it's a good day or a bad one. I refuse to give up. I face fear every day. Understanding that courage does not mean you are without fear but that you press on in spite of the fear. Every day is a gift. On a physical level, my strength is my strength. I'm just physically pretty strong for my size.

What is your biggest challenge?

My biggest challenge is having so many ambitions all at one time and being so detailed and organized. Sometimes I have to remind myself it's okay to fly by the seat of my pants. It's okay not to have all the dots and slashes. Just live life and be joyful. Trying to always remain focused when I have so many ideas and my hands in so many things is hard. Balancing every aspect of my life as a mother, wife, housekeeper, business owner and athlete is also a huge challenge.

Are the non-vegans in your industry supportive or not?

Yes. In fact, four of my sponsors are non-vegan and they are some of my biggest supporters and love me so very much. Clark's Nutrition and Natural Foods Markets, Stark Nutraceuticals, Sapphire Swim and TRUElicious superfood bar owners are all omnivores and respect me as a vegan 100% and support me every step of my fitness career and journey, and I am so grateful. I don't want to leave our Vegan Biceps who are vegan but also a huge support.

Are your family and friends supportive of your vegan lifestyle?

Yes. My family and friends are very supportive of my choice to live compassionately. It is awesome to see friends eat less flesh, or choose family chickens for eggs as even a small step, or have my Mom tell me she baked something without eggs or dairy.

What is the most common question/comment that people ask/say when they find out that you are a vegan and how do you respond?

The most common question/comment I get is "OMG! You don't eat meat - Isn't that hard?" "How do you build muscle without meat?" and "I can't give up meat, but good for you." I respond by letting them know that being a vegan is actually easier than eating animal flesh. I don't have to worry about keeping my chicken cold or my stomach aching from too much whey protein. I aim to educate that every living thing contains amino acids, and that instead of eating chicken, I eat tofu, tempeh, nuts, seeds, edamame etc etc etc and thus I have no problem building or maintaining muscle without the senseless slaughtering of a defenseless animal. If I'm lucky, I get the chance to share some of what I've experienced in the way of peace through veganism. I sometimes point to my bicep - that one always gets them!

Who or what motivates you?

This might sound conceited but I'm one of the most grateful and humble people you will ever meet. "Who has been forgiven much, loves much." I am my best motivator. I've been fighting my way through life my whole life. There have been times in my life that I've been alone and abandoned. I've been in some really dark holes. To make it out alive (literally and figuratively) has never been easy. I just keep going. Although when I see photos of some of my favorite athletes or get challenged by something someone says that I can't do, that also motivates me. My children are another huge motivator for me. Knowing that they are watching for how I respond to situations, how determined I am, and that I never give up. I want them to know whatever they can dream, they can achieve. Living authentic to who they are as individuals as I do the same.

FOOD & SUPPLEMENTS

What do you eat for Breakfast?

Pancakes! Or seeds, nuts and chocolate.

What do you eat for Lunch?

Tofu with BBQ sauce, veggies, and yams with coconut oil, or Beyond chick'n with romaine, kimchi and veganise.

What do you eat for Dinner?
Tempeh, veggies and avocado, or something like beefy crumble tacos.

What do you eat for Snacks - healthy & not-so healthy?
My favorite snack is almond butter right off the spoon with a few chocolate chips. I also love a pink lady apple with some mixed raw nuts or edamame. High protein pudding and a banana with peanut butter.

What is your favorite source of Protein?
Tofu, roasted edamame, soy flour, Beyond Meat products that are gluten-free, hemp seeds, quinoa, nutritional yeast and Now Foods plain pea protein.

What is your favorite source of Calcium & Iron?
Greens.

What foods give you the most energy?
I love a smoothie with a ton of greens and fruit for natural energy. Also fresh cold pressed raw juice and a TRUElicious bar. (It's filled with dates, maca, cacao, nuts and seeds).

Do you take any supplements?
Yes. Stark Nutraceuticals BCAAS, Jarrow Formulas B12, MRM D3, creatine and algae omegas.

ADVICE

What is your top tip for gaining muscle?
Make sure your macros line up with your goals. Don't be afraid of carbs and be sure you're taking in enough protein. Lift heavy weights - all the weights!

What is your top tip for losing weight?
Expend more calories than you take in. Don't neglect hydration. DONT spend your life on a cardio machine. And lift those weights.

What is your top tip for maintaining weight?
Eat well, be well, stay well.

What is your top tip for improving metabolism?
Drink water first thing in the morning, add in some cayenne and lemon juice. Eat within the first hour upon waking if possible. Be sure you're getting good sleep.

What is your top tip for toning up?
Lift, lift, lift!

How do you promote veganism in your daily life?
Social Media, in my gym, at my sponsor store, by supporting cruelty-free companies as a consumer, and whenever someone asks. I lead by example. With kindness and grace. If someone would have been in my path way back when, I'd have been vegan a long time ago. Preaching at someone never gets their attention. I'm not always quiet in my beliefs... ok I'm never quiet, but I don't lead with anger.

How would you suggest people get involved with what you do?
Go to my current website, new website Elevated Fitness coming soon, and find me on Social Media.

"Motivate others, inspire from your heart, and live life alive and with compassion with every single breath that you take. Be authentic to who you are and live with intention. Don't let anyone steal your sparkle. Every single day is a gift!"

Zac Anstee
VEGAN TRIATHLETE

Melbourne, Victoria, Australia
Vegan since: 2012

tarianpantry.com.au
SM: *FaceBook, Google+, Pinterest, Twitter*

Zac Anstee is an IT Managing consultant by day and athlete by night. He grew up with sand and surf as a nipper and then surf lifesaver, who always had a love for water - the fitness side of it was just a bonus. Now fitness - with the addition of food - is an important part of his overall wellbeing. His job is often very stressful, with long days - not to mention business trips away. With everything in life, there has to be a balance. It's important for Zac to manage his work responsibilities with training, and of course keeping a happy home - and wife! When he's not working or training, Zac enjoys spending time in the kitchen and watching motor sports.

WHY VEGAN?

How and why did you decide to become vegan?
Was vegetarian for 10 years, and through learning and experience, I decided a completely animal-free diet aligned with my ethos towards anti-animal cruelty.

How long have you been vegan?
Over 3 years.

What has benefited you the most from being vegan?
Mental wellbeing.

What does veganism mean to you?
An animal-free diet.

TRAINING

What sort of training do you do?
Cross-train due to triathlon goals: swim, ride, run, stretch.

How often do you (need to) train?
Approximately 10-12 hours per week.

Do you offer your fitness or training services to others?
No, my only training is to motivate by example.

What sports do you play?
Triathlons.

STRENGTHS, WEAKNESSES & OUTSIDE INFLUENCES

What do you think is the biggest misconception about vegans and how do you address this?
That we eat nothing but carrots and lettuce! I just explain to people what I ate last night which no doubt was a delicious meal. This helps people understand further what is served up on my dinner plate.

What are your strengths as a vegan athlete?
Quick recovery.

What is your biggest challenge?
I travel interstate for work, which can be difficult to find clean healthy food. This can be particularly challenging when with a group of work colleagues who all want to eat out together, and there are not many restaurants to choose from other than a steak house & Nando's.

Are the non-vegans in your industry supportive or not?
Yes, mostly curious.

Are your family and friends supportive of your vegan lifestyle?
Yes.

What is the most common question/comment that people ask/say when they find out that you are a vegan and how do you respond?
"Where do you get your protein?" Often I explain we don't need much protein (0.8g per body weight kg) and that even our greens contain some levels of protein. I use big animals such as cows as an example of getting enough protein even from grass.

Who or what motivates you?
My wife, Amanda Meggison, who runs Tarian Pantry - she is a huge source of information about good healthy living and eating.

FOOD & SUPPLEMENTS

What do you eat for Breakfast?
Porridge.

What do you eat for Lunch?
Beans and rice, pasta and noodles.

What do you eat for Dinner?
Curries, pasta, salads, pizza and Mexican food.

What do you eat for Snacks - healthy & not-so healthy?
Bliss balls, fruit and homemade bars.

What is your favourite source of Protein?
Tofu and tempeh (served with a satay sauce, yum.)

What is your favourite source of Calcium?
Walnuts and broccoli.

What is your favourite source of Iron?
Kale and spinach.

What foods give you the most energy?
Anything with high carbohydrates: potatoes, pasta and rice.

Do you take any supplements?
B12 oral spray.

ADVICE

What is your top tip for gaining muscle?
Pump iron.

What is your top tip for losing weight?
Run and eat well.

What is your top tip for Maintaining weight & Improving metabolism?
Eat well.

What is your top tip for toning up?
Join a triathlon club!

How do you promote veganism in your daily life?
I don't stuff it down people's throats. If they find out I am vegan and ask me why, I answer their questions without trying to push my morals or views. The main way I promote veganism is through leading by example.

How would you suggest people get involved with what you do?
Go straight to Tarian Pantry online and explore the wealth of information.

"People eat meat and think they will become as strong as an ox, forgetting that the ox eats grass."

- Pino Caruso

Dreams don't work, unless you do.

WANT TO SEE THE PHOTOS?

FaceBook

Google+

Pinterest

About Viva la Vegan!

Viva la Vegan! started in 2005 to promote Leigh-Chantelle's recipe calendars, and educate others about the vegan lifestyle. 2015 sees the 10th anniversary of this oft-shared and much-loved Australian site, that has grown to be an interactive, multimedia community for vegans all over the world, focusing on positive education, information and vegan outreach. Through the vivalavegan.net website, Leigh-Chantelle's focus is on educating people about ethical lifestyle choices, proving that through compassion we can heal ourselves and each other.

Vivalavegan.net focuses on easy-to-prepare recipes, blogs, articles, podcasts, informative and how-to videos, interviews with inspiring vegans, eBooks, print books and much more. The 10th anniversary of Viva la Vegan! sees a complete overhaul of the website, with more focus on Leigh-Chantelle's passions – Speaking, Consulting, Training and Coaching.

You can find Viva la Vegan! on FaceBook, Google+, Instagram, Pinterest, Twitter, and YouTube.

Podcasts on: iTunes, ScatterRadio, SoundCloud, and Stitcher.

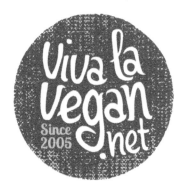

About Leigh-Chantelle

Leigh-Chantelle is a Published Author, International Speaker & Consultant, Singer/ Songwriter and Blogger who lives mostly in Brisbane, Australia. She gives lectures, workshops, consultations, and coaching for Understanding Social Media, Staging Effective Events, and Vegan Health & Lifestyle.

She has run the online vegan community Viva la Vegan! since 2005, bringing positive education, information and vegan outreach to a worldwide audience. Leigh-Chantelle previously founded and ran the not-for-profit environmental awareness Green Earth Group from 2009-2013, which put on two successful all-vegan environmental festivals in Brisbane.

Leigh-Chantelle is an accredited naturopath, nutritionist and Western herbalist (no longer practicing) who combines her passion for vegan health along with her natural therapies and healing skills. She has released three Viva la Vegan! recipe calendars, a plant-based detox diet eBook, various other recipe eBooks, re-released her recipe calendars as recycled recipe cards, and has published many other print books.

Over the past 19 years since Leigh-Chantelle has been vegan, she has been involved as a sponsor, performer, speaker, MC and stallholder for various animal rights, vegan, vegetarian, environmental and cruelty-free fundraisers, forums, conferences, festivals and events throughout Australia and Internationally.

Leigh-Chantelle is available for select speaking engagements, seminars, panel discussions and readings worldwide.

To enquire about a possible appearance, please contact email@leigh-chantelle.com

About the Illustrator

Weronika Kolinska has been drawing since she was a little girl. And since she was a child, she's also been fascinated with nature and animals. She spent days observing lives of insects and other small creatures in her garden or watching David Attenborough's documentaries.

It was not until she was 23 years old that she became vegetarian and got interested in animal rights, which soon led her to become vegan. She now volunteers at a Polish animal rights organization Otwarte Klatki (Open Cages). Their goal is to prevent the suffering of animals by implementing systemic social change, to document the conditions of factory farming, and to educate people along with promoting positive attitudes towards animals.

Weronika creates gloomy, detailed illustrations maintained in gray scale, but also likes to use her art to promote animal rights and veganism by creating more approachable and colorful pieces.

Find her artwork at veganmisanthrope.tumblr.com

Other Books by Leigh-Chantelle

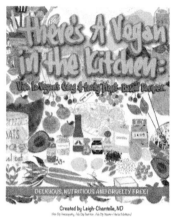

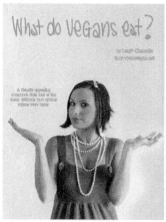

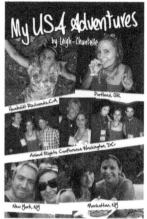

There's A Vegan in the Kitchen
ISBN 978-0-9808484-4-1
Digital ISBN 978-0-9808484-5-8
2014

What Do Vegans Eat?
ISBN 978-0-9808484-0-3
Digtial ISBN 978-0-9808484-1-0
2012

My USA Adventures
ISBN 978-0-9808484-2-7
Digital ISBN 978-0-9808484-3-4
2012

EBOOKS

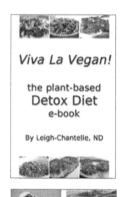

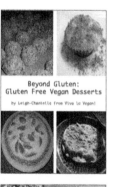

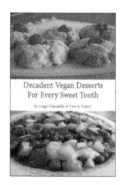

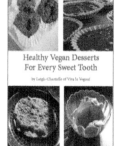

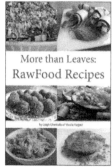

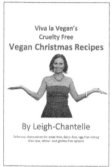

vivalavegan.net/community/store.html

Lightning Source UK Ltd.
Milton Keynes UK
UKOW06f0141141016

285187UK00004B/143/P